Study Guide to Accompany

Introductory Clinical Pharmacology

SEVENTH EDITION

Bonnie J. Smith, BSN, RN
Former Coordinator, Educational Researcher
Practical Nurse Program
Sikeston Public Schools, Health Occupations
Hayti, MO

Sally S. Roach, MSN, RN
Associate Professor
University of Texas at Brownsville and Texas Southmost College
Brownsville, TX

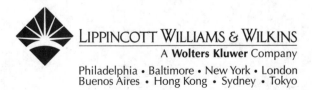
LIPPINCOTT WILLIAMS & WILKINS
A **Wolters Kluwer** Company

Philadelphia • Baltimore • New York • London
Buenos Aires • Hong Kong • Sydney • Tokyo

Acquisitions Editor: Lisa Stead
Managing Editor: Joseph Morita
Senior Production Editor: Debra Schiff
Senior Production Manager: Helen Ewan
Managing Editor /Production: Erika Kors
Art Director: Brett MacNaughton
Manufacturing Manager: William Alberti
Compositor: Lippincott Williams & Wilkins
Printer: Victor

7th Edition

ISBN: 0-7817-3697-8

Care has been taken to confirm the accuracy of the information presented and to
describe generally accepted practices. However, the authors, editors, and publisher
are not responsible for errors or omissions or for any consequences from application
of the information in this book and make no warranty, express or implied, with
respect to the content of the publication.

The authors, editors, and publisher have exerted every effort to ensure that drug
selection and dosage set forth in this text are in accordance with the current
recommendations and practice at the time of publication. However, in view of
ongoing research, changes in government regulations, and the constant flow of
information relating to drug therapy and drug reactions, the reader is urged to check
the package insert for each drug for any change in indications and dosage and for
added warnings and precautions. This is particularly important when the
recommended agent is a new or infrequently employed drug.

Some drugs and medical devices presented in this publication have Food and Drug
Administration (FDA) clearance for limited use in restricted research settings. It is the
responsibility of the health care provider to ascertain the FDA status of each drug or
device planned for use in his or her clinical practice.

LWW.com

Preface

This *Study Guide* is designed to help the nursing student obtain the most benefit from the revised and updated seventh edition of *Introductory Clinical Pharmacology*. The textbook gives current and comprehensive coverage of the newest pharmacological aspects, as well as basic nursing skills needed in administering medications and caring for the patient.

The *Study Guide to Accompany Introductory Clinical Pharmacology* will help you, the student, learn vocabulary, identify and master the most important content in the textbook, and help prepare you for the various examinations you will take. As you read the textbook, this *Study Guide* will be an important tool that you can use to verify that your reading and study habits are allowing you to identify the most important ideas in each chapter.

The *Study Guide to Accompany Introductory Clinical Pharmacology* has been designed around the following elements:

- Each chapter of the study guide corresponds to the exact same chapter in the textbook.
- Each question and exercise is based on the information found within the text, and only as a learning tool will the student be asked to identify information found in other sources.
- Each chapter contains NCLEX-style, multiple-choice questions that follow the currently used format for the CAT-PN examination, allowing the student to practice and learn test-taking skills.
- Critical thinking questions are presented that encourages the student to identify all aspects of the problem and formulate nursing actions that may be needed to resolve the situation involved. Critical thinking is a necessary component of the nursing process and true comprehension develops with learning and understanding. These exercises provide the student with the opportunity to practice problem-solving techniques he or she will need as a practicing nurse. It would be in the student's best interest to be very detailed in his or her response to each of the critical thinking questions. The solution each student identifies will not always be the same for each problem, but the end result should be based on the patient's needs and the nursing process.
- The answers for each section of questions or exercises are found in the Answer Key. The Answer Key is arranged by chapter number and allows the student easy identification of all answers to each of the exercises or question. The student is encouraged to complete each chapter and then verify their answers with the Answer Key. This will allow the student to identify which areas of the content matter need further study.
- No answers are provided for the critical thinking questions, as the answers should vary depending on each student and his or her knowledge base.

Each activity in the *Study Guide* was carefully thought out and developed to accommodate different learning styles. Each chapter contains one or more of the following elements:

Crossword Puzzles provide a unique way to recall important key terms, drugs, or adverse reactions included in the chapter.

Fill in the Blank questions correlate almost word-for-word with the textbook and point out important information in the chapter.

Matching allows the student to distinguish among several key terms, drugs, or adverse reactions.

Dosage Problems provided at the end of each chapter give the student practice in solving common medication dosage problems related to the specific medication studied in the chapter. This reinforces the ability to continually solve dosage problems and gives the student practice in solving problems that may come up in the clinical setting.

Internet Exercises are included in a number of chapters and the student is encouraged to take advantage of the Internet addresses provided to discover other Internet sites that may offer valuable pharmacological information to the student. These exercises are optional and the instructor may or may not choose to make use of them.

I truly hope that this *Study Guide* will provide you, the student, with a tool that will help you to better understand and comprehend the complicated and sometimes world of pharmacology. Try to give yourself time to study and learn. There will be a tremendous amount of material you will have to learn, but you will find that the more you learn, the easier it becomes to learn.

Bonnie J. Smith, RN, BSN

Contents

CHAPTER 1

General Principles of Pharmacology

I. Matching

Match each term in Column A with the correct definition or statement in Column B.

COLUMN A

_____ 1. anaphylactic shock

_____ 2. controlled substances

_____ 3. additive drug reaction

_____ 4. pharmacology

_____ 5. teratogenic

_____ 6. angioedema

_____ 7. toxic reaction

_____ 8. pharmacokinetic

_____ 9. half-life

_____ 10. orphan drug

COLUMN B

A. The study of drugs and their actions on living organisms.

B. Products developed and marketed for the treatment of rare diseases.

C. A substance that causes abnormal development of the fetus, leading to severe deformity of the fetus.

D. Drugs that have a high potential for abuse and may cause physical or psychological dependence.

E. Activities occurring within the body after a drug is administered. These include absorption, distribution, metabolism, elimination, and half-life.

F. An extremely serious allergic drug reaction, which can be fatal and requires immediate medical attention.

G. Time required for the body to eliminate 50% of a drug.

H. Type of allergic reaction identified by swelling of eyelids, lips, mouth, and throat.

I. Reaction produced when blood concentration levels of a drug exceed therapeutic levels.

J. The combined effect of two drugs that equals the sum of each drug given alone.

II. Multiple Choice

Circle the letter of the most appropriate answer.

1. A new nurse is using a drug guide to identify a patient's medications that have been ordered by the physician. Estrone, a hormone classified as Pregnancy Category X, is to be given daily. What is the most important question to ask a female patient during your drug history?

   a. "How many children do you have?"

   b. "Have you experienced nausea and vomiting?"

   c. "Is there a possibility you might be pregnant?"

   d. "Have you noticed a sudden weight gain?"

2. While checking your patient's medications, you find that Ecotrin (enteric-coated aspirin) has been ordered. You remember that dissolution of enteric-coated drugs occurs in the small intestine. A drug will dissolve during the:

   a. pharmacodynamic phase.

   b. pharmaceutic phase.

   c. pharmacokinetic phase.

   d. biotransformation.

3. A doctor writing orders for a new patient states to the nurse, "I want this medicine to work as quickly as possible." The nurse is aware that the fastest absorption route for medication is:

   a. orally.

   b. subcutaneously.

   c. intramuscularly.

   d. intravenously.

4. While interviewing Ms. Jones, a newly admitted patient to the medical unit, the nurse discovers Ms. Jones has a history of hepatitis C (a liver disease). In planning the care for this patient, the nurse must consider that liver disease may result in a(n):

a. increase in the excretion rate of a drug.

b. need to increase the dosage of a drug.

c. impaired ability to metabolize or detoxify a drug.

d. decrease in the excretion rate of a drug.

5. Your patient is showing signs of respiratory depression because of the morphine he has been receiving for severe pain. The doctor has ordered Narcan, an antagonist of morphine, administered intramuscuarly. Monitoring the patient for the antagonist response, you would expect to see:

a. increased response to pain control.

b. increase in rate and depth of respirations.

c. decrease in the level of pain because of Narcan.

d. decrease in rate and depth of respirations.

6. A nurse is taking a drug history on a newly admitted patient. The patient states the last time she took penicillin she felt a fullness in her throat, and her eyes and lips became slightly swollen. These symptoms describe an allergic reaction identified as:

a. urticaria (hives).

b. severe skin rash.

c. decreased cardiac function.

d. possible angioedema.

7. Herbal therapy and nutritional supplements are parts of complementary/alternative therapy. Complementary therapy may also include:

a. relaxation techniques.

b. radiological tests.

c. hematologic studies.

d. prescription drugs.

8. A nurse working in the emergency department is caring for a patient with a high alcohol blood level. The doctor has ordered Ativan (lorazepam) to control the symptoms of alcohol withdrawal. The nurse is aware of the possibility of a(n)_____ due to the combination of these two drugs.

a. synergistic drug reaction

b. adverse drug reaction

c. antagonistic drug reaction

d. drug–food interaction

9. The physician has written orders for a medication to be given in smaller dosages than usual. The patient has a history of kidney and liver disease. As the nurse, you understand the lowered dosage is to prevent the possibility of a(n):

a. development of drug tolerance.

b. cumulative drug effect.

c. severe adverse drug reaction.

d. idiosyncratic drug reaction.

10. Anaphylactic shock is an extremely serious allergic drug reaction that can be fatal if not identified and treated quickly. A nurse would recognize the signs and symptoms of this allergic reaction as:

a. elevated blood pressure, low heart rate.

b. wheezing respirations, elevated heart rate.

c. warm, dry skin; regular respirations.

d. dizziness, elevated blood pressure.

III. Crossword Puzzle

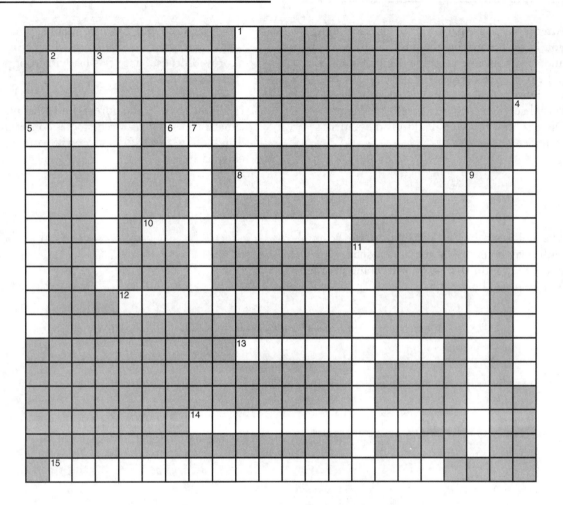

ACROSS CLUES

2. Patients usually recognize drugs by their
   _____ name.
5. Occurs when blood concentration levels of
   drugs exceed the therapeutic level.
6. Phase when drug dissolution occurs.
8. Therapy that includes herbal therapy and
   nutritional supplements.
10. Decreased response to drug requiring an
    increased dosage.
12. Refers to an allergic reaction.
13. Drug that interacts and produces effects greater
    than its separate action.
14. Effect produced when drugs cannot be
    metabolized and excreted effectively.
15. Body process by which drugs are metabolized.

DOWN CLUES

1. Nonproprietary drug name.
3. Allergic drug reaction manifested by excess fluid
   in subcutaneous tissue.
4. Taking numerous drugs, usually seen in the
   elderly.
5. Substance that causes abnormal development of
   the fetus.
7. Time required for the body to eliminate 50% of
   drug.
9. An extremely serious allergic reaction.
11. Drug that interferes with the action of another
    drug.

IV. Critical Thinking

1. After admitting a patient to the medical unit, you begin performing the physical assessment and ask about any nutritional supplements the patient may be taking. The patient asks you why this information is necessary because these herbal supplements aren't really medicine. Discuss how you would address the patient's statements.

2. Ms. Smith is being discharged from the hospital with several new medications that she is unfamiliar with. Discuss your teaching plan for Ms. Smith and her family.

V. Internet Exercise

1. Using the following Internet address, www.centerwatch.com, obtain a listing of newly approved drugs. Share this list with your classmates.

2. Using the same Web address, find a listing of clinical trials and research studies concerning drugs. Share this information with your classmates.

CHAPTER 2

The Administration of Drugs

I. Matching

Match each term in Column A with the correct definition or statement in Column B.

COLUMN A

_____ 1. infiltration

_____ 2. drug error

_____ 3. Z-track

_____ 4. standard precautions

_____ 5. extravasation

_____ 6. sublingual

_____ 7. intradermal

_____ 8. parenteral

_____ 9. unit dose

_____ 10. intravenous

COLUMN B

A. Special technique used for intramuscular injections of medication that may stain the skin or cause severe irritation to the subcutaneous tissue.

B. Administration of medication directly into the blood by inserting a needle into a vein.

C. Escape of fluid from a blood vessel into surrounding tissues while the needle or catheter remains in the vein.

D. Type of injection used for tuberculin test or allergy skin testing.

E. Administration of a drug by the subcutaneous, intramuscular, intravenous, or intradermal methods.

F. Collection of fluid in the tissue surrounding the area where an intravenous catheter has accidentally slipped out of the vein but continues to flow into the subcutaneous tissue.

G. Medication packaged and labeled with each package containing one tablet or capsule, a premeasured amount of liquid drug, a prefilled syringe, or one suppository.

H. Administering an incorrect dose of a medication.

I. Wearing gloves to protect against exposure to blood and body fluids.

J. Route of medication administration where the drug is allowed to dissolve under the tongue.

II. Multiple Choice

Circle the letter of the most appropriate answer.

1. Your patient has been prescribed an inhalation-type medication. The primary nursing responsibility for this patient is to:
   a. demonstrate how to deposit the medication to the tongue.
   b. teach the patient how to breath out when dispensing the drug.
   c. provide the correct and necessary instructions for administering the drug.
   d. explain that the instructions accompanying the device are not helpful.

2. When preparing a drug for administration, the nurse should:
   a. remove tablets or capsules by shaking them from their container into his or her hand.
   b. ask another nurse to prepare some of the doses for your patient when you're in a hurry.
   c. remove all wrappings from the unit doses to be administered before you take them to your patient.
   d. always check the written orders, verifying all information and questions you may have with the primary health care provider.

3. A nurse can prevent drug errors by always:

   a. verifying calculations with another nurse.

   b. reciting the six "patient rights" at least once daily.

   c. asking another nurse to prepare the medications.

   d. administering the drugs, then answering questions.

4. In order to be certain you have the "right" patient when administering medication, the nurse should:

   a. ask the patient, "Is your name Mr. Jones?"

   b. check the patient wristband lying on the nightstand.

   c. ask the alert and oriented patient to identify himself.

   d. be assured that the patient in the room is always the right patient.

5. Nursing responsibilities for administering drugs using the transdermal delivery system would include:

   a. applying all doses to the same site to ensure uninterrupted delivery of the medication.

   b. rotating sites for the transdermal patches to prevent skin irritation.

   c. applying the patches to the lower legs, which are the most common sites.

   d. shaving the area to be used for the patch to provide a hairless area.

6. When preparing a drug for subcutaneous injection, the nurse would be aware that the usual volume of medication injected by this route is:

   a. less than 0.2 milliliter.

   b. 0.1 milliliter.

   c. 2 to 5 milliliters.

   d. 0.5 to 1 milliliter.

7. A patient asks the nurse how long it will take for her intravenous antibiotic to start working. As this patient's nurse, you would explain that the medicine should start to work:

   a. almost immediately.

   b. in a few hours.

   c. in 24 to 48 hours.

   d. in 12 to 24 hours.

8. A new nurse is having a difficult time differentiating between extravasation and infiltration. Extravasation is best described as:

   a. escape of fluid from a vein into the surrounding tissues while the catheter remains in the vein.

   b. fluid seeping from the subcutaneous tissue to the surface of the skin.

   c. collection of fluid in the subcutaneous tissue caused by an intravenous catheter that has moved out of the vein.

   d. collection of large amounts of fluid in the vein.

9. An intravenous therapy is initiated by inserting the appropriate size catheter into the patient's vein. One of the first steps in this process is:

   a. placing a tourniquet below the selected vein site.

   b. inserting the catheter bevel down at a steep angle.

   c. reusing the same catheter if the first attempt is unsuccessful.

   d. placing a tight tourniquet above the selected vein site.

10. A physician has written an order for Valium, 10 mg, IVP @ 10:00 A.M. This is an example of a:

    a. STAT order.

    b. single order.

    c. PRN order.

    d. standing order.

11. To administer drugs safely by the intravenous route, an infusion pump may be used by the nurse to:

    a. intermittently deliver 2 to 5 milliliters of a drug.

    b. calculate the time required for 1000 milliliters to infuse.

    c. deliver a large amount of drug over a short time.

    d. deliver the desired number of drops per minute accurately.

12. When administering a medication, the nurse:
    a. is alert for drugs with similar names.
    b. checks drug labels two times before administration.
    c. administers drugs prepared by another nurse.
    d. may crush all tablets the patient is unable to swallow.

III. Fill in the Blanks

1. List six "rights" of drug administration.
    a) _____
    b) _____
    c) _____
    d) _____
    e) _____
    f) _____

2. Name four types of medication orders and give an example of each.
    a) _____
    b) _____
    c) _____
    d) _____

3. List the five different routes used for drug administration.
    a) _____
    b) _____
    c) _____
    d) _____
    e) _____

4. List four nursing responsibilities following the administration of medication to a patient.
    a) _____
       _____
       _____
    b) _____
       _____
    c) _____
       _____
    d) _____
       _____
       _____

5. Medication errors occur when the patient receives the _____ _____, the _____ _____, or an incorrect _____ of the drug by the _____ _____, or if the _____ is given at the _____ time.

6. Drugs administered by the _____ _____ are readily absorbed from the skin and have _____ effects. This type of drug system maintains a _____ _____ _____ _____ and _____ the possibility of _____.

7. Drug droplets, vapors, or gases are administered through the _____ _____ of the _____ tract with the use of a _____ or a _____ _____ _____ _____. Examples of drugs administered through inhalation include _____, _____, and some _____ drugs.

IV. Crossword Puzzle

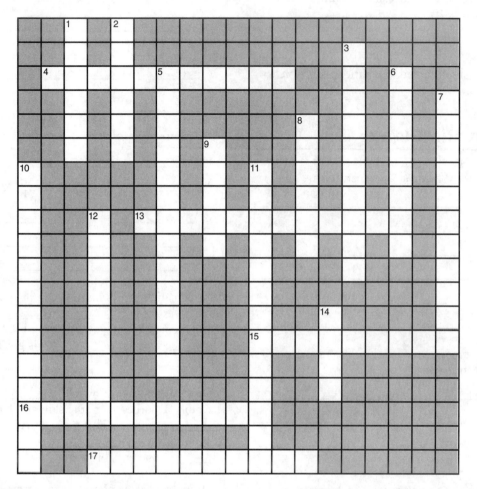

ACROSS CLUES

4. Route used when drugs are readily absorbed by the skin for a systemic effect.
13. Collection of fluid into subcutaneous tissue when the intravenous catheter moves from the vein, but remains in the tissue.
15. Will help prevent drug errors if consistently practiced (two words).
16. Route commonly used for tuberculin test or allergy skin testing.
17. Giving a drug by the subcutaneous, intramuscular, intravenous, or intradermal route.

DOWN CLUES

1. Technique for administering injections when drug may be irritating to subcutaneous tissue.
2. Order for a drug to be given only one time.
3. Route where drugs are administered through the mucous membrane of the respiratory tract.

5. The "right" that is extremely important when administering PRN narcotic drugs.
6. Type of order given when drug is given on a regular basis.
7. Route that requires a suitable vein for venipuncture.
8. Route where the drug is placed against the mucous membrane of the cheek and jaw.
9. Computerized dispensing systems used by hospitals to dispense drugs.
10. Escape of fluid from a blood vessel into surrounding tissues while intravenous catheter is in the vein.
11. Route used to inject drug into the ventrogluteal or dorsogluteal muscles.
12. Occurrence that can cause a patient to receive a wrong drug (two words).
14. Route most frequently used for drug administration.

IV. Critical Thinking

1. While the nurse administers a Z-track injection, the patient questions the nurse about the technique being used. Discuss the rationale you would give the patient for the method used for Z-track injections.

2. Mr. Dennis, a patient with newly diagnosed type 1 diabetes, is to start insulin injections. Insulin is administered by subcutaneous injections. Describe how you would teach Mr. Dennis the proper technique for these injections.

3. You have just completed your medication administration rounds and realize you have given the wrong drug to one of your patients. Describe how you would respond to this situation.

4. Discuss the process for reporting medication errors.

Review of Arithmetic and Calculation of Drug Dosages

The following list is provided to help the reader locate various topics covered in the questions in this chapter. These questions are based on the review of mathematical principles and the mathematics of pharmacology discussed in Chapter 3, **A Review of Arithmetic and Calculation of Drug Dosages.**

I. Review of Arithmetic

A. Fractions
B. Mixed Numbers and Improper Fractions
C. Adding Fractions with Like Denominators
D. Adding Fractions with Unlike Denominators
E. Adding Mixed Numbers or Fractions with Mixed Numbers
F. Comparing Fractions
G. Multiplying Fractions
H. Multiplying Whole Numbers and Fractions
I. Multiplying Mixed Numbers
J. Multiplying a Whole Number and a Mixed Number
K. Dividing Fractions
L. Dividing Fractions and Mixed Numbers
M. Ratios
N. Percentage
O. Proportion
P. Decimals

II. Calculation of Drug Dosages

A. Systems of Measurement
B. Conversion Between Systems
C. Converting Within a System
D. Oral Dosages of Drugs
E. Parenteral Dosages of Drugs

F. Calculating IV Flow Rates
G. Oral or Parenteral Drug Dosages Based on Weight
H. Temperatures

III. Review of Arithmetic

A. FRACTIONS

1. Name the two parts of a fraction.

   _____   _____

2. Define the following:
   a. Proper fraction _____

   b. Improper fraction _____

3. In the blank provided, write the letters designating an *improper fraction.*

   _____

   a. $\dfrac{4}{5}$ f. $\dfrac{2}{3}$

   b. $\dfrac{3}{1000}$ g. $\dfrac{5}{8}$

   c. $\dfrac{8}{6}$ h. $\dfrac{5}{4}$

   d. $\dfrac{20}{3}$ i. $\dfrac{500}{3}$

   e. $\dfrac{13}{19}$ j. $\dfrac{3}{4}$

4. Briefly explain why the following is incorrectly expressed as a fraction.

   $\dfrac{3 \text{ grains}}{8 \text{ ounces}}$

   Explanation: _____

   _____

B. MIXED NUMBERS AND IMPROPER FRACTIONS

1. What is a mixed number?

_____

2. Change the following mixed numbers to improper fractions.

   a. $1\frac{5}{8}$ = _____

   b. $2\frac{2}{3}$ = _____

   c. $4\frac{1}{2}$ = _____

   d. $12\frac{1}{6}$ = _____

   e. $5\frac{1}{3}$ = _____

   f. $7\frac{1}{2}$ = _____

   g. $9\frac{1}{8}$ = _____

   h. $20\frac{1}{2}$ = _____

   i. $8\frac{1}{3}$ = _____

3. Change the following improper fractions to mixed numbers.

   a. $\frac{16}{7}$ = _____

   b. $\frac{14}{9}$ = _____

   c. $\frac{31}{3}$ = _____

   d. $\frac{17}{4}$ = _____

   e. $\frac{12}{5}$ = _____

   f. $\frac{30}{13}$ = _____

   g. $\frac{8}{3}$ = _____

   h. $\frac{14}{3}$ = _____

   i. $\frac{9}{5}$ = _____

C. ADDING FRACTIONS WITH LIKE DENOMINATORS

1. Add the following fractions. When necessary, reduce the answer to the lowest possible terms.

   a. $\frac{1}{4} + \frac{1}{4}$ = _____

   b. $\frac{1}{5} + \frac{3}{5}$ = _____

   c. $\frac{2}{7} + \frac{3}{7}$ = _____

   d. $\frac{1}{8} + \frac{3}{8}$ = _____

   e. $\frac{2}{3} + \frac{1}{3}$ = _____

   f. $\frac{7}{10} + \frac{1}{10}$ = _____

   g. $\frac{4}{9} + \frac{2}{9}$ = _____

   h. $\frac{1}{3} + \frac{2}{3} + \frac{1}{3}$ = _____

   i. $\frac{1}{6} + \frac{1}{6} + \frac{1}{6}$ = _____

D. ADDING FRACTIONS WITH UNLIKE DENOMINATORS

1. Add the following fractions. When necessary, reduce the answer to the lowest possible terms.

   a. $\frac{2}{3} + \frac{4}{5}$ = _____

   e. $\frac{1}{5} + \frac{1}{2}$ = _____

   b. $\frac{1}{7} + \frac{1}{14}$ = _____

   c. $\frac{2}{7} + \frac{2}{5}$ = _____

   d. $\frac{3}{8} + \frac{2}{3}$ = _____

   f. $\frac{1}{5} + \frac{3}{10}$ = _____

   g. $\frac{1}{32} + \frac{1}{64}$ = _____

   h. $\frac{1}{3} + \frac{1}{6}$ = _____

2. Add the following fractions and change the improper fraction to a mixed number.

   a. $\frac{2}{3} + \frac{5}{6}$ = _____

   b. $\frac{1}{3} + \frac{8}{9}$ = _____

   c. $\frac{3}{5} + \frac{5}{9}$ = _____

   d. $\frac{3}{4} + \frac{7}{8}$ = _____

   e. $\frac{10}{11} + \frac{1}{2}$ = _____

   f. $\frac{4}{5} + \frac{2}{3}$ = _____

E. ADDING MIXED NUMBERS OR FRACTIONS WITH MIXED NUMBERS

1. Add the following mixed numbers or fractions and mixed numbers.

   a. $2\frac{1}{5} + 1\frac{1}{4}$ = _____

   b. $1\frac{2}{3} + \frac{1}{2}$ = _____

   c. $4\frac{1}{4} + 2\frac{1}{2}$ = _____

   d. $3\frac{1}{3} + \frac{1}{3}$ = _____

   e. $\frac{1}{4} + 2\frac{1}{8}$ = _____

   f. $1\frac{1}{2} + 3\frac{1}{8}$ = _____

F. COMPARING FRACTIONS

1. Which is the largest fraction?

   a. $\frac{4}{5}$ or $\frac{2}{3}$ _____

   b. $\frac{5}{8}$ or $\frac{3}{8}$ _____

   c. $\frac{2}{3}$ or $\frac{1}{10}$ _____

   d. $\frac{5}{16}$ or $\frac{3}{8}$ _____

   e. $\frac{2}{5}$ or $\frac{1}{2}$ _____

   f. $\frac{1}{4}$ or $\frac{1}{2}$ _____

2. You read an older textbook that discusses drugs and their administration. The text states that the average dose of morphine is grain $^{1}/_{6}$ to grain $^{1}/_{4}$. Which is the larger of the two doses? _____

G. MULTIPLYING FRACTIONS

1. Multiply the following fractions. When necessary, reduce the answer to the lowest possible terms.

   a. $\frac{1}{2} \times \frac{1}{4}$ = _____

   b. $\frac{2}{3} \times \frac{1}{2}$ = _____

   c. $\frac{2}{3} \times \frac{4}{5}$ = _____

   d. $\frac{5}{6} \times \frac{7}{8}$ = _____

   e. $\frac{1}{10} \times \frac{4}{5}$ = _____

   f. $\frac{1}{3} \times \frac{1}{3}$ = _____

H. MULTIPLYING WHOLE NUMBERS AND FRACTIONS

1. Multiply the following whole numbers and fractions. When necessary, change an improper fraction to a mixed number or a whole number. Reduce all answers to the lowest possible terms.

   a. $4 \times \frac{2}{3} =$ _____

   b. $2 \times \frac{3}{10} =$ _____

   c. $5 \times \frac{1}{2} =$ _____

   d. $7 \times \frac{6}{7} =$ _____

   e. $5 \times \frac{2}{3} =$ _____

   f. $9 \times \frac{2}{3} =$ _____

I. MULTIPLYING MIXED NUMBERS

1. Multiply the following mixed numbers. When necessary, change an improper fraction to a mixed number or a whole number. Reduce all answers to the lowest possible terms.

   a. $3\frac{3}{4} \times 1\frac{1}{2} =$ _____

   b. $2\frac{1}{2} \times 3\frac{1}{4} =$ _____

   c. $4\frac{1}{2} \times 5\frac{1}{2} =$ _____

   d. $2\frac{2}{3} \times 3\frac{1}{2} =$ _____

   e. $4\frac{1}{2} \times 6\frac{1}{3} =$ _____

   f. $7\frac{1}{2} \times 1\frac{2}{3} =$ _____

J. MULTIPLYING A WHOLE NUMBER AND A MIXED NUMBER

1. Multiply the following whole numbers and mixed numbers. When necessary, change an improper fraction to a mixed number or a whole number. Reduce all answers to the lowest possible terms.

   a. $3 \times 4\frac{5}{8} =$ _____

   b. $4 \times 1\frac{1}{2} =$ _____

   c. $2 \times 4\frac{1}{4} =$ _____

   d. $1 \times 3\frac{1}{3} =$ _____

   e. $5 \times 1\frac{1}{2} =$ _____

   f. $2 \times 2\frac{3}{8} =$ _____

2. Mr. Wilson has been advised to drink extra fluids. The glass he uses holds 8 ounces. He tells you he drank 2½ glasses of water. How many ounces did he drink? _____

3. Ms. Adams has been advised to drink a protein supplement. Each container holds 3½ ounces of fluid. She drank three containers in the past 5 hours. How many ounces of the protein supplement did Ms. Adams drink? _____

4. Mr. Brent received 1½ containers of intravenous fluid. Each container held 500 milliliters. How many milliliters did Mr. Brent receive? _____

K. DIVIDING FRACTIONS

1. Divide the following fractions. When necessary, change an improper fraction to a mixed number or a whole number. Reduce all answers to the lowest possible terms.

   a. $\frac{2}{3} \div \frac{1}{3} =$ _____

   b. $\frac{1}{6} \div \frac{1}{3} =$ _____

   c. $\frac{9}{10} \div \frac{1}{3} =$ _____

   d. $\frac{2}{3} \div \frac{1}{6} =$ _____

   e. $\frac{1}{5} \div \frac{2}{3} =$ _____

   f. $\frac{5}{6} \div \frac{2}{3} =$ _____

   g. $\frac{1}{100} \div \frac{1}{1000} =$ _____

   h. $\frac{1}{250} \div \frac{1}{2} =$ _____

L. DIVIDING FRACTIONS AND MIXED NUMBERS

1. Divide the following fractions and mixed numbers. When necessary, change an improper fraction to a mixed number or a whole number.

   a. $2\frac{1}{2} \div \frac{1}{2} =$ _____

   b. $2\frac{1}{3} \div \frac{1}{4} =$ _____

   c. $5\frac{1}{2} \div \frac{1}{4} =$ _____

   d. $3\frac{5}{8} \div \frac{3}{5} =$ _____

   e. $\frac{1}{5} \div 2\frac{2}{3} =$ _____

   f. $\frac{4}{5} \div 2\frac{1}{2} =$ _____

2. Divide the following mixed numbers. When necessary, reduce the answer to the lowest possible terms and change an improper fraction to a mixed number or a whole number.

   a. $1\frac{1}{2} \div 2\frac{1}{2} =$ _____

   b. $2\frac{3}{4} \div 1\frac{5}{8} =$ _____

   c. $8\frac{1}{2} \div 4\frac{1}{2} =$ _____

   d. $6\frac{2}{3} \div 1\frac{2}{3} =$ _____

   e. $8\frac{1}{2} \div 4\frac{1}{4} =$ _____

   f. $1\frac{3}{8} \div 2\frac{1}{2} =$ _____

3. Divide the following whole numbers and fractions. When necessary, reduce the answer to the lowest possible terms.

   a. $2 \div \frac{2}{4} =$ _____

   b. $\frac{1}{16} \div 2 =$ _____

   c. $\frac{1}{8} \div 3 =$ _____

   d. $\frac{2}{3} \div 2 =$ _____

   e. $\frac{1}{6} \div 2 =$ _____

   f. $3 \div \frac{1}{8} =$ _____

4. Divide the following whole numbers and mixed numbers. When necessary, reduce the answer to the lowest possible terms and change an improper fraction to a mixed number or a whole number.

   a. $4 \div 5\frac{1}{2} =$ ___

   b. $1\frac{1}{2} \div 2 =$ ___

   c. $5 \div 4\frac{3}{4} =$ ___

   d. $4 \div 2\frac{1}{10} =$ ___

   e. $3\frac{1}{3} \div 2 =$ ___

   f. $6 \div 2\frac{1}{2} =$ ___

M. RATIOS

1. Define a ratio. _____

   _____

2. Write the following as both a ratio and a fraction. When necessary, reduce to the lowest possible terms.

	Ratio	Fraction
a. one part to four parts	_____	_____
b. one part to one hundred parts	_____	_____
c. five parts to fifty parts	_____	_____
d. One hundred parts to two hundred parts	_____	_____

3. Write the following ratios as fractions.

   a. 1:200 = _____

   b. 1:1000 = _____

   c. 1:5 = _____

   d. 1:120 = _____

4. Express the following fractions as ratios.

   a. $\frac{1}{10}$

   b. $\frac{1}{250}$

   c. $\frac{3}{400}$

   d. $\frac{1}{2000}$

5. If one solution is labeled as ½ strength and another is labeled as ¼ strength, which is the stronger solution? _____

6. If a solution is labeled as 1:2000, is it stronger or weaker than a solution labeled as 1:200? _____

7. If one drug is labeled as grain $\frac{1}{32}$ and another drug is labeled as grain $\frac{1}{64}$, which is the strongest drug? _____

N. PERCENTAGE

1. Define the term *percent*.

   _____

   _____

2. Express the following percents as parts per hundred.

   a. 54% _____

   b. 35% _____

   c. 80% _____

   d. 25% _____

3. Liz received 87% on a nursing examination. If there were 100 questions on the test, how many questions did Liz answer correctly? _____

4. Express Liz's grade as parts per hundred. _____
   Express Liz's grade as a fraction. _____

5. Change each of the following percents to a fraction. When necessary, reduce the answer to the lowest possible terms.

   a. 22% _____

   b. 50% _____

   c. 37% _____

   d. 90% _____

   e. 10% _____

   f. 41% _____

6. Change the following fractions to percents.

   a. $\frac{4}{5} =$ ___

   b. $\frac{2}{3} =$ ___

   c. $\frac{1}{10} =$ ___

   d. $\frac{3}{8} =$ ___

   e. $\frac{1}{4} =$ ___

   f. $\frac{1}{6} =$ ___

7. Change the following ratios to percents.

   a. 1:500 = _____

   b. 1:50 = _____

   c. 1:250 = _____

   d. 1:8 = _____

   e. 1:1000 = _____

   f. 1:200 = _____

8. Change the following percents to ratios.

   a. 5% = _____

   b. 25% = _____

   c. 30% = _____

   d. 1% = _____

   e. .3% = _____

   f. .8% = _____

9. A solution applied to Ms. Bartel's leg is labeled as 1:250. What is the percentage of the solution? _____

10. A solution used for irrigating the bladder is labeled as 1:4000. What is the percentage of the solution? _____

11. Mr. Jennings has an irrigating solution labeled as 10%. Express 10% as a ratio. _____

O. PROPORTION

1. Solve the following proportions.

   a. 5:10: : 10:X   X = _____

   b. $\frac{4}{X} = \frac{5}{20}$ X = _____

   c. 2:9: : X:18   X = _____

   d. 1:8: : 10:X   X = _____

   e. $\frac{15}{5} = \frac{30}{X}$ X = _____

   f. 7:14: : 14:X   X = _____

2. Set up and solve the following questions as proportions.

   a. If it takes 30 minutes to drive 20 miles, how many miles can be driven in 1 hour?
   Proportion: _____   Solution: X = _____

   b. If it takes 15 minutes to walk 1 mile, how many miles can you walk in 30 minutes?
   Proportion: _____   Solution: X = _____

   c. Using the same figures as in the previous problem but substituting medical terminology, if 15 grains equals 1 gram, how many grams are there in 30 grains?
   Proportion: _____   Solution: X = _____

   d. If 2.2 pounds equals 1 kilogram, how many pounds are there in 45 kilograms?
   Proportion: _____   Solution: X = _____

   e. If 30 milligrams equals 1/2 grain, how many grains are there in 90 milligrams?
   Proportion: _____   Solution: X = _____

   f. If 1 milligram equals 1/60 grain, how many grains are there in 5 milligrams?
   Proportion: _____   Solution: X = _____

P. DECIMALS

1. What is a decimal? _____
   _____

2. Both decimal fractions and mixed fractions are commonly referred to as decimals.

   a. What is a decimal fraction? _____
   _____

   b. What is a mixed decimal?_____
   _____

3. Write the following as decimals.
   a. nine tenths _____
   b. five hundredths _____
   c. three and four tenths _____
   d. one tenth _____

4. Write out the following decimals.
   a. 0.3 is read as _____
   b. 1.7 is read as _____
   c. 0.07 is read as _____
   d. 6.9 is read as _____

5. Add the following decimals.
   a. 1.5 + 1.5 = _____
   b. 100.6 + 50.4 = _____
   c. .7 + 1.9 = _____
   d. 12.4 + 22.3 = _____

6. Subtract the following decimals.
   a. 15.0 − 6.4 = _____
   b. 12.5 − 0.5 = _____
   c. 7.2 − 5.9 = _____
   d. 27.4 − 18.2 = _____

7. Multiply the following whole numbers and decimals.
   a. 2 × 0.5 = _____
   b. 16 × 0.2 = _____
   c. 2 × 3.25 = _____
   d. 12 × 2.4 = _____

8. Multiply the following decimals.

    a. $1.2 \times 3.6 = $ _____

    b. $4.8 \times 1.5 = $ _____

    c. $17.5 \times 0.4 = $ _____

    d. $0.3 \times 6.6 = $ _____

    e. $4.4 \times 6.5 = $ _____

    f. $6.2 \times 2.4 = $ _____

9. Divide the following decimals.

    a. $1.3 \div 2.5 = $

    b. $2.5 \div 1.2 = $

    c. $0.6 \div 0.2 = $

    d. $5.5 \div 7.2 = $

    e. $6.5 \div 9.2 = $

    f. $0.7 \div 10.6 = $

10. Change the following decimals to a fraction. When necessary reduce the answer to the lowest possible terms.

    a. 0.3   c. 0.006

    b. 0.35   d. 0.5

IV. Calculation of Drug Dosages

A. SYSTEMS OF MEASUREMENT

1. Name the three systems of measurement.

    a. _____

    b. _____

    c. _____

2. Which system is most commonly used for the dosage of drugs? _____

3. The unit of weight in the metric system is the _____

4. The unit of volume in the metric system is the _____

5. The unit of length in the metric system is the _____

B. CONVERSION BETWEEN SYSTEMS

1. Although the apothecaries' system and household measurements are rarely used today, nurses may, on occasion, need to use this system. The following problems give practice in converting from the apothecaries' system to the metric system. Label each answer with the correct abbreviation for the metric equivalent.

    a. 30 grains to 30 grams _____

    b. 2 milligrams to grains _____

    c. 2 fluid ounces to milliliters _____

    d. 500 milliliters to pints _____

    e. 30 minims to milliliters _____

    f. 60 grains to grams _____

    g. 1 quart to milliliters _____

C. CONVERTING WITHIN A SYSTEM

1. Convert the following metric measurements. Label the answer with the correct abbreviation.

    a. 2000 mL to liters _____

    b. 30 mg to grams _____

    c. 650 mg to grams _____

    d. 500 mcg to milligrams _____

    e. 0.2 mg to micrograms _____

    f. 100 mg to grams _____

    g. 0.1 g to milligrams _____

    h. 500 mg to grams _____

D. ORAL DOSAGES OF DRUGS

1. Using D/H or any other method, find the correct dosage of the following solid oral drugs. Label each answer correctly—for example, 2 *capsules,* 1 *tablet,* and so on.

   a. Ordered: erythromycin stearate 500 mg
      Have available: erythromycin stearate 250 mg
      Give: _____

   b. Ordered: V-Cillin K 0.5 g
      Have available: V-Cillin K 500 mg tablets
      Give: _____

   c. Ordered: oxacillin sodium 0.25 g
      Have available: oxacillin sodium 250 mg tablets
      Give: _____

   d. Ordered: Feldene 20 mg
      Have available: Feldene 10 mg capsules
      Give: _____

   e. Ordered: Cipro 0.5 g
      Have available: Cipro 250 mg tablets
      Give: _____

   f. Alkeran 4 mg
      Have available: Alkeran 2 mg tablets
      Give: _____

   g. Ordered: Dipentum 1 g/day in two equally divided doses
      Have available: Dipentum 250 mg capsules
      Give: _____

2. Using proportion or any other method, answer the following questions. Note that some of these problems may require conversion within a system.

   a. If the total daily dose of a drug is 0.9 g and the drug is to be given in three equally divided doses each day, what is the amount of each dose in milligrams? _____

   b. If a drug is available as 250 mg tablets and 0.5 g is given bid (twice a day) what is the total number of tablets given each day? _____

   c. If 500 mg of a drug is given qid (four times a day), what is the total amount of the drug given each day in milligrams? _____ In grams? _____

   d. A patient is to receive a total of 1.5 g of a drug each day in three equally divided doses. How much of the drug is given each time? _____

   e. If the usual daily dose of Zantac is 300 mg and the drug is normally given bid, what is the dosage given each time? _____

3. Using D/H × Q = X or any other method, find the correct dosage of the following liquid oral drugs.

   a. Ordered: Pentids "400" 200,000 units
      Have available: Pentids "400" 400,000 units/5 mL
      Give: _____

   b. Ordered: Retrovir syrup 200 mg
      Have available: Retrovir syrup 50mg/5 mL
      Give: _____

   c. Ordered: ampicillin 125 mg
      Have available: ampicillin 250 mg/5 mL
      Give: _____

   d. Ordered: Spectobid 250 mg
      Have available: Spectobid 125 mg/5 mL
      Give: _____

E. PARENTERAL DOSAGES OF DRUGS

1. Using D/H × Q = X or any other method, determine the amount of drug (liquid volume) to be given for the following parenteral preparations. Label each answer.

   a. Ordered: Demerol 50 mg IM
      Have available: Demerol 75 mg/mL
      Give: _____

   b. Ordered : Dilaudid 1 mg SC
      Have available: Dilaudid 2 mg/mL
      Give: _____

   c. Ordered: Levo-Dromoran 3 mg SC
      Have available: Levo-Dromoran 2 mg/mL
      Give: _____

   d. Ordered: Valium 10 mg IM
      Have available: Valium 5 mg/mL
      Give: _____

   e. Ordered: hydroxyzine 25 mg IM
      Have available: hydroxyzine 50 mg/mL
      Give: _____

   f. Ordered: Zantac 150 mg added to an IV infusion
      Have available: Zantac 25 mg/mL
      Give: _____

   g. Ordered: Vancomycin 500 mg added to IV infusion
      Have available: Vancomycin 1 g/10 mL
      Give: _____

h. Ordered: Rocephin 1 g/day in two divided doses IM
   Have available: Rocephin 1 g vial; when reconstituted according to directions 250 mg/mL
   Give: _____

2. Using proportion or any other method, answer the following questions.

   a. A multiple dose vial of cimetidine contains 8 mL. If the usual dose of this drug is 300 mg and the vial is labeled 300 mg/2 mL, how many 300 mg doses are contained in the vial? _____

   b. A patient is to receive 60 mL of 5% dextrose in water IV each hour. The IV fluid is available in 500 mL and 1000 mL containers. How many containers should be on hand to provide a 24-hour supply of IV fluid? _____

   c. The directions for reconstitution of a drug read: Reconstitute each gram of ticarcillin with 2 mL sterile water for injection or sodium chloride injection. Ticarcillin is available in 1 g, 3 g, and 6 g vials. How much diluent would you add to each of these vials?
      1 g vial _____; 3 g vial _____; 6 g vial _____

F. CALCULATING IV FLOW RATES

1. Using any method, calculate the following.

   a. 1000 mL to infuse in 8 hours. The drop factor is 14. The IV is to infuse at _____ drops per minute.

   b. If 1000 mL of IV fluid is to be infused over a period of 12 hours, how many milliliters are infused each hour? _____

   c. 1000 mL to infuse in 12 hours. The drop factor is 15. The IV is to infuse at _____ drops per minute.

   d. An IV solution is to infuse at 120 mL/h. The drop factor is 15. The IV is to infuse at _____ drops per minute.

   e. The physician orders a continuous IV infusion to run at 90 mL/h. How many milliliters will be infused in 24 hours? _____

   f. A patient is to receive 2500 mL of IV fluid infused over 24 hours. How many milliliters are infused each hour? _____

   g. A child is to receive 400 mL of IV fluid over 24 hours. How many milliliters are infused each hour? _____

h. 1000 mL to infuse in 8 hours. The drop factor is 12. The IV is to infuse at _____ drops per minute.

G. ORAL OR PARENTERAL DRUG DOSAGES BASED ON WEIGHT

1. Convert the following weights given in pounds to kilograms.

   a. 10 pounds = _____ kg

   b. 165 pounds = _____ kg

   c. 123 pounds = _____ kg

   d. 140 pounds = _____ kg

   e. 22 pounds = _____ kg

   f. 60 pounds = _____ kg

2. Convert the following weights given in kilograms to pounds.

   a. 100 kilograms = _____ lb

   b. 40 kilograms = _____ lb

   c. 20 kilograms = _____ lb

   d. 55 kilograms = _____ lb

3. Calculate the following drug dosages.

   a. A child weighing 40 pounds is to receive oral oxacillin. The recommended dose is 50 mg/kg/d in four equally divided doses. What dose of the drug is given each time? _____ If oxacillin is available as an oral solution labeled as 250 mg/5 mL, how many mL are given each time? _____

   b. A patient with a body surface area of 1.9 m² is to receive Pentostatin. The dose of Pentostatin is 4 mg/m². The dose to be given is _____.

   c. A patient is to receive a parenteral drug whose dose is 6 mg/kg/d in four equally divided doses q6h. The patient weighs 135 pounds. What is the total daily dosage of the drug? _____ What is the dose given each time? _____

   d. A patient is to receive Ativan IV. The recommended dose is 0.044 mg/kg. The patient weighs 145 pounds. What is the dose given to this patient? _____ If the drug is available in 10 mL vials labeled as 2 mg/mL, how many milliliters are withdrawn from the vial? _____

H. TEMPERATURES

1. Convert the following temperatures written in Fahrenheit to Celsius.

    a. 92° F = _____   c. 102° F = _____

    b. 101° F = _____   d. 99.2° F = _____

2. Convert the following temperatures written in Celsius to Fahrenheit.

    a. 37.5° C = _____   c. 38.4° C = _____

    b. 38° C = _____   d. 38.9° C = _____

CHAPTER 4

The Nursing Process

I. Matching

Match each term in Column A with the correct definition or statement in Column B.

COLUMN A

_____ 1. objective data

_____ 2. initial assessment

_____ 3. nursing diagnosis

_____ 4. NANDA

_____ 5. subjective data

_____ 6. implementation

_____ 7. evaluation

_____ 8. planning

_____ 9. ongoing assessment

_____ 10. expected outcome

COLUMN B

A. Carrying out a plan of action.

B. The expected behavior of the patient or family that indicates the problem is being resolved or progress is occurring.

C. Completed when the patient is first seen in the hospital.

D. An organization formed to define, explain, classify, and research summary statements about health problems related to nursing.

E. Facts observed by the nurse during the physical assessment or physical examination.

F. Identifies problems that can be solved or prevented by independent nursing actions.

G. Steps for carrying out nursing activities or interventions that will meet expected outcomes.

H. Phase of the nursing process that determines the effectiveness of nursing interventions in meeting expected outcomes.

I. Information supplied by the patient or patient's family.

J. Performed at the time of every patient contact.

II. Multiple Choice

Circle the letter of the most appropriate answer.

1. The nurse performing a physical assessment is told by the patient, "I have headaches every day." This patient information would be considered:

   a. subjective data.   c. medical data.

   b. personal data.   d. objective data.

2. The nurse will use the information obtained during the initial assessment to:

   a. evaluate the patient's need for a certain type of medication.

   b. provide a database from which present and future decisions can be made.

   c. aid the physician in selecting the correct drug and dosage.

   d. evaluate the effectiveness of a drug the patient has been taking.

3. A nurse caring for an incontinent patient prevents skin breakdown by keeping him clean and dry. This nursing task is referred to as:

   a. an independent nursing action.

   b. an unexpected outcome.

   c. a nursing diagnosis.

   d. an evaluation of the plan.

4. When a nurse documents subjective data in the patient chart, the information has been obtained from:

   a. the physician's notes.

   b. other health care team members.

   c. past entries in the patient chart.

   d. information given by the patient or family.

5. After completing an assessment of the patient, the nurse uses the data to develop a nursing diagnosis that will be based on:

   a. the physician's medical diagnosis.

   b. the identified problems of the patient.

   c. the cause of the patient's illness.

   d. a description of subjective data.

6. The nursing process includes establishing expected outcomes. These goals should be:

   a. patient oriented.   c. physician oriented.

   b. staff oriented.   d. nurse oriented.

7. The nurse uses the evaluation phase of the nursing process to:

   a. make sure nursing procedures have been performed.

   b. make a list of all nursing tasks that have been performed.

   c. make decisions regarding the effectiveness of nursing interventions.

   d. make notations regarding the patient's response to medical treatment.

8. A patient tells you, "I'm afraid to take the medicine. My sister was taking the same kind of medicine and it made her really sick." Which nursing diagnosis will be most appropriate for this patient?

   a. Noncompliance

   b. Effective Therapeutic Regimen Management

   c. Deficient Knowledge

   d. Anxiety

9. A patient is receiving a blood pressure medication for high blood pressure. His blood pressure has decreased from 172/104 to 130/82. The nurse must decide what actions she must take in regard to administering the medication. Which phase of the nursing process does this involve?

   a. Implementation   c. Diagnosis

   b. Evaluation   d. Planning

10. A patient tells the nurse, "I know I should be taking my pills three times a day, but I can't afford to take more than two a day." The nurse decides that the most appropriate nursing diagnosis would be:

    a. Effective Therapeutic Regimen Management

    b. Anxiety

    c. Ineffective Therapeutic Regimen Management

    d. Deficent Knowledge

III. Fill in the Blanks

1. List the five phases of the nursing process.

   a) _____
   b) _____
   c) _____
   d) _____
   e) _____

2. List the two components of assessment.

   a) _____
   b) _____

3. List the two types of data collected during an assessment.

   a) _____
   b) _____

4. List the four nursing diagnoses most commonly used when administering medications.

   a) _____
   b) _____
   c) _____
   d) _____

5. List six possible causes of Ineffective Management of the Health Care Regimen.

   a) _____
   b) _____
   c) _____
   d) _____
   e) _____
   f) _____

IV. Crossword Puzzle

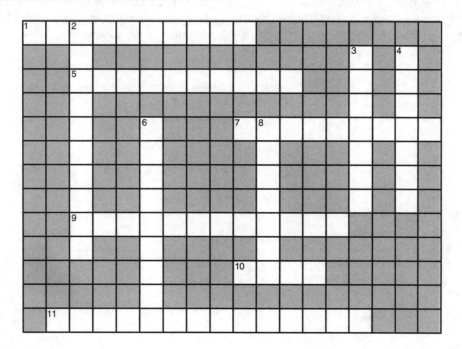

ACROSS CLUES

1. Process used to determine effectiveness of nursing interventions.
5. Facts supplied by the patient or the patient's family.
7. A description of the patient's problems and their related causes.
9. Not complying with the treatment regimen.
10. Lays the groundwork for carrying out nursing interventions.
11. Carrying out a plan of action.

DOWN CLUES

2. Collecting objective and subjective data.
3. Assessment made at the time of each patient contact.
4. A vague uneasiness.
6. Data obtained during the physical examination.
8. Assessment made when patient is first seen in the health care setting.

V. Critical Thinking

1. A new nurse tells her coworker that she is having difficulty deciding between the nursing diagnoses of Noncompliance and Ineffective Therapeutic Regimen Management. What information should the nurse look for to make this decision?

2. A nurse working with you states she has difficulty understanding and using the nursing process. Discuss examples you could give to show that the parts of the nursing process are often used in our daily lives.

3. Several nurses on your unit are having difficulty with setting patient goals. Explain how you would help these nurses better to understand this step in the nursing process.

4. Discuss the possible causes that could lead to the nursing diagnosis of Ineffective Therapeutic Regimen Management. How would the nurse respond to these causes?

CHAPTER 5

Patient and Family Teaching

I. Matching

Match each term in Column A with the correct definition or statement in Column B.

COLUMN A

_____ 1. affective domain

_____ 2. teaching

_____ 3. motivation

_____ 4. evaluation

_____ 5. planning

_____ 6. learning

_____ 7. nursing diagnosis

_____ 8. implementation

_____ 9. cognitive domain

_____10. assessment

COLUMN B

A. Development of strategies to be used in the teaching plan.

B. Acquiring new skills.

C. Attitudes, feelings, beliefs, and opinions.

D. Method used to determine the effectiveness of a teaching plan.

E. Thought, recall, decision-making, and drawing conclusions.

F. Interactive process that promotes learning.

G. Desire or seeing the need to learn.

H. Formulated after analyzing the data obtained during the assessment.

I. Data-gathering phase of the nursing process.

J. Actual performance of interventions identified in the teaching plan.

II. Multiple Choice

Circle the letter of the most appropriate answer.

1. Mr. Smith comments to the nurse, "One of my home medications has changed color and smells bad." The nurse best replies by telling Mr. Smith:
   a. to place the drug in a different container.
   b. to call his pharmacist and ask if he should keep taking the drug.
   c. the drug may have deteriorated.
   d. this may be a normal chemical change in the drug.

2. The nurse is preparing a teaching plan for a patient who has mild dementia and has suffered a stroke, which has left her dominant hand paralyzed. Which two domains of learning have been impaired?
   a. Cognitive and affective
   b. Psychomotor and affective
   c. Cognitive and psychomotor
   d. Affective and cognitive

3. The nurse should inform patients that their medications should not be exposed to heat, sunlight, or moisture because:
   a. it may cause a color change.
   b. a poisonous residue will form.
   c. the printing on the label will fade.
   d. a chemical change may occur.

4. A patient who has been prescribed bright orange-colored tablets asks if they can be chewed before swallowing. The best response from the nurse would be:
   a. as long as it's a tablet, you can chew it.
   b. you may never chew a tablet.
   c. only drugs labeled "chewable" should be chewed.
   d. it is always safe to chew white tablets.

5. A nurse preparing a teaching plan for a 62-year-old patient who is being released from the hospital considers the adult learning process. The nurse should remember:

   a. adults learn only when they feel the need to learn.

   b. most adults prefer an informal environment.

   c. a large percentage of adults are visual learners.

   d. all of the above describe adult learners.

6. Implementation of a teaching plan can be most effective if the nurse initiates the teaching:

   a. a day or more before discharge, when the patient is alert and comfortable.

   b. when the patient has several visitors from out of town to help him remember.

   c. while several other health care providers are in the room bathing the patient.

   d. by providing written, standard material and saying, "If you have any questions, let me know."

7. If there are no specific instructions on the medication label, the best instructions from the nurse would be to take the medication with:

   a. fruit juice.   c. water.

   b. milk.   d. food.

8. Teaching and learning are interactive processes. When developing a teaching plan, the nurse should remember:

   a. only the patient must be actually involved in the teaching process.

   b. when learning occurs, there will be a change in the patient's behavior.

   c. a patient does not have to be motivated for learning to occur.

   d. a therapeutic nurse–patient relationship is only a minor prerequisite to learning.

9. Mr. Billings tells the nurse that the antibiotic prescribed for him is to be taken for 2 weeks. After 6 days, his symptoms are gone and he asks if he can stop taking the drug. The best response from the nurse would be:

   a. "If you want, stop taking the medication and call the physician."

   b. "Check with your pharmacist and ask if you can stop taking the drug."

   c. "Do not stop taking the drug until you check with your physician."

   d. "Stop the drug and let your physician know at your next office visit."

10. Some of the important information the nurse should include in a teaching plan for medication is:

   a. dosage of the drug and route of administration.

   b. therapeutic response expected from the drug.

   c. adverse reactions to expect when taking this drug.

   d. all of the above are important for the patient to learn.

III. Fill in the Blanks

1. Assessment allows the nurse to gather data that will identify the patient's individual needs. List the three areas these needs stem from.

   a) _____

   b) _____

   c) _____

2. List the basic information to consider when developing a teaching plan for medication.

   a) _____

   b) _____

   c) _____

   d) _____

   e) _____

   f) _____

3. List the three domains of learning and give a brief definition of each.

   a) _____

   b) _____

   c) _____

IV. Critical Thinking

1. A new nurse on your unit is preparing a teaching plan for a patient who is to be discharged in 2 days with several new medications. This nurse has asked your help in preparing the teaching for the patient. Discuss how you could assist this nurse to develop the skills necessary for this process.

2. Mr. Jones is to be dismissed within the next 2 days. He will be taking several oral medications after discharge from the hospital. Mr. Jones is very forgetful and the nurse caring for him is unsure if he can take his medications correctly when he gets home. Discuss what suggestions you can make to assist Mr. Jones in taking his medications as prescribed.

3. Ms. Gates is scheduled for dismissal from the hospital tomorrow. Her physician has prescribed two new oral medications daily. You are going to develop a teaching plan for Ms. Gates, but first you must assess her motivation and ability to learn. Discuss methods you could use to assess a patient's motivation and ability to learn.

V. Crossword Puzzle

ACROSS CLUES

3. Psychomotor domain involves learning new _____ skills.
4. Acquiring new knowledge or skills.
7. Teaching plans are _____ to meet specific patient needs.
8. The area of a prescription bottle where dosage instructions are written.
9. Domain of learning associated with thought, recall, decision-making, and drawing conclusions.
10. Having the desire or seeing the need to learn.

DOWN CLUES

1. Under most circumstances, it is the fluid of choice for taking medications.
2. Domain of learning associated with attitudes, feelings, beliefs, and opinions.
5. Type of bracelet worn when taking certain medications.
6. Interactive process that promotes learning.

VI. Internet Exercise

Use one of the following Web addresses,
www.rxlist.com, www.healthatoz.com, or
www.mayoclinic.com (or any other comparable Web
site), to find information concerning a specific drug.
Use the information to develop a patient education
plan.

CHAPTER 6

Sulfonamides

I. Matching

Match each term in Column A with the correct definition or statement in Column B.

COLUMN A

_____ 1. antibacterial

_____ 2. prophylaxis drug treatment

_____ 3. agranulocytosis

_____ 4. stomatitis

_____ 5. sulfonamides

_____ 6. anorexia

_____ 7. crystalluria

_____ 8. bacteriostatic

_____ 9. thrombocytopenia

_____ 10. photosensitivity reaction

COLUMN B

A. The first antibiotic that effectively treated infections.

B. Decrease in number of platelets.

C. Slows or retards the multiplication of bacteria.

D. Reaction similar to severe sunburn.

E. Loss of appetite.

F. Inflammation of the mouth.

G. Crystals in the urine.

H. Receiving a drug to prevent an infection.

I. Active against bacteria.

J. Decrease in or lack of granulocytes.

II. Multiple Choice

Circle the letter of the most appropriate answer.

Mr. Lawrence, a patient in a clinic treating urological diseases, is being treated for repeated urinary tract infections. His physician has prescribed a sulfonamide preparation for his most recent infection. Questions 1–3 pertain to Mr. Lawrence's case.

1. Mr. Lawrence asks how the sulfonamides control an infection. The nurse would correctly answer that these drugs:
   a. make the urine alkaline, which eliminates bacteria.
   b. cause a decrease in urine output.
   c. interfere with the action of PABA, a substance some bacteria need to multiply.
   d. encourage the production of antibodies that fight off the bacteria.

2. While teaching Mr. Lawrence about the sulfonamides, the nurse stresses the importance of:
   a. taking the drug with a full glass of water.
   b. limiting his fluid intake while taking these drugs.
   c. drinking fruit juice.
   d. taking the drug at mealtime with a glass of milk.

3. When Mr. Lawrence returns to the clinic, the nurse can evaluate his response to treatment by asking him if:
   a. he completed taking all the medication.
   b. his symptoms have been relieved.
   c. he has noticed blood in his urine.
   d. he has had any further tests on his urine.

4. A patient asks why it is important to take the entire antibiotic during a course of therapy. The nurse would be correct to respond that taking all of the medicine is necessary to:

   a. maintain adequate blood levels of the drug for 3 to 4 weeks.

   b. ensure all the infecting microorganisms have been eradicated.

   c. prevent crystalluria and albuminuria from occurring in the urine.

   d. prevent a superimposed infection in the urinary tract.

5. Patients who are prescribed sulfasalazine (Azulfidine) for ulcerative colitis are told that the drug:

   a. is to be taken with food.

   b. rarely causes adverse effects.

   c. may cause hair loss.

   d. may turn the urine a yellow-orange color.

6. When mafenide, a topical sulfonamide, is used in the treatment of burns, it is applied to the burned area:

   a. with a sterile gloved hand.

   b. immediately before debridement.

   c. with cotton wads or balls.

   d. every 1 to 2 hours.

7. When mafenide (Sulfamylon) is applied to a burn area, the nurse:

   a. uses a sterile gauze pad to apply the drug.

   b. uses the mafenide to cleanse and debride the area.

   c. warns the patient that stinging or burning may occur.

   d. instructs the patient to drink large amounts of water.

8. A patient who has been prescribed an oral sulfonamide is experiencing gastrointestinal irritation. The nurse would be correct to tell the patient to:

   a. discontinue taking the medication.

   b. take the drug with food or right after meals.

   c. keep the drug refrigerated, which will prevent this.

   d. take the drug 1 hour before or 2 hours after a meal.

9. A nurse is assessing a patient who is taking a sulfonamide for a urinary tract infection. The patient has red blisters on the face and in the mouth. These symptoms would alert the nurse to the possibility of:

   a. thrombocytopenia.

   b. Stevens-Johnson syndrome.

   c. aplastic anemia.

   d. leukopenia.

10. A nurse educating a patient taking a sulfonamide teaches that crystalluria may be prevented by:

   a. drinking large amounts of cranberry juice.

   b. limiting the amount of fluid intake.

   c. limiting the amount of salt intake.

   d. increasing fluid intake to 2000 mL a day.

III. Crossword Puzzle

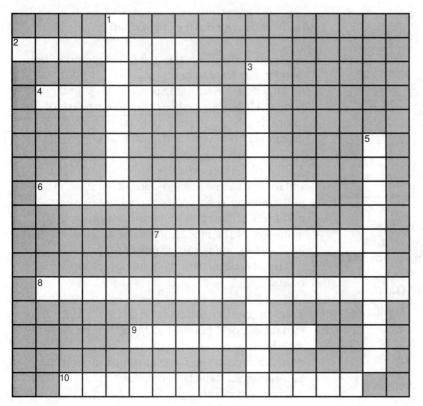

ACROSS CLUES

2. Hypersensitivity.
4. Loss of appetite.
6. Crystals in the urine.
7. A decrease in the number of white blood cells.
8. A decrease in the number of platelets.
9. Type of anemia that occurs because of deficient red blood cell production in the bone marrow.
10. Active against bacteria.

DOWN CLUES

1. Itching
3. Slows the multiplication of bacteria.
5. Inflammation of the mouth.

IV. Fill in the Blanks

1. Sulfonamide therapy can be associated with these hematologic changes:

   a) _____

   b) _____

   c) _____

   d) _____

2. Define each of the four hematologic changes associated with sulfonamide therapy.

   a) _____
   _____

   b) _____
   _____

   c) _____
   _____

   d) _____
   _____

3. List and define the three terms used to describe the sulfonamides.

   a) _____
   _____

   b) _____
   _____

   c) _____
   _____

4. List the two topical sulfonamides used in the treatment of second- and third-degree burns.

   a) _____

   b) _____

5. The sulfonamides are used with caution in patients:

a) _____

b) _____

c) _____

d) _____

e) _____

f) _____

V. Critical Thinking

1. Ms. Smith is being treated prophylactically with sulfasalazine (Azulfidine) for ulcerative colitis. She will need to learn how to monitor for adverse and allergic reactions associated with this medication. Discuss how you would teach Ms. Smith to identify hematologic changes that might occur.

2. Anorexia and stomatitis have occurred in your patient who is taking an oral sulfonamide. Discuss nursing interventions that could be used to assist this patient in dealing with these adverse reactions.

3. Mr. Stevens is receiving sulfisoxazole (Gantrisin) for a recurrent bladder infection. He tells you he feels like he has the flu. He describes his symptoms as feeling warm and achy, with a headache. Discuss how you would determine if Mr. Stevens might have a problem more serious than the flu.

4. Ms. Evans is a diabetic taking tolbutamide (Orinase). Her physician has prescribed the combination drug sulfamethoxazole and trimethoprim (Septra) for a low-grade, recurrent bladder infection. Discuss how you would explain the drug interaction that might occur and any special instructions you would give to Ms. Evans.

VI. Dosage Problems

Solve the following dosage calculations.

1. A doctor orders sulfasalazine (Azulfidine), initial dose of 2 grams, then 2 grams daily in four divided doses. Azulfidine comes in 500-milligram tablets. How many tablets should be given for the initial dose?_____ How many tablets should be given every 6 hours for the daily dose?_____

2. The combination drug sulfamethoxazole–trimethoprim contains 200 milligrams of sulfamethoxazole in each 5 milliliters of liquid. The doctor has ordered 10 milliliters of the medication to be given every 12 hours. How many milligrams of sulfamethoxazole will the patient receive every 24 hours? _____

3. Your patient has sulfadiazine ordered. After the initial dose of 2 grams, orally, he will be receiving maintenance doses of 3 grams in six divided doses each day. The medication is available in 500-milligram tablets. How many tablets will he receive each dose? _____ How often will the doses be given? _____

4. The doctor's order reads, "1000 milligrams of sulfamethizole in 4 divided doses." The medication is available in 500-milligram tablets. How many tablets are to be given at each dose?

_____

VII. Internet Exercise

Go to http://www.mylifeguardforhealth.com. Find information about the sulfonamides. Print the information and discuss in class why this Web site is or is not a reliable source for information about the sulfonamide drugs.

CHAPTER 7

Penicillins

I. Matching

Match each term in Column A with the correct definition or statement in Column B.

COLUMN A

_____ 1. superinfection

_____ 2. normal flora

_____ 3. culture and sensitivity tests

_____ 4. bacteriostatic

_____ 5. glossitis

_____ 6. cross-sensitivity

_____ 7. bacterial resistance

_____ 8. urticaria

_____ 9. anaphylactic shock

_____10. *Candida* fungal superinfection

_____11. bactericidal

_____12. hypersensitivity

_____13. pseudomembranous colitis

_____14. phlebitis

_____15. penicillinase

COLUMN B

A. Ability of bacteria to produce substances that inactivate or destroy the penicillins.

B. An enzyme that inactivates penicillin.

C. Destroys bacteria.

D. Determines if a specific type of bacteria is sensitive to penicillin.

E. A secondary infection that occurs during antibiotic therapy.

F. Allergy to drugs in the same or related groups.

G. Nonpathogenic microorganisms found in the body.

H. A bacterial superinfection occurring in the intestinal tract.

I. Inflammation of the tongue.

J. Inflammation of a vein.

K. Hives.

L. Slows or retards the multiplication of bacteria.

M. A severe form of hypersensitivity reaction.

N. Allergic.

O. Signs and symptoms include lesions in the mouth and around the anal and genital areas.

II. Multiple Choice

Circle the letter of the most appropriate answer.

1. Your patient has been prescribed penicillin G potassium prophylactically. Your teaching would include how to recognize the symptoms of pseudomembranous colitis, the most prominent of which is:

   a. urticaria.   c. bloody diarrhea.

   b. glossitis.   d. anorexia.

2. Mr. Brown is in the clinic complaining of severe diarrhea, abdominal cramping, and blood and mucus in his stool. Five weeks ago, Mr. Brown was treated with penicillin for an upper respiratory infection. His present symptoms may indicate:

   a. cross-sensitivity.

   b. candidiases or moniliasis.

   c. glossitis and stomatitis.

   d. pseudomembranous colitis.

3. While obtaining an allergy history from Mr. Burns, the nurse discovers that he has had an allergic reaction to penicillin in the past. This information alerts the nurse to the fact that Mr. Burns may also be allergic to:

   a. cephalosporins.   c. macrolides.

   b. tetracyclines.   d. erythromycins.

4. When reviewing your patient's culture and sensitivity test, you learn that the bacteria causing the patient's infection are sensitive to penicillin. According to a laboratory test reference book, this test result indicates:

   a. the patient is highly allergic to penicillin.

   b. penicillin is a likely treatment for this infection.

   c. the patient is not allergic to any penicillin

   d. the bacteria are highly resistant to penicillin.

5. Your new patient, Mary Bullis, age 14 years, tells you she has been prescribed penicillin G potassium orally on a continuous basis for the prevention of a repeat episode of rheumatic fever. This type of treatment is called:

   a. prophylactic therapy.

   b. ongoing therapy.

   c. initial therapy.

   d. recurring therapy.

6. Patients receiving penicillin are observed for signs and symptoms of a bacterial superinfection. The most common sign would be:

   a. anorexia.　　　c. glossitis.

   b. urticaria.　　　d. diarrhea.

7. Alice More, a 19-year-old patient, asks the nurse if it matters what time she takes her penicillin medication. The nurse would be correct in stating:

   a. "Just be sure to take it three times a day."

   b. "Take it every time you eat a meal."

   c. "Space your doses evenly throughout a 24-hour day."

   d. "Take it morning, noon, and at bedtime."

8. In preparing to administer a dosage of penicillin in the parenteral form, a nurse would:

   a. be careful not to shake the container and cause bubbles to form.

   b. carefully shake the vial to ensure even distribution throughout the solution.

   c. allow the sediment to settle to the bottom of the medication vial.

   d. allow the penicillin to set for 10 minutes to enhance the rate of absorption.

9. Ms. Thomas, who is receiving oral penicillin for a soft tissue infection, complains of a sore mouth. On inspection, you identify she has a black, furry tongue and bright red oral mucous membranes. The physician is immediately notified because these symptoms may indicate:

   a. a vitamin C deficiency.

   b. severe dehydration.

   c. poor oral hygiene.

   d. a superinfection.

10. A severe, sometimes fatal anaphylactic reaction to penicillin can occur. A nurse must be able to recognize the signs and symptoms of the reaction, which would include:

    a. acute abdominal pain.

    b. severe hypotension and respiratory distress.

    c. loss of consciousness and hypertension.

    d. dry skin and diffuse rash.

11. In order for the nurse properly to administer a penicillin-type drug, he should be aware that:

    a. absorption of most penicillins is affected by food.

    b. penicillins should be given 1 hour before or 2 hours after meals.

    c. some penicillins need to be refrigerated.

    d. all of the above are important properties of penicillins.

12. Which of the following patients will most need information about drug interactions while taking penicillin for their medical treatment?

    a. A 50-year-old man with soft tissue infection who works out daily

    b. A 32-year-old woman with pneumonia who is taking a birth control drug

    c. A 17-year-old boy with upper respiratory infection who plays sports

    d. A 62-year-old woman with a urinary tract infection who takes a multivitamin daily

III. Crossword Puzzle

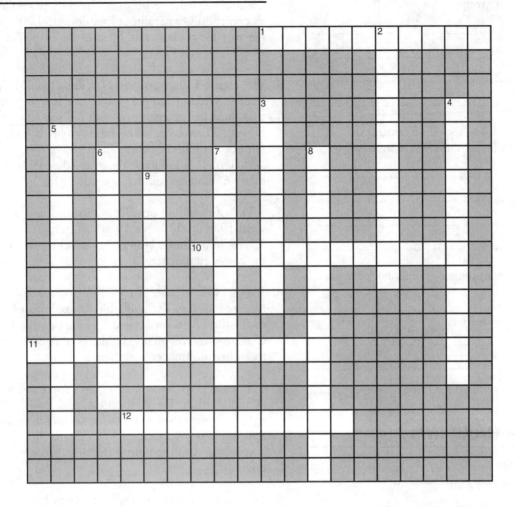

ACROSS CLUES

1. Low white blood cell count.
10. Destroys bacteria.
11. Enzyme that inactivates penicillin.
12. Disease producing.

DOWN CLUES

2. Preventive.
3. Inflammation of a vein.
4. A severe form of hypersensitivity reaction is called _____ shock.
5. Normal flora found in the mouth.
6. Laboratory examination used to determine the appropriate antibiotic to treat an infection.
7. Inflammation of the mouth.
8. A secondary infection that occurs during antibiotic treatment.
9. Inflammation of the tongue.

IV. Fill in the Blanks

1. Before the nurse administers the first dose of penicillin, a health history should be completed. The health history should contain:

   a) _____

   b) _____

   c) _____

   d) _____

2. List four nursing diagnoses that may be used for patients taking penicillin antibiotics.

   a) _____

   b) _____

   c) _____

   d) _____

3. List the four groups of penicillins and give names of drugs in each group.

    a) _____

    b) _____

    c) _____

    d) _____

4. List four examples of the combinations of penicillins with beta-lactamase inhibitors.

    a) _____

    b) _____

    c) _____

    d) _____

5. List signs and symptoms of pseudomembranous colitis.

    a) _____

    b) _____

    c) _____

    d) _____

V. Dosage Problems

Solve the following dosage calculations.

1. The physician's order reads, "Amoxicillin, 0.5 g, PO, q 6 hours." The drug is available as: Amoxicillin oral suspension 125 mg per 5 mL. How many milliliters would you administer each dose? _____

2. The physician's order reads, "V-Cillin K suspension, 500,000 U, PO, QID." The drug is available as V-Cillin K oral solution, 200,000 U per 5 mL. How many milliliters would you administer? _____

3. The physician's order reads, "penicillin G, 250,000 U, IM, q 6 hours." The drug is available as penicillin G procaine suspension, 300,000 U per mL. How many milliliters of the penicillin would you give? _____

4. The physician has ordered Nafcillin, 1 g, IM, q 6 hours. Nafcillin sodium is available in a 2-g vial that must be reconstituted with 6.6 mL of diluent. The reconstituted solution yields 8 mL, with each milliliter containing 250 mg of Nafcillin. To administer the ordered dose, how many milliliters would you need? _____

5. A vial of penicillin powder is reconstituted to yield 10,000,000 U per 10 mL. A patient is to receive 600,000 U. How many milliliters should the nurse administer? _____

6. The nurse is to administer 600 mg amoxicillin (Amoxil) orally. The available Amoxil must be reconstituted and will yield 250 mg per milliliter of solution. How many milliliters of Amoxil will the nurse administer? _____

7. The nurse is to prepare 250 mg of Augmentin for administration. The Augmentin label reads, "125 mg per 5 mL of solution." One teaspoon contains approximately 125 mg of Augmentin. How many teaspoons would the nurse instruct the patient to take? _____

8. Your pediatric patient has been prescribed amoxicillin, 125 mg, PO, q 8 hours. Your patient weighs 16 pounds. The Amoxil label reads, "when reconstituted, each 5 mL of solution yields 125 mg amoxicillin." The label also states, "usual dosage for children is 20–40 mg/kg/day in divided doses every 8 hours." What would be the recommended dosage range for your patient? Is the ordered dosage safe? _____

CHAPTER 8

Cephalosporins

I. Matching

Match each term in Column A with the correct definition or statement in Column B.

COLUMN A

_____ 1. Stevens-Johnson syndrome

_____ 2. cephalosporins

_____ 3. nephrotoxicity

_____ 4. thrombophlebitis

_____ 5. aplastic anemia

_____ 6. cefaclor

_____ 7. diarrhea

_____ 8. Hemoccult

_____ 9. Rocephin

_____ 10. fungal superinfection

COLUMN B

A. Anemia due to deficient red blood cell production.

B. Symptom that may indicate pseudomembranous colitis.

C. Test used to detect occult blood in the stool.

D. Structurally and chemically related to penicillin.

E. Inflammation of a vein with formation of a blood clot in the vein.

F. Infection that may occur in the mouth, vagina, and anogenital area when taking the cephalosporins.

G. Damage to the kidneys by a toxic substance.

H. Serious hypersensitivity reaction sometimes seen with cephalosporins.

I. Third-generation cephalosporin.

J. Second-generation cephalosporin.

II. Fill in the Blanks

1. Cephalosporins may be differentiated according to the _____ that are _____ to them.

2. Cephalosporins are valuable in treating _____ that have become _____ to penicillin.

3. Cephalosporins affect the _____ ___ ____, making it _____ and _____, resulting in the destruction of the _____.

4. The most common adverse reactions seen with cephalosporins are _____, _____, and _____.

5. Because of the close relation of the cephalosporins to penicillin, a patient who is allergic to _____ may also be allergic to the _____.

III. Multiple Choice

Circle the letter of the most appropriate answer.

A team conference is held to discuss the drug therapy being used to treat Ms. Yates' infection. One of the drugs used belongs to the group of drugs called cephalosporins. Questions 1–4 pertain to Ms. Yates' care.

1. A nurse asks why Ms. Yates received a cephalosporin preoperatively. The most correct answer is that preoperative use may help prevent infection in those having surgery:
   a. on the lower extremities.
   b. that require a general anesthetic.
   c. in or near the abdominal cavity.
   d. on a contaminated or potentially contaminated area.

2. A nurse asks why it is important to determine if Ms. Yates is allergic to penicillin before the first dose of cephalosporins is given. Another nurse correctly answers that a person who is allergic to penicillin:
   a. is usually allergic to most other antibiotics.
   b. requires higher doses of the cephalosporins.
   c. is more likely to be allergic to cephalosporins.
   d. responds poorly to antibiotic treatment.

3. Two nurses reviewing the adverse reactions associated with cephalosporins agree that the most common are:
   a. hypotension, dizziness, urticaria.
   b. vomiting, nausea, diarrhea.
   c. skin rash, constipation, headache.
   d. bradycardia, pruritus, insomnia.

4. While the cephalosporin is administered, Ms. Yates is observed for signs and symptoms of a mild hypersensitivity reaction, one of which is:
   a. pruritus.   c. psoriasis.
   b. cardiac arrhythmia. d. nephrotoxicity.

5. During the ongoing assessment of a patient being treated with cephalosporins, he tells you that he has been experiencing abdominal cramping and has seen blood in his stool. The nurse would be correct in notifying the primary health care provider immediately because these symptoms may indicate:
   a. a fungal infection.   c. a gastric ulcer.
   b. ulcerative colitis.   d. a parasitic infection.

6. When a cephalosporin is given by the intramuscular route, the drug is injected into:
   a. the deltoid muscle.   c. the gluteus muscle.
   b. the abdominal area.   d. the triceps muscle.

7. Cephalosporin medication can be administered as an intramuscular injection. The nurse should explain to the patient that:
   a. a stinging, burning sensation will be felt and the site will be sore.
   b. the injection site will be red for several days.
   c. all injections will be given in the same area.
   d. the injection should not cause any discomfort.

8. When cephalosporins are administered as a continuous intravenous drip, nursing responsibilities would include:
   a. keeping the infusion bottle 12 inches above the bed.
   b. inspecting the catheter insertion site for extravasation or infiltration.
   c. placing the extremity being used higher than the patient's head.
   d. changing the dressing over the catheter insertion site every 2 hours.

9. A patient receiving a cephalosporin intravenously is complaining of redness in the arm above the intravenous catheter insertion site. The nurse would be aware that this symptom could indicate:
   a. endocarditis.   c. hypovolemia.
   b. phlebitis.   d. arteriospasm.

10. The nurse must be aware of the possibility for Stevens-Johnson syndrome to occur in the patient taking a cephalosporin. Signs and symptoms that could indicate this syndrome is occurring include:
   a. hypertension, fast heart rate, increased respirations.
   b. swelling of the hands and feet.
   c. pain in the joints of the hands and feet.
   d. red wheals and blisters on the skin or mucous membranes.

IV. Dosage Problems

Solve the following dosage calculations.

1. Cephalexin (Keflex) is available in oral suspension and is often prescribed for children. The vial label contains the following information:

   125 mg cephalexin per 5 mL of solution
   Usual pediatric dosage: 25–50 mg/kg/day in four divided doses

   1 teaspoon contains approximately 125 mg cephalexin

   The physician has prescribed 150 mg cephalexin, PO, q 6 hours for your pediatric patient, who weighs 35 pounds.

   a. What is the recommended safe dose in mg/kg/day? _____

   b. What is the safe dose range for your patient? _____

   c. Is the ordered dose safe for your patient? _____

   d. How many milliliters will be administered each dose? _____

2. Cefotetan 500 mg, IM, is prescribed for your patient. The medication vial is prepared to contain 1 gram cefotetan per 2 mL solution. You would administer how many milliliters of solution? _____

3. The physician has ordered ceftazidine, a third-generation cephalosporin. The order reads, ceftazidine, 250 mg, IM, q 12 hours. The medication label reads, ceftazidine 600 mg. Directions for IM use state, add 1.5 mL of appropriate diluent to provide 300 mg per 1 mL of solution. How many milliliters would you administer? _____

4. A patient is to receive 500 mg of cephalexin orally. The drug is available in 250-mg capsules. The nurse would administer how many capsules? _____

5. Tazicef, 1.5 gram is prescribed. Tazicef must be reconstituted for use. The amount of diluent can be adjusted to yield different concentrations of solution:

   26 mL of diluent yields 1 gram per 5 mL solution

   56 mL of diluent yields 1 gram per 10 mL solution

   How many milliliters of Tazicef solution would you administer if 26 mL of diluent is used? _____

6. The physician's order reads, "Cefixime (Suprax), 400 mg, PO, q day." Suprax is available in a reconstituted form that yields 100 mg per 5 mL of solution. Using an oral syringe, how many milliliters would you administer? _____

V. Crossword Puzzle

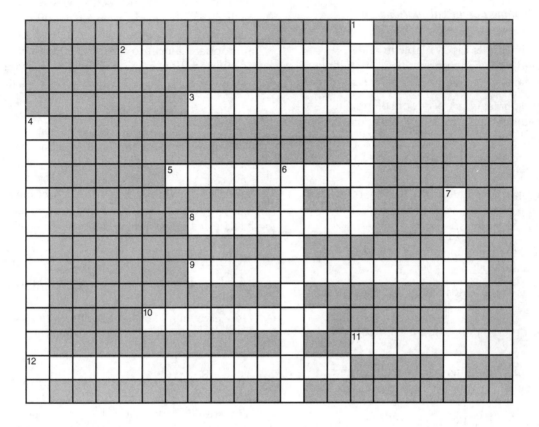

ACROSS CLUES

2. Inflammation of a vein with formation of a blood clot within the vein.
3. Damage to the kidneys by a toxic substance.
5. Test used to detect occult blood in the stool.
8. A third-generation cephalosporin.
9. One route by which the cephalosporins may be administered.
10. Symptom that may indicate pseudomembranous colitis.
11. Symptom of the Stevens-Johnson syndrome.
12. A group of drugs effective in the treatment of almost all strains of bacteria affected by the penicillins.

DOWN CLUES

1. One of the cephalosporins.
4. Type of bacteria susceptible to the cephalosporins.
6. A cephalosporin that is administered orally.
7. A second-generation cephalosporin.

VI. Critical Thinking

1. Ms. Rose has returned to the clinic for the third time in 3 months. Each time, her diagnosis is urinary tract infection. You suspect that she is not completing her prescribed medication, allowing the infecting bacteria to continue the infectious process. Discuss how you would approach this situation and what teaching Ms. Rose will need.

2. Your 86-year-old patient has been receiving a cephalosporin for treatment of septicemia. You are concerned about nephrotoxicity with this patient. Discuss how you would monitor this patient and what signs and symptoms you would watch for.

3. The mother of your pediatric patient states this is the second time he has had tonsillitis in 2 months. She states that the antibiotic doesn't seem to be working. How would you approach this parent to be sure she is administering the medication appropriately?

4. Mr. Addison, age 84, has a urinary tract infection and is prescribed cefpodoxime (Vantin), 100-milligram tablets that he must take every 12 hours for 7 days. Discuss suggestions you could give this patient to help him to remember to take his medicine as prescribed.

CHAPTER 9

Tetracyclines, Macrolides, and Lincosamides

I. Matching

Match each term in Column A with the correct definition or statement in Column B.

COLUMN A

_____ 1. *Helicobacter pylori*

_____ 2. rickettsiae

_____ 3. photosensitivity reaction

_____ 4. kaolin, aluminum salts, or magaldrate

_____ 5. tetracyclines

_____ 6. calcium

_____ 7. myasthenia gravis

_____ 8. lincosamides

_____ 9. macrolides

_____ 10. *Chlamydia trachomatis*

COLUMN B

A. Group of anti-infectives composed of natural and semisynthetic compounds.

B. A microorganism responsible for Rocky Mountain spotted fever that is susceptible to the tetracyclines.

C. A microorganism that is associated with some urethral, endocervical, or rectal infections.

D. A bacterium in the stomach that can cause peptic ulcer.

E. Reaction manifested by an exaggerated sunburn when the skin is exposed to sunlight even for brief periods.

F. A mineral that impairs the absorption of tetracycline.

G. Used as a prophylaxis before dental or other procedures in patients allergic to penicillin.

H. Causes a decreased gastrointestinal absorption of the macrolides.

I. Used only for the treatment of serious infections in which penicillin or erythromycin (a macrolide) is not effective.

J. An autoimmune disease manifested by extreme weakness and exhaustion of the muscles.

II. Multiple Choice

Circle the letter of the most appropriate answer.

Mr. Baynes is prescribed azithromycin (Zithromax) for lower respiratory tract infection. The physician tells Mr. Baynes to be sure he takes the drug on an empty stomach. Azithromycin is available in 250-milligram capsules. Questions 1–3 pertain to Mr. Baynes' case.

1. The physician tells Mr. Baynes that he should take 500 milligrams of the medication as soon as he has the prescription filled. The nurse explains to Mr. Baynes that his first dose of medication will be:

   a. 1 capsule.

   b. 2 capsules.

   c. 1 capsule now and 1 capsule in 2 hours.

   d. 3 capsules.

2. Mr. Baynes tells the nurse that he would rather take his medication before he leaves for work at 2:00 PM. To instruct Mr. Baynes properly, the nurse should ask:

   a. when he arrives at work.

   b. what he eats for breakfast.

   c. when he eats his biggest meal.

   d. the times of day he eats his meals.

3. It is very important that the nurse instruct Mr. Baynes to:

    a. take Imodium A-D if diarrhea develops.

    b. complete the full course of therapy.

    c. take an antacid if nausea develops.

    d. take his temperature every 2 hours.

4. Your patient taking tetracycline has been complaining of constipation. The physician has ordered a laxative to be given at bedtime. What does the nurse need to know about administering laxatives with tetracycline?

    a. It is correct to give tetracycline and the laxative at the same time.

    b. Give the laxative just before administering the tetracycline.

    c. Give the laxative 2 hours before or 2 hours after the tetracycline.

    d. If given together, the laxative will cause rapid absorption of the tetracycline.

5. Ms. Tanner is taking erythromycin for a severe respiratory infection. She tells the nurse that she has started having painful abdominal cramping. The nurse would be correct in telling Ms. Tanner:

    a. "Try lying on your side and relaxing."

    b. "I'll notify your physician immediately."

    c. "This is a normal reaction to erythromycin."

    d. "Take a walk in the hall and maybe the cramps will stop."

6. Ms. Shaw asks the nurse why her physician prescribed an antibiotic when she was told she has a viral infection. The most correct response is that antibiotics may be used to prevent a:

    a. primary fungal infection.

    b. repeat viral infection.

    c. secondary bacterial infection.

    d. breakdown of the immune system.

7. A 38-year-old female patient is receiving erythromycin gluceptate, IV, for acute pelvic inflammatory disease. Her vital signs are being monitored every 4 hours. Her temperature, which has been normal, is now elevated. As her nurse, you would anticipate:

    a. checking her temperature, pulse, and respirations every hour until temperature returns to normal.

    b. continuing to monitor her vital signs every 4 hours.

    c. discontinuing the IV antibiotic and notifying the primary care physician.

    d. maintaining an accurate intake and output record while the temperature is elevated.

8. A 12-year-old male patient is receiving azithromycin (Zithromax) for a severe episode of pharyngitis/tonsillitis. His mother has reported that he is allergic to penicillin. His first dose of medication was administered at 12:00 noon today. As this patient's nurse, you would be correct in:

    a. reporting all adverse reactions to the primary care physician at the end of your shift.

    b. monitoring the patient at frequent intervals for the first 48 hours of therapy.

    c. checking the patient's vital signs at least once during your 12-hour shift.

    d. giving the drug with an antacid if gastrointestinal upset occurs.

9. Nurses caring for patients receiving azithromycin or clarithromycin should monitor for the common adverse reactions associated with these two drugs, which are:

    a. skin rash, urinary retention.

    b. sores in the mouth, hypertension.

    c. related to the nervous system.

    d. related to the gastrointestinal tract.

10. Mr. Sharp is receiving minocycline (Minocin), a tetracycline. His response to antibiotic therapy can best be evaluated by:

    a. monitoring his vital signs every 12 hours.

    b. comparing initial and current signs and symptoms.

    c. measuring fluid intake and output every 12 hours.

    d. asking him if he is feeling better.

11. When asked at a team conference to describe a photosensitivity reaction, the nurse correctly states that this reaction may be described as a(n):

    a. tearing of the eyes on exposure to bright light.

    b. aversion to bright lights and sunlight.

    c. sensitivity to products in the environment.

    d. exaggerated sunburn reaction when the skin is exposed to sunlight.

12. Before administering the first dose of any antibiotic, it is important for the nurse to:

    a. take and record vital signs.

    b. obtain a through allergy history.

    c. identify and record signs and symptoms of the infection.

    d. complete all of the above.

III. Crossword Puzzle

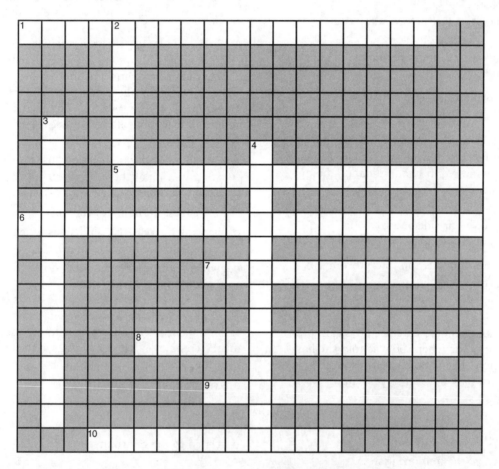

ACROSS CLUES

1. A bacteria in the stomach that can cause peptic ulcer and is susceptible to tetracycline (two words).
5. An autoimmune disease manifested by extreme weakness and exhaustion of the muscles (two words).
6. Microorganism susceptible to the tetracyclines (two words).
7. Azithromycin, clarithromycin, erythromycin.
8. Seems to cause the most serious photosensitivity reaction.
9. Clindamycin, lincomycin
10. Microorganisms causing Rocky Mountain spotted fever.

DOWN CLUES

2. Prevents the absorption of the tetracyclines if ingested concurrently.
3. A microorganism susceptible to the lincosamides.
4. Doxycline, minocycline

IV. Fill in the Blanks

1. List the three groups of broad-spectrum antibiotics discussed in this chapter and give examples of each.

   a) _____
      1. _____
      2. _____
      3. _____
   b) _____
      1. _____
      2. _____
      3. _____
   c) _____
      1. _____
      2. _____

2. Gastrointestinal reactions that may occur during tetracycline administration include:

   a) _____
   b) _____
   c) _____
   d) _____
   e) _____
   f) _____
   g) _____
   h) _____

3. Tetracyclines are contraindicated in _____ because they may cause permanent _____ of the teeth.

4. Foods high in _____ impair absorption of the tetracyclines.

5. The macrolides are particularly effective against infections of the _____ and _____ tracts.

6. _____ are used as prophylaxis treatment before dental and other procedures in patients allergic to _____.

7. Macrolides are primarily eliminated from the body by the _____ and should be used with caution in patients with _____ _____.

8. Use of antacids _____ the absorption of most macrolides.

9. _____ have a high potential for toxicity.

10. The _____ _____ _____ of _____ poses a danger to patients with myasthenia gravis.

V. Critical Thinking

1. Discuss the teaching plan you would use for a 17-year-old male patient who is prescribed a tetracycline for severe acne vulgaris. He plays outdoor sports and has a summer job as a lifeguard.

2. Discuss nursing interventions you would use for the patient with pseudomembranous colitis with severe abdominal cramping and diarrhea.

3. The physician has ordered Zithromax for your patient. Discuss your preadministration assessment for this patient.

VI. Dosage Problems

Solve the following dosage calculations.

1. The physician has ordered clindamycin, 0.3 gram, IM, every 6 hours. The vial label reads, "Cleocin Phosphate 150 mg/mL." How many milliliters will you administer at each dose? _____

2. The label on the bottle of erythromycin ethylsuccinate for oral suspension reads:

   Directions for preparation: add 140 mL water; shake vigorously to make 200 mL of suspension. Keep tightly closed, store in refrigerator, discard unused portion after 10 days. After reconstitution, 200 mg of erythromycin activity per 5 mL.

   a. How much diluent must be added to prepare the solution? _____

   b. What is the volume of the solution after it is mixed? _____

   c. What is the dose strength of the prepared solution? _____

   d. How long is the reconstituted solution good? _____

3. The physician's order is for doxycycline calcium (Vibramycin) oral suspension, 100 mg, PO, every 12 hours. The drug is available in a dose strength of 50 mg/5 mL. How many milliliters will be administered in 24 hours? _____ How many milliliters will be administered at each dose? _____

4. A patient is prescribed 200 mg, minocycline (Minocin) oral suspension initially, followed by 100 mg PO every 12 hours. Minocin is available as an oral suspension of 50 mg per 5 mL. How many milliliters would the nurse administer for the first dose? _____

5. A patient is prescribed 500 mg of azithromycin PO on the first day, followed by 250 mg PO on days 2 through 5. What is the total dosage the patient is to receive? _____

6. A patient is prescribed 600 mg of lincomycin every 12 hours IM. The drug is available as 300 mg/mL. How many milliliters will the nurse administer? _____

CHAPTER 10

Fluoroquinolones and Aminoglycosides

I. Matching

Match each term in Column A with the correct definition or statement in Column B.

COLUMN A

_____ 1. kanamycin (Kantrex)

_____ 2. norfloxacin

_____ 3. ototoxicity

_____ 4. hepatic coma

_____ 5. proteinuria

_____ 6. neuromuscular blockade

_____ 7. neurotoxicity

_____ 8. hematuria

_____ 9. nephrotoxicity

_____ 10. bowel prep

COLUMN B

A. Damage to the nervous system by a toxic substance.

B. A fluoroquinolone available in ophthalmic form.

C. Preoperative procedure that reduces the number of bacteria normally present in the intestine.

D. Oral aminoglycoside used for bowel prep.

E. Damage to the kidneys by a toxic substance.

F. Protein in the urine.

G. Blood in the urine.

H. Damage to the organs of hearing by a toxic substance.

I. Acute muscular paralysis and apnea.

J. Route of medication administration where the drug is allowed to dissolve under the tongue.

II. Multiple Choice

Circle the letter of the most appropriate answer.

Mr. Allison has been admitted to your unit for a severe gram-negative infection. Culture and sensitivity tests have identified the causative microorganism as E. coli and the drug most likely to control the infection is the aminoglycoside, gentamicin (Garamycin). The physician orders the drug to by given by intermittent IV infusion. Questions 1–4 pertain to Mr. Allison's case.

1. Mr. Allison has many problems and complaints. Which of the following may be related to the development of ototoxicity?

    a. Complains that he is unable to hear the television

    b. Episodes of anorexia and nausea

    c. Changes in his ability to remember and mental status

    d. Periodic episodes of diarrhea

2. As Mr. Allison's nurse, you will monitor him for signs and symptoms of nephrotoxicity by:

    a. measuring his fluid intake and output.

    b. testing his urine for glucose.

    c. offering him fluids to drink often.

    d. taking his vital signs every 4 hours.

3. Mr. Allison's plan of care will also include observing him for signs and symptoms of neurotoxicity, which could include:

    a. anorexia, diarrhea, abdominal pain.

    b. muscle spasms, nausea, constipation.

    c. muscular twitching, numbness, muscle weakness.

    d. headache, agitation, memory loss.

4. Mr. Allison's medication, gentamicin, is to be administered by intermittent infusion over a period of ½ hour to 2 hours. As his nurse, you would:

   a. caution him to expect redness at the IV insertion site.

   b. check the infusion rate at least once an hour.

   c. keep the patient in bed and the head of the bed flat.

   d. inspect the IV insertion site for signs of extravasation.

5. Your patient is scheduled for bowel surgery. The doctor has ordered kanamycin (Kantrex) orally every hour for 4 hours followed by 1 gram every 6 hours for 36 to 72 hours. The patient asks why he is taking an antibiotic before his surgery. You would be correct in replying:

   a. abdominal surgery requires starting antibiotic therapy 2 to 3 days before surgery.

   b. the microorganisms found in the bowel cannot be destroyed after surgery.

   c. the antibiotic reduces the number of bacteria in the bowel, decreasing the risk of postoperative infection.

   d. anesthesia makes the bowel resistant to an antibiotic after surgery.

6. Ms. Long is being treated for liver failure. She asks the nurse why the doctor has ordered the antibiotic kanamycin for her. As her nurse, you could best explain the doctor's action as a:

   a. precaution to prevent a buildup of liver enzymes.

   b. way to destroy ammonia-producing bacteria that could cause hepatic coma.

   c. way of changing the pH of the blood and lowering blood ammonia levels.

   d. way of preventing the liver from producing too much ammonia.

7. Ms. Davis is being seen in the clinic for a urinary tract infection that has been difficult to treat. The physician has ordered ciprofloxacin (Cipro). It is very important to get a complete drug history of the current medications she is taking to enable the nurse to identify:

   a. a workable dosing schedule for all her medications.

   b. if Ms. Davis is taking any drugs that could interact with Cipro.

   c. any of the medications that might need to have a new prescription written.

   d. if Ms. Davis is taking all her medications as prescribed.

8. Patients receiving kanamycin as part of the treatment for hepatic coma are:

   a. given the drug along with a protein supplement.

   b. closely observed for difficulty swallowing the drug.

   c. given extra fluids after administration of the drug.

   d. closely monitored for sudden weight loss or gain.

9. When administering an aminoglycoside before surgery as a bowel prep, it is important for the nurse to remember:

   a. the dosing schedule is usually every 4 hours.

   b. to tell the patient he will be placed on a fluid restriction.

   c. the timing of the administration of the drug is very important.

   d. the bowel prep usually is only one dose of medication.

10. Patients prescribed a fluoroquinolone are encouraged to:

    a. decrease their fluid intake.

    b. eat a high-protein diet.

    c. avoid high-carbohydrate foods.

    d. increase their fluid intake.

11. Mr. Reynolds is receiving a fluoroquinolone. The nurse must observe him for signs and symptoms of a superinfection or pseudomembranous colitis by:

    a. monitoring his blood pressure.

    b. weighing him daily.

    c. checking his stools.

    d. checking his tray after meals.

12. The fluoroquinolones can be responsible for severe adverse reactions that can include:

    a. hypotension, headache, anxiety.

    b. low tolerance to cold.

    c. constipation, increased appetite.

    d. pain, inflammation, ruptured tendon.

III. Fill in the Blanks

1. Examples of the fluoroquinolones include (*list the generic and trade name*):

   a)_____ _____

   b)_____ _____

   c)_____ _____

   d)_____ _____

   e)_____ _____

   f)_____ _____

   g)_____ _____

2. The more common adverse reactions seen with the fluoroquinolones include:

   a) _____

   b) _____

   c) _____

   d) _____

   e) _____

3. Examples of the aminoglycosides include (*list the generic and trade name where applicable*):

   a)_____ _____

   b)_____ _____

   c)_____ _____

   d)_____ _____

   e)_____ _____

   f)_____ _____

   g)_____

4. List the drugs that can interact with the fluoroquinolones. Include the drug name or type and the action expected.

   a) _____ _____

   b) _____ _____

   c) _____ _____

   d) _____ _____

   e) _____ _____

   f) _____ _____

5. _____, _____, and _____ are used orally in the management of hepatic coma.

6. Serious adverse reactions causing damage that may be permanent are seen with the aminoglycosides. List them below.

   a) _____

   b) _____

   c) _____

7. An aminoglycoside used for long-term treatment of tuberculosis is _____.

8. Signs of neurotoxicity would include:

   a) _____

   b) _____

   c) _____

   d) _____

   e) _____

   f) _____

   g) _____

   h) _____

   i) _____

9. Before administering a fluoroquinolone or aminoglycoside, the nurse should:

   a) _____

   b) _____

   c) _____

10. When kanamycin or neomycin is given for hepatic coma, the nurse must evaluate the patient's:

    a) _____

    b) _____

IV. Crossword Puzzle

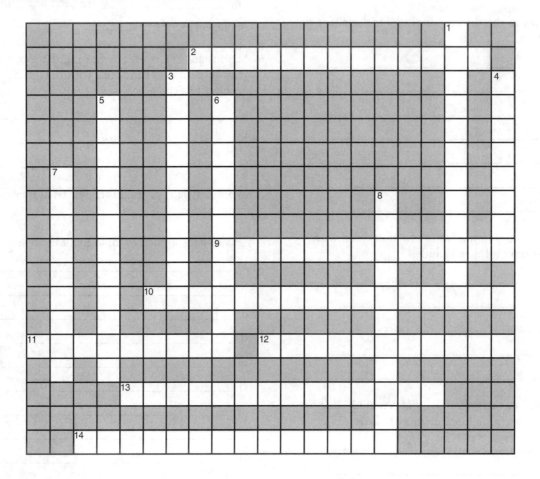

ACROSS CLUES

2. Word used to describe damage to the nervous system by a toxic substance.
9. Fluoroquinolone that may be given on an empty stomach.
10. Drug class that is not administered intramuscularly.
11. Blood in the urine.
12. Protein in the urine.
13. Drug class capable of causing a neuromuscular blockade.
14. Damage to the kidneys by a toxic substance.

DOWN CLUES

1. Drug that can cause a photosensitivity reaction.
3. Around the mouth.
4. Drug used to suppress intestinal bacteria.
5. Bacteria destroying
6. A disorder created by ammonia-forming bacteria that is treated with aminoglycosides (two words).
7. Tendon particularly vulnerable to rupture with fluoroquinolone administration.
8. Damage to the organs of hearing by a toxic substance.

V. Critical Thinking

1. Discuss the information you would give to the patient taking fluoroquinolones to promote an optimal response to the therapy.

2. Your nursing responsibilities include the monitoring and managing of adverse drug reactions. Discuss the nursing actions you would perform to care for your patient who is taking a fluoroquinolone or an aminoglycoside.

3. Mr. Jones has been admitted to your unit with a serious gram-negative infection. The physician has prescribed an aminoglycoside. As his nurse, you would be responsible for monitoring him for any adverse reactions, including nephrotoxicity. Discuss the nursing actions needed that will enable you to identify nephrotoxicity in this patient.

VI. Dosage Problems

Solve the following dosage calculations.

1. A patient is prescribed 20 mg tobramycin IM. The drug is available as 10 mg/mL. How many milliliters would the nurse administer? _____

2. Ciprofloxacin 750 mg, PO, is prescribed for a patient. The drug is available in 250-mg tablets. The nurse would administer how many tablets? _____

3. The primary health care provider prescribes norfloxacin, 200 mg, PO, for a urinary tract infection. The drug is available in scored, 400-mg tablets. The nurse would administer how many tablets? _____

4. The physician has ordered kanamycin (Kantrex), 750 mg, IM, q 12 hour. The drug is available as 0.5 g/2 mL. The safe recommended adult dose is 7.5 mg/kg every 12 hours. The patient weighs 220 pounds.

   a. Is this a safe dose for the patient? _____

   b. How many milliliters would the nurse give? _____

5. Streptomycin is available in powdered form that must be reconstituted before use. The instructions on the label read:

   Adult average single injection—0.5 to 1.0 g

   Milliliters diluent added—9 mL

   Solution strength—400 mg/mL

   The physician's order reads, "streptomycin 0.5 g, IM, q 6 hours."

   a. What is the volume of diluent used for reconstituting the drug? _____

   b. What is the dose strength of the reconstituted streptomycin? _____

   c. How many milliliters will the nurse administer? _____

CHAPTER 11

Miscellaneous Anti-infectives

I. Matching

Match each term in Column A with the correct definition or statement in Column B.

COLUMN A

_____ 1. hypoglycemia

_____ 2. vancomycin (Vancocin)

_____ 3. VRE

_____ 4. linezolid

_____ 5. anaerobic

_____ 6. metronidazole

_____ 7. hypotension

_____ 8. pentamidine isethionate

_____ 9. oxazolidinone

_____ 10. blood dyscrasias

_____ 11. meropenem

_____ 12. NebuPent

_____ 13. intravenous route

_____ 14. MRSA

_____ 15. spectinomycin

COLUMN B

A. Pathologic condition of blood; disorder of cellular elements of blood.

B. A drug used in treatment of VRE and MRSA.

C. Vancomycin-resistant *Enterococcus* bacteria.

D. Methicillin-resistant *Staphylococcus aureus* bacteria.

E. A drug effective against bacterial meningitis caused by *Neissseria meningitides*, *Streptococcus pneumoniae*, and *Haemophilus influenzae*.

F. Able to live and grow without oxygen.

G. Low blood sugar

H. Low blood pressure

I. Aerosol form of pentamidine isethionate used to prevent *Pneumocystis carinii* pneumonia.

J. Anti-infective used to treat gonorrhea.

K. May see the adverse reaction of a sudden drop in blood pressure with parenteral administration of this drug.

L. This drug needs to be protected from light by leaving the overwrap in place until ready to administer.

M. The only route used for administration of meropenem.

N. May produce an unpleasant metallic taste during therapy.

O. Aerosol form of this drug is administered with the use of a special nebulizer.

II. Fill in the Blanks

1. List the anti-infective along with their trade names discussed in the chapter:

   a)_____ _____

   b)_____ _____

   c)_____ _____

   d)_____ _____

   e)_____ _____

   f)_____ _____

   g)_____ _____

2. Administration of _____ is recommended to be done in a hospital setting because of the serious and sometimes fatal _____ _____ that can occur.

3. _____ is an anti-infective that is effective in treating VRE and MRSA.

4. The two most serious adverse reactions caused by linezolid are:

    a) _____

    b) _____

5. _____ is contraindicated in patients allergic to cephalosporins and penicillin.

6. The most serious adverse reactions associated with metronidazole are associated with the _____, and include _____ and _____ of the _____.

7. Pentamidine isethionate is used to treat *Pneumocystis carinii* pneumonia. Severe and sometimes life-threatening reactions that occur with the parenteral form include:

    a) _____

    b) _____

    c) _____

    d) _____

8. The two, possibly irreversible, adverse reactions that may be seen with vancomycin are _____ and _____.

III. Multiple Choice

Circle the letter of the most appropriate answer.

1. When giving pentamidine isethionate (Pentam 300), the nurse must monitor for any adverse reactions, which may include:

    a. hypertension.   c. urticaria.

    b. hypoglycemia.   d. insomnia.

2. Your patient is receiving pentamidine isethionate by the IV route. After the infusion has been completed, you assess the patient and find the patient weak and diaphoretic. As a nurse, you should recognize the symptoms as a possible:

    a. hypertensive episode.

    b. anxiety attack.

    c. hyperglycemic episode.

    d. hypoglycemic episode.

3. When monitoring the IV infusion of vancomycin (Vancocin), the nurse monitors the infusion every 15 minutes or less to protect against rapid infusion, which can result in a:

    a. fluid deficit and dehydration

    b. sudden rise in blood pressure.

    c. sudden, profound fall in blood pressure.

    d. fluid overload and respiratory distress.

4. Mr. Jackson is being treated for a complicated case of gonorrhea. He is receiving spectinomycin as treatment for the infection. The nurse would be correct in advising Mr. Jackson:

    a. to keep his follow-up appointment to check elimination of infection.

    b. that there should not be any soreness at the injection site.

    c. there is no need to notify his sexual partners.

    d. to limit his fluid intake over the next 24 hours.

5. When giving a drug that is potentially neurotoxic, the nurse should be particularly concerned about patient complaints of:

    a. headache, feeling chilly.

    b. blurred vision, poor appetite.

    c. lightheadedness, abdominal pain.

    d. numbness of extremities, dizziness.

6. The weekly team conference is planned for tomorrow. Your supervisor asks you to be able to define the term *anaerobic*. You would be correct in your definition to the team if you stated:

    a. "Able to live without oxygen."

    b. "Requires oxygen to live."

    c. "Requires carbon dioxide to live."

    d. "Able to live without carbon dioxide."

7. Ms. Blade is receiving vancomycin (Vancocin) orally for a serious gram-positive infection that has not responded to treatment with other antibiotics. During your shift, Ms. Blade has a fluid intake of 900 mL and an output of 300 mL. Her urine color has become much darker. Your best nursing action would be to:

   a. encourage Ms. Blade to immediately drink 1000 mL of fluid.

   b. notify the primary care physician immediately.

   c. keep monitoring the intake and output during your shift.

   d. check the vital signs and ask about her appetite.

8. Mr. Allen is receiving linezolid (Zyvox) for a serious *S. aureus* infection. The patient has been on an 81-mg aspirin per day treatment regimen. The nurse will closely monitor Mr. Allen for:

   a. numbness around the mouth.

   b. skin rash and pruritus.

   c. decrease in urine output.

   d. any unusual bruising.

9. Your patient teaching for a patient being treated with metronidazole should include telling him to avoid:

   a. drinking alcohol.

   b. eating foods containing tyramine.

   c. taking the drug on a full stomach.

   d. exposure to sunlight or tanning lamps.

10. When assessing the patient receiving chloramphenicol (Chloromycetin), the nurse must remember that the chief adverse reaction associated with this drug is:

   a. nausea, vomiting.   c. abdominal pain.

   b. blood dyscrasias.   d. bloody diarrhea.

IV. Crossword Puzzle

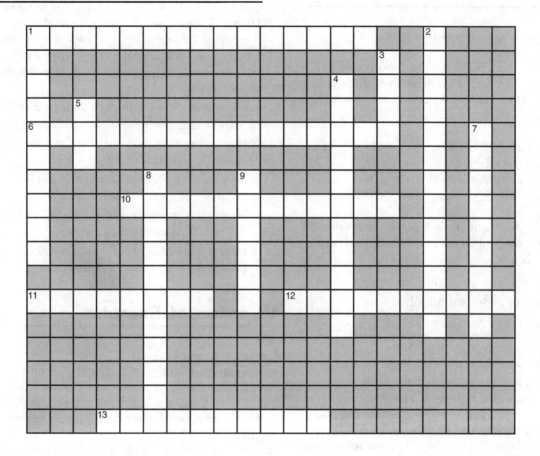

ACROSS CLUES

1. Phenobarbital or rifampin decreases blood levels of this drug.
6. A serious adverse reaction caused by linezolid.
10. Low blood sugar.
11. Aerosol form of pentamidine isethionate used to prevent *P. carinii* pneumonia.
12. Patients allergic to meropenem may also be allergic to _____.
13. Drug used to treat serious susceptible gram-positive infections not responding to other antibiotics.

DOWN CLUES

1. Metabolism of metronidazole may decrease when administered with this drug.
2. A severe reaction may occur if this anti-infective is administered with alcohol.
3. Methicillin-resistant *S. aureus*.
4. Aerosol administration of this drug may cause a metallic taste in the mouth, shortness of breath, or anorexia.
5. Vancomycin-resistant *Enterococcus*.
7. Able to live without oxygen.
8. Adverse reaction seen with the administration of pentamidine isethionate.
9. Brand name of metronidazole.

V. Dosage Problems

Solve the following dosage calculations.

1. A patient is prescribed 500 mg vancomycin, PO, q 6 hours. The drug is available in 250-mg capsules. The nurse would administer how many capsules? _____

2. Metronidazole 250 mg, IV, is ordered. The drug is available in solution with dose strength of 500 mg/2 mL. How many milliliters will be administered? _____

3. Vancomycin is available in a powder form that must be reconstituted for use in IV fluid. The label reads:

   Vancocin HCL

   IV equivalent to 500 mg/10 mL

   Usual adult dose 2-gram daily

   Dilute with 10 mL of sterile water

   After dilution—Refrigerate

   The physician's orders read: "Vancomycin, 1 gram, IV, every 12 hours." How many milliliters of solution will the pharmacist add to the IV soulution? Can the ordered dose be obtained from one vial? _____ How many vials will the pharmacist need? _____

4. Your patient is being treated for an anaerobic bacterial infection. The physician has ordered Flagyl, IV, first dose 15 mg/kg, infused over 1 hour, then 7.5 mg/kg, infused over 1 hour, every 6 hours for 7 days. Your patient weighs 132 pounds. Reconstitution yields a dosage strength of 100 mg/mL:

   a. How many kilograms does your patient weigh? _____

   b. How many milligrams of Flagyl will be added to the IV solution for the first dose? _____

   c. How many milliliters of solution will be needed? _____

   d. How many milligrams of Flagyl will be added for each of the remaining doses? _____

   e. How many milliliters of solution will be needed for each remaining dose? _____

VI. Internet Exercise

Use the Web address www.fda.gov, www.centerwatch.com, or www.rxlist.com to discover any newly approved anti-infectives (or antibiotics). Obtain as much information as you can, such as drug name(s), classification, use, adverse reactions, special considerations, and so forth, and share this information with your classmates.

CHAPTER 12

Antitubercular Drugs

I. Matching

Match each term in Column A with the correct definition or statement in Column B.

COLUMN A

_____ 1. extrapulmonary

_____ 2. isoniazid

_____ 3. gout

_____ 4. anaphylactoid reaction

_____ 5. *Mycobacterium tuberculosis*

_____ 6. retreatment

_____ 7. directly observed therapy (DOT)

_____ 8. fluoroquinolones

_____ 9. peripheral neuropathy

_____ 10. optic neuritis

_____ 11. rifampin

_____ 12. tuberculosis

_____ 13. hepatotoxicity

_____ 14. primary antitubercular drugs

_____ 15. second-line drugs

COLUMN B

A. World's leading cause of death from infectious disease.

B. Bacillus causing the infectious disease tuberculosis.

C. Tuberculosis affecting the lungs caused by tuberculosis found in other organs of the body (i.e., liver, kidneys, spleen, uterus).

D. Drugs used to treat extrapulmonary tuberculosis or drug-resistant organisms.

E. Drugs that have proven to be effective against tuberculosis and are considered second-line drugs.

F. Only antitubercular drug used alone.

G. Necessary when treatment fails and usually includes the use of four or more antitubercular drugs.

H. Ethambutol, isoniazid, pyrazinamide, rifampin, streptomycin.

I. A decrease in visual acuity and changes in color perception.

J. Unusual or exaggerated allergic reactions.

K. Numbness and tingling of the extremities.

L. Principal adverse reaction seen with pyrazinamide use, identified by abnormal liver function test results and jaundice.

M. A metabolic disorder resulting in increased levels of uric acid.

N. Drug causing a red-orange discoloration of body fluids (i.e., urine, tears, saliva, sweat, and sputum).

O. When patients must take their antituberculosis drugs in the presence of a health care professional.

II. Multiple Choice

Circle the letter of the most appropriate answer.

1. Which of the following would the nurse include in a teaching plan for a patient being treated for tuberculosis? Antituberculosis drugs are:

   a. administered at weekly intervals.

   b. rarely necessary unless symptoms are present.

   c. given for an extended period.

   d. administered only when the bacillus is present in sputum.

2. The nurse explains to the patient that to slow bacterial resistance to an antitubercular drug, the physician may initially prescribe:

   a. at least three drugs.

   b. an antibiotic to be given with the drug.

   c. that the drug be given every second or third day.

   d. that the drug to be given once a week.

3. When teaching the patient who is taking an antitubercular drug on an outpatient basis, the nurse should tell the patient:

   a. to take aspirin if a fever is present.

   b. not to increase or decrease the dose unless instructed by the physician.

   c. to double the next dose when one dose is missed.

   d. not to take the drug when symptoms improve.

4. The nurse administering isoniazid to a patient with tuberculosis knows that one adverse reaction that can occur with the administration of isoniazid is:

   a. usually serious and even fatal hepatitis.

   b. related to the genitourinary tract.

   c. related to the gastrointestinal tract.

   d. often due to the location of the tubercular lesion.

5. Which is the only antitubercular drug used alone?

   a. pyrazinamide   c. isoniazid

   b. streptomycin   d. rifamycin

6. The nurse monitors the patient taking isoniazid for toxicity. The most common symptom of toxicity is:

   a. peripheral edema.

   b. hypersensitivity reaction.

   c. circumoral edema.

   d. peripheral neuropathy.

7. The principal adverse reaction seen with pyrazinamide is:

   a. ototoxicity.   c. neurotoxicity.

   b. nephrotoxicity.   d. hepatotoxicity.

8. Pyrazinamide is contraindicated in the patient with a history of:

   a. hypertension.   c. visual disturbance.

   b. gout.   d. hearing loss.

9. The physician will discontinue streptomycin if the patient experiences:

   a. hearing loss.   c. hypertension.

   b. visual disturbances.   d. hepatotoxicity.

10. When ethambutol is prescribed for treatment of tuberculosis, the nurse must monitor for adverse reactions that can include:

    a. peripheral neuropathy.

    b. ototoxicity.

    c. psychic disturbances.

    d. gout.

III. Fill in the Blanks

1. What are the primary antitubercular drugs discussed in this chapter?

   a. _____

   b. _____

   c. _____

   d. _____

   e. _____

2. What are the secondary antitubercular drugs discussed in this chapter?

   a. _____

   b. _____

   c. _____

   d. _____

3. The drugs used to treat tuberculosis do not _____ the disease, but they render the patient _____ to _____.

4. Second-line tuberculosis drugs are used to treat _____ _____ and _____ _____.

5. Some patients treated with ethambutol experience

_____, which appears to be dose

related and usually disappears with

_____ of the drug.

6. Severe and sometimes fatal _____

has been associated with isoniazid therapy.

7. Isoniazid toxicity may develop and can be

identified by the common symptom of

_____ _____.

8. List the adverse reactions associated with
streptomycin:

a. _____

b. _____

c. _____

d. _____

e. _____

f. _____

g. _____

h. _____

i. _____

IV. Dosage Problems

Solve the following dosage calculations.

1. A patient is prescribed isoniazid syrup 300 mg,
PO. The isoniazid is available in a solution
strength of 50 mg/mL. How many milliliters
would the nurse administer? _____

2. Ethambutol 200 mg, PO, is ordered. The drug is
available in 100-mg tablets. How many tablets
will the nurse administer? _____

3. Rifampin 600 mg, PO, is prescribed. The drug is
available in 150-mg tablets. The nurse would give
how many tablets? _____

4. The physician has prescribed rifampin, 600 mg,
PO, for your pediatric patient, who weighs 66
pounds. The safe dose range for children is 10 to
20 mg/kg in one daily dose.

a. What is the safe dosage range for your patient?
_____

b. Is the ordered dosage safe for your patient?
_____

c. How many kilograms does your patient weigh?
_____

5. The physician has ordered streptomycin, 1 gram,
IM daily. Streptomycin is available in a solution
for injection with a dosage strength of 400
mg/mL. How many milliliters will you administer
at each dose? _____

6. A patient with tuberculosis is on a drug regimen
that includes three antitubercular drugs. The
physician has ordered pyrazinamide as a fourth
drug. The dose ordered is 3 grams daily.
Pyrazinamide is available in 500-mg tablets. The
ordered dose will need how many tablets each
day? _____

V. Crossword Puzzle

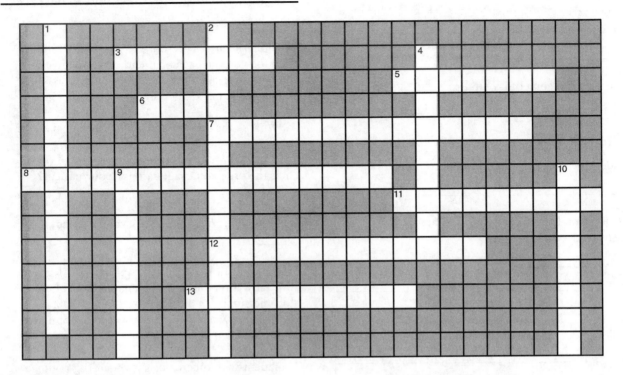

ACROSS CLUES

3. First-line drugs used to treat tuberculosis.
5. Dizziness.
6. A metabolic disorder resulting in increased levels of uric acid.
7. Outside of the respiratory system (lungs).
8. Class of second-line drugs used to treat tuberculosis.
11. Only antitubercular drug used alone.
12. Infectious disease primarily affecting the lungs.
13. Causes the dose-related adverse reaction of optic neuritis.

DOWN CLUES

1. Severe hypersensitivity reaction.
2. To slow or retard the growth of bacteria.
4. Destruction of the red blood cells.
9. Drug that may cause red-orange discoloration of body fluids.
10. Ringing in the ears.

VI. Internet Exercise

Compare the information available on these Web sites and decide which offers the best teaching information to the patient with tuberculosis: www.cdc.gov, www.lungusa.org, www.Columbia.edu. Print out the material you choose and bring to class for discussion.

VII. Critical Thinking

1. Using the information you have acquired from the Internet exercise, develop a plan to help Mr. Schwartz understand the necessary prophylactic treatment for tuberculosis.

2. With the use of antitubercular drugs, bacterial resistance can develop, making a multidrug therapy necessary. Discuss how you would explain DOT (directly observed therapy) and why it may be necessary in some cases to ensure patient compliance with multidrug treatment.

3. Mr. Moore has been started on a four-drug treatment regimen for tuberculosis. One of the drugs is streptomycin. Discuss the side effects he should be aware of and symptoms he must watch for and report.

CHAPTER 13

Leprostatic Drugs

I. Matching

Match each term in Column A with the correct definition or statement in Column B.

COLUMN A

_____ 1. clofazimine

_____ 2. leprostatic drugs

_____ 3. dapsone

_____ 4. leprosy

_____ 5. hemolysis

_____ 6. *Mycobacterium leprae*

COLUMN B

A. A chronic, communicable disease spread by prolonged intimate contact.

B. Bacterium causing leprosy.

C. Drug used to treat leprosy that may cause pigmentation of the skin.

D. Drug used to treat leprosy that may cause a hemolytic reaction.

E. Destruction of red blood cells.

F. Important to give these drugs with food to minimize gastric upset.

II. Multiple Choice

Circle the letter of the most appropriate answer.

1. A patient who visits the clinic has been diagnosed with leprosy. One of your nursing responsibilities is to perform a thorough skin assessment. You have already identified lesions on the patient's face, and he tells you these are the only lesions he has. Why must you check all skin surfaces for lesions?

   a. Lesions are always widespread over the entire body.

   b. You will need accurate baseline data to use for comparison during therapy.

   c. You need to check only his face because he states these are his only lesions.

   d. You won't need to check because the lesions last only for a few days.

2. Mary Smith, age 28, has just been diagnosed with leprosy. The physician has ordered clofazimine for her drug treatment. During your teaching about the drug regimen, Ms. Smith asks, "If I get pregnant, how will this medicine affect my baby?" You would be correct in replying:

   a. "This drug is perfectly safe for the fetus."

   b. "This drug is in Pregnancy Category A and is safe."

   c. "There will be no effects if taken during early pregnancy."

   d. "This drug may cause the infant to be born with pigmented skin."

3. You are attending a seminar on caring for the patient with leprosy. These patients will be faced with long-term medical and drug therapy and possibly disfigurement. With this in mind, what would be an important and necessary nursing intervention for these patients?

   a. Spend time with the patients and allow them to verbalize their fears and anxieties.

   b. Explain that the leprostatic drugs will need to be taken on an empty stomach.

   c. Describe the skin pigmentation that may occur but assure them it disappears quickly after treatment stops.

   d. Discuss that the long-term therapy used for treatment of leprosy usually only lasts for three months.

4. Patients being treated with clofazimine must be told to expect the adverse reaction of:

   a. hair loss.   c. skin pigmentation.

   b. vertigo.   d. hemolysis.

5. A serious adverse reaction that can occur with the leprostatic drug dapsone is hemolysis. This reaction is identified by:

   a. increase in red blood cells.

   b. destruction of red blood cells.

   c. increase in white blood cells.

   d. decrease in white blood cells.

III. Critical Thinking

1. Compliance with treatment is a very important aspect for the patient diagnosed with leprosy. Discuss the teaching plan you would use for a patient being treated with a leprostatic drug.

2. As a nurse, you will be responsible for educating your patient about the disease of leprosy and the treatment regimen. Discuss how you will know if the patient is receptive to your teaching. If the patient shows no interest in learning, discuss ways you would encourage him to learn.

IV. Internet Exercise

www.hhs.gov
Use information found on this site to write an information sheet about leprosy and the treatment recommendations used in the United States.

V. Crossword Puzzle

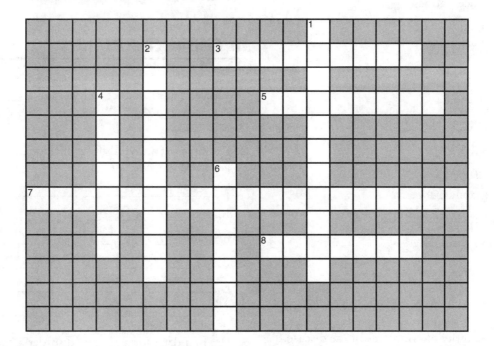

ACROSS CLUES

3. Destruction of red blood cells.
5. Drug that may be administered with the leprostatic drugs to minimize drug resistance to the leprostatic drugs.
7. Bacterial organism causing leprosy (two words).
8. Another term that identifies leprosy.

DOWN CLUES

1. Drug used to treat leprosy that may cause pigmentation of the skin.
2. Absolutely necessary if the long-term treatment regimen is to be effective.
4. A leprostatic drug that may cause hemolysis.
6. Chronic communicable disease spread by prolonged intimate contact.

CHAPTER 14

Antiviral Drugs

I. Matching

Match each term in Column A with the correct definition or statement in Column B.

COLUMN A

_____ 1. remissions

_____ 2. erythema

_____ 3. ribavirin

_____ 4. respiratory syncytial virus

_____ 5. exacerbations

_____ 6. retinitis

_____ 7. jaundice

_____ 8. pancreatitis

_____ 9. asthenia

_____ 10. peripheral neuropathy

_____ 11. crystalluria

_____ 12. viruses

_____ 13. granulocytopenia

_____ 14. anticholinergic effects

_____ 15. antiviral drugs

COLUMN B

A. Reproduce only by using the body's cellular material.

B. Increase in severity of symptoms of the disease.

C. Periods of partial or complete disappearance of the signs and symptoms of a disease.

D. Are effective against only a small number of specific viral infections.

E. Inflammation of the retina of the eye.

F. A severe lower respiratory tract infection.

G. Presence of crystals in the urine.

H. Weakness or loss of strength.

I. Redness of the skin.

J. Low levels of granulocytes, a type of white blood cell, in the blood.

K. A Pregnancy Category X drug.

L. Dry mouth, blurred vision, and constipation, adverse reactions seen when amantadine is administered with an antihistamine.

M. Nausea, vomiting, abdominal pain, jaundice, and elevated liver enzymes are symptoms of _____.

N. Numbness, tingling, or pain in the hands or feet.

O. Yellowish discoloration of the skin or eyes.

II. Fill in the Blanks

1. Viruses can reproduce only within a _____ _____.

2. Examples of antiviral drugs include (*list the generic and trade name*):

   a. _____ _____

   b. _____ _____

   c. _____ _____

   d. _____ _____

   e. _____ _____

   f. _____ _____

3. Use of a drug for a specific disorder a condition that is not officially approved by the Food and Drug Administration (FDA) is called an _____ _____.

4. General uses of antiviral drugs include treatment of:

   a. _____

   b. _____

   c. _____

   d. _____

   e. _____

   f. _____

   g. _____

5. Antiviral drugs are given _____ or as _____ drugs.

6. Preadministration assessment of the patient who will be receiving an antiviral drug may include the nurse:

   a. _____
   _____
   _____ .

   b. _____
   _____
   _____ .

   c. _____
   _____
   _____ .

   d. _____
   _____
   _____ .

7. A nurse caring for a patient requiring antiviral therapy may encourage and promote an optimal response to the therapy by:

   a. _____
   _____
   _____ .

   b. _____
   _____
   _____ .

   c. _____
   _____
   _____ .

   d. _____
   _____
   _____ .

   e. _____
   _____
   _____ .

   f. _____
   _____
   _____ .

8. List four nursing diagnoses that may be valid for the patient receiving antiviral therapy.

   a. _____
   _____
   _____ .

   b. _____
   _____
   _____ .

   c. _____
   _____
   _____ .

   d. _____
   _____
   _____ .

III. Multiple Choice

Circle the letter of the most appropriate answer.

1. Which of the following adverse reactions should the nurse expect in patients receiving acyclovir by the oral route?
   a. Nausea, vomiting
   b. Constipation, urinary retention
   c. Conjunctivitis, blurred vision
   d. Burning, stinging

2. A nurse administering acyclovir should encourage the patient to:

   a. limit fluid intake.

   b. eat a diet high in bulk-producing food.

   c. drink 2000 to 3000 mL of fluid daily.

   d. avoid a diet of highly spiced food.

3. Your 3-month-old patient has an admitting diagnosis of RSV infection. The physician has ordered treatment with ribavirin. Which of the following would you report immediately to the primary care physician?

   a. Refusal to take fluid or food

   b. No bowel movement in the last 24 hours

   c. Drowsiness

   d. Worsening of the respiratory status

4. The physician has ordered didanosine to be administered to your patient. When receiving the administration information, you find:

   a. tablets are crushed and mixed with 1 ounce of water.

   b. drug is prepared for subcutaneous injection.

   c. tablets are swallowed with a full glass of water.

   d. the buffered powder is mixed with fruit juice.

5. Ms. Davis is receiving acyclovir, IV. As her nurse, you would know that IV administration of this drug can result in:

   a. hypovolemic shock.   c. cardiac arrest.

   b. crystalluria.   d. hypertensive crisis.

6. A 23-year-old female patient has been admitted to your unit and assigned to you. The physician has ordered treatment with zidovudine. During your assessment, you learn the patient is breast-feeding her 2-month-old baby. Your nursing action would be:

   a. administer the drug as prescribed.

   b. withhold the drug and notify the physician.

   c. document the patient is lactating and give the drug cautiously.

   d. tell the patient she will have to stop breast-feeding the infant.

7. Patients taking antiviral drugs must be able to identify the symptoms of pancreatitis, an adverse reaction that can occur with this type of drug. The nurse would instruct the patient to watch for:

   a. sore throat, difficulty breathing.

   b. numbness or pain in hands and feet.

   c. orthostatic hypotension.

   d. nausea, vomiting, abdominal pain, jaundice.

8. A patient receiving zidovudine (AZT) is experiencing symptoms of gastrointestinal upset, anorexia, nausea, and vomiting. Your nursing actions would include:

   a. keeping the room clean and free of odors.

   b. immediately notifying the physician.

   c. ordering the patient NPO until symptoms diminish.

   d. providing aromatic food to stimulate appetite.

9. Mr. Burns is being discharged from the hospital and is being prescribed acyclovir for recurrent episodes of herpes simplex. The nurse instructs Mr. Burns:

   a. the drug will prevent the spread of the disease.

   b. severe burning and worsening of lesions is common.

   c. topical application is not to exceed prescribed frequency.

   d. used as directed the drug will cure the disease.

10. When administering ribavirin, the nurse must remember:

    a. to give the drug with large quantities of water.

    b. women of childbearing age having direct contact with patient should observe respiratory precautions.

    c. patients receiving this drug should avoid activities requiring alertness until effects of the drug are known.

    d. to crush the tablets and mix with 1 ounce of water before administering the drug.

IV. Crossword Puzzle

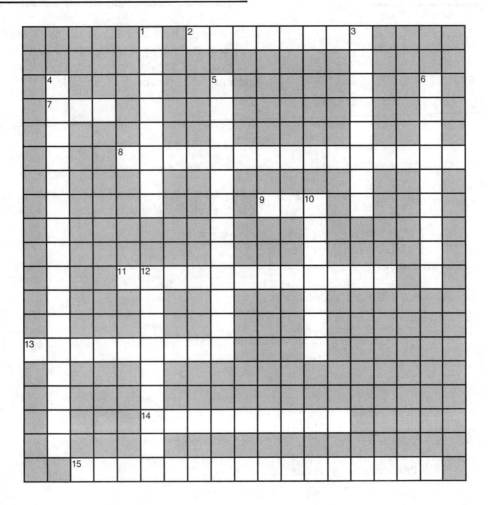

ACROSS CLUES

2. Yellowish discoloration of the skin and/or eyes.
7. Viral infection transmitted through an infected person's bodily secretions.
8. Drug effects causing dry mouth, blurred vision, and constipation.
9. A severe lower respiratory tract infection treated with ribavirin.
11. Presence of crystals in the urine.
13. Pregnancy Category X antiviral drug.
14. Acute respiratory illness caused by influenza viruses A and B.
15. Low levels of granulocytes in the blood.

DOWN CLUES

1. Weakness, loss of strength.
3. Redness of the skin.
4. Sensitivity to light.
5. Increase in severity of the symptoms.
6. Inflammation of the retina.
10. Reproduce only within a living cell.
12. Partial or complete disappearance of the signs and symptoms.

V. Dosage Problems

Solve the following dosage calculations.

1. The physician's order reads: Zanamivir 10 mg, inhalation, q 12 hours. You have available zanamivir in diskhaler form, with 5-mg blisters. How many blisters would be used for each dose? _____

2. Acyclovir 200 mg is prescribed. The drug is available in 400-mg tablets. The nurse will administer how many tablets? _____

3. The patient is prescribed 200 mg didanosine. The drug is available in 100-mg tablets. The nurse will administer how many tablets? _____

4. Didanosine, buffered powder, 200 mg is ordered. Instructions for mixing are: mix dose with 4 oz water, dissolve completely and drink immediately. How many milligrams of didanosine are in each ounce of water? _____

5. Your patient has been admitted to the hospital with a severe, initial outbreak of genital herpes. The physician has ordered acyclovir, 1200 mg, IV, each day, in three divided doses q 8 hours. Dosage instructions on the vial are 15 mg/kg per day. Diluted concentrate will be 50 mg/mL. Dilute further for IV to 7 mg/mL or less. Your patient weighs 176 pounds.

   a. What is the recommended milligram dose on the vial for your patient? _____
   b. How many milliliters of drug concentrate must be added to a 100-mL bag of IV fluid to meet the dose ordered? _____
   c. Is this diluted strength of the drug in the IV fluid 7 mg/mL or less? _____
   d. What is the diluted strength of the drug in the IV fluid? _____

VI. Critical Thinking

1. Discuss the instructions you would include with patient and family teaching that would be appropriate for the patient prescribed antiviral drugs. Be as thorough as possible.

2. Prepare a patient education plan specific to each of the following antiviral drugs:

   a. Acyclovir

   b. Ribavirin

   c. Zidovudine

CHAPTER 15

Antifungal Drugs

I. Matching

*Match each term in Column A with the correct
statement or definition in Column B.*

COLUMN A

_____ 1. onychomycosis

_____ 2. fungicidal

_____ 3. tinea corporis

_____ 4. mycotic infections

_____ 5. fungus

_____ 6. tinea cruris

_____ 7. fungistatic

_____ 8. tinea pedis

_____ 9. miconazole

_____ 10. systemic

_____ 11. hypokalemia

_____ 12. superficial

_____ 13. flucytosine

_____ 14. amphotericin B

_____ mn   15. *Candida albicans*

COLUMN B

A. Athlete's foot.

B. Jock itch.

C. Nail fungus.

D. Yeast infection affecting women in the vulvovaginal area.

E. Ringworm.

F. Able to slow down or retard the multiplication of fungi.

G. Low potassium level.

H. Fungal infections that occur when fungi gain entrance into the interior of the body.

I. Fungal infections.

J. A colorless plant that lacks chlorophyll.

K. Mycotic infections occurring on the surface of, or just below, the skin or nails.

L. Able to destroy fungi.

M. Representative of all of the vaginal antifungal agents.

N. Most effective drug available for the treatment of most systemic fungal infections.

O. Dosage of this antifungal drug is determined according to the patient's weight.

II. Fill in the Blanks

1. List the antifungal drugs discussed in this chapter (*list the generic and trade name*).

   a) _____ _____

   b) _____ _____

   c) _____ _____

   d) _____ _____

   e) _____ _____

   f) _____ _____

2. Antifungal drugs may be _____ or

   _____.

3. Antifungal drugs are used to treat _____

   and _____ _____ infections.

4. Amphotericin B often results in these serious adverse reactions: _____,

_____, _____,

_____, _____,

_____, _____,

_____, _____, and

_____.

5. Fluconazole administration may result in abnormal _____ _____.

6. Flucytosine administration requires periodic

_____ _____ _____.

7. Miconazole, a Pregnancy Category C antifungal, is used during the _____

_____ of pregnancy only when essential.

8. A preadministration assessment completed before giving the first dose of an antifungal drug would include:

a. _____
   _____
   _____ .

b. _____
   _____
   _____ .

c. _____
   _____
   _____ .

d. _____
   _____
   _____ .

e. _____
   _____
   _____ .

f. _____
   _____
   _____ .

g. _____
   _____
   _____ .

9. List the nursing diagnoses that may be valid for a patient being administered antifungal drugs.

a. _____
   _____
   _____ .

b. _____
   _____
   _____ .

c. _____
   _____
   _____ .

d. _____
   _____
   _____ .

10. Amphotericin B is reconstituted with

_____ _____ because any other diluent may cause _____.

III. Multiple Choice

Circle the letter of the most appropriate answer.

1. Miconazole is given with caution to patients who are pregnant because it is classified in Pregnancy Category:

   a. A.   c. C.
   b. B.   d. D.

2. There is an increased risk of elevated digoxin levels if the patient taking digoxin is also prescribed:

   a. ketoconazole.   c. itraconazole.
   b. miconazole.   d. flucytosine.

3. When administering amphotericin B, the nurse must be aware of an adverse reaction that can occur within 15 to 20 minutes of initiation of treatment, which is:

    a. fever (sometimes with shaking chills).

    b. abnormal hepatic function.

    c. renal impairment or renal failure.

    d. flushing of the skin.

4. A patient has been prescribed flucytosine to be administered as six capsules at each dose. The patient is experiencing minor gastrointestinal distress. The nurse would give the capsules:

    a. all six at one time.

    b. one at a time every 10 minutes.

    c. two at a time every 30 minutes.

    d. one or two at a time over 15 minutes.

5. When a patient is receiving griseofluvin, the nurse should notify the primary health care provider if the following occurs:

    a. fever, sore throat, skin rash.

    b. drowsiness or dizziness.

    c. anorexia or nausea.

    d. headache or malaise.

6. When educating a patient receiving miconazole for chronic, recurrent *Candida albicans* infection, the nurse would advise the patient to monitor for signs and symptoms of:

    a. renal impairment.

    b. diabetes.

    c. abnormal liver function.

    d. hypokalemia.

7. Nursing actions that may help the patient achieve an optimal response to antifungal therapy would include explaining:

    a. that all fungal infections respond quickly to therapy.

    b. all fungal infections can be controlled easily.

    c. treatments are inexpensive and will not require hospitalization.

    d. therapy must be continued until the infection is under control.

8. When a patient is taking an antifungal drug and begins to show signs of renal impairment, the nurse would:

    a. reduce the dosage of the drug until renal function improves.

    b. notify the primary care provider of any abnormal laboratory results.

    c. place the patient on strict bed rest and restrict all fluids.

    d. order more laboratory tests to rule out other problems.

9. During treatment of a child with ringworm, the parent will be instructed on how to apply griseofulvin ointment. The nurse would be correct in stating:

    a. apply as often as necessary to keep area moist.

    b. increase the amount used if no improvement is seen.

    c. apply as directed by the primary care physician.

    d. do not clean the area each time the medication is applied.

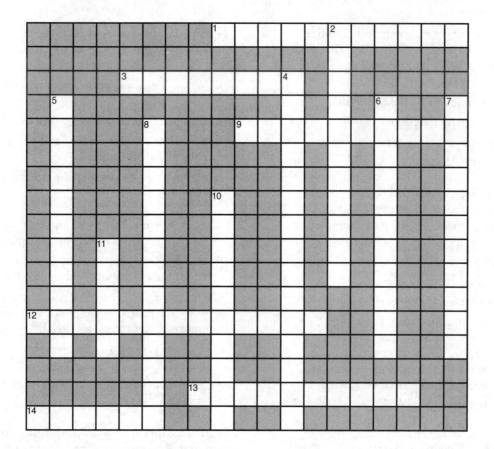

10. Patients receiving miconazole for a vaginal yeast infection should not use the drug if the following is present:

    a. abdominal or pelvic pain.

    b. anorexia, nausea.

    c. drowsiness, dizziness.

    d. diarrhea, headache.

IV. Crossword Puzzle

ACROSS CLUES

1. Mycotic infections occurring on the surface of or just below the skin or nails.
3. Fungal infection that occurs when fungi gain entrance into the interior of the body.
9. Able to destroy fungi.
12. Ringworm (two words).
13. Representative of all of the vaginal antifungal agents.
14. A colorless plant that lacks chlorophyll.

DOWN CLUES

2. Able to slow down or retard the multiplication of fungi.
4. Yeast infection affecting women in the vulvovaginal area (two words).
5. Low potassium level.
6. Jock itch (two words).
7. Antifungal drug that may cause abnormal liver function.
8. Nail fungus.
10. Athlete's foot (two words).
11. Adverse reaction possible within the first few minutes after amphotericin B administration.

V. Dosage Problems

Solve the following dosage calculations.

1. The physician has ordered miconazole, IV, 1200 mg per day in three divided doses. The initial dose is to be 200 mg, administered with the

physician in attendance. How many milligrams of the drug should be administered in each of the remaining two doses? _____

2. A patient has been ordered amphotericin B, 150 mg, IV, q day. The drug information identifies the safe dosage range for this drug as 0.25 mg/kg per day, not to exceed 1.5 mg/kg per day. The patient's weight is 176 pounds.

   a. What is the patient's weight in kilograms? _____

   b. What is the safe dosage range for this patient? _____

   c. Is the dosage ordered within the safe range? _____

3. A patient diagnosed with aspergillosis has been prescribed itraconazole (Sporanox), 100 mg, PO, daily with dosage to increase 100 mg per day until a maximum dosage of 400 mg per day is reached. The patient can swallow only liquid medication. Sporanox is available in 100-mg capsules and in 100 mg/mL solution. The medication is to be started on Monday.

   a. Which form of the medication will the patient receive? _____

   b. What is the initial dose amount? _____

   c. How many milliliters of medication will the patient receive on Thursday? _____

4. The physician's order is for ketoconazole (Nizoral), 400 mg, PO, daily. The drug is available in 200-mg and 400-mg tablets. Treatment can last from 3 to 6 weeks.

   a. How many milligrams of Nizoral will be administered each week? _____

   b. The pharmacist has given the patient enough medication for a 4-week treatment regimen. How many tablets should the patient have? _____

   c. If treatment must be continued for the 6 weeks, how many more tablets will the patient need? _____

   d. What type of toxicity is the patient at risk for developing with this drug? _____

5. The physician has prescribed flucytosine, 150 mg/kg per day, PO, for a patient who weighs 176 pounds. Dosage schedule is every 6 hours. The drug is available in 500-mg capsules.

   a. What is the total milligrams ordered per day? _____

   b. How many milligrams of drug will be administered at each dose? _____

   c. How many capsules will be administered at each dose? _____

VI. Critical Thinking

1. A patient is hospitalized with a severe fungal infection of the skin and nails. One of the patient's nursing diagnoses is Impaired Skin Integrity. Discuss the nursing interventions that would be appropriate for this patient.

2. Your patient is being discharged from the hospital with a prescription for miconazole (Monistat) cream. Discuss the information that needs to be provided during your patient teaching for this

CHAPTER 16

Antiparasitic Drugs

I. Matching

Match each term in Column A with the correct definition or statement in Column B.

COLUMN A

_____ 1. anthelmintics

_____ 2. quinine

_____ 3. amebicides

_____ 4. cinchonism

_____ 5. treatment

_____ 6. malaria

_____ 7. suppression

_____ 8. chloroquine

_____ 9. helminths

_____ 10. pyrantel

_____ 11. mebendazole

_____ 12. parasite

_____ 13. ameba

_____ 14. pinworm

_____ 15. amebiasis

COLUMN B

A. Invasion of the body by the ameba *Entamoeba histolytica*.

B. An infectious disease caused by a protozoan and transmitted to humans through a bite from an infected mosquito.

C. Organism that lives in or on another organism (the host) without contributing to the survival or well-being of the host.

D. First antimalarial drug.

E. Drugs used to treat helminth infections whose prime purpose is to kill the parasite.

F. Roundworms, pinworms, whipworms, hook-

worms, tapeworms.

G. Helminth infection that is universally common.

H. A group of symptoms associated with quinine.

I. Using an antimalarial drug to prevent malaria.

J. One-celled organism found in soil and water.

K. Drugs that kill amebas.

L. Taking this drug with high-fat foods increases absorption.

M. Irreversible retinal damage has occurred in patients on long-term therapy with these drugs.

N. Using an antimalarial drug to manage a malarial attack.

O. Drug used to treat roundworm and pinworm.

II. Fill in the Blanks

1. List the anthelmintic drugs discussed in this chapter. Include the generic as well as the trade name.

   a) _____ _____

   b) _____ _____

   c) _____ _____

   d) _____ _____

2. List the antimalarial drugs discussed in this chapter. Include the generic as well as the trade name.

   a) _____ _____

   b) _____ _____

   c) _____

3. List the amebicides discussed in this chapter. Include the generic as well as the trade name.

   a) _____ _____

   b) _____ _____

   c) _____ _____

   d) _____ _____

4. Diagnosis of a helminth infection is made by examination of the _____ for _____ and all or part of the _____.

5. When pinworm infection is suspected, the nurse takes a specimen from the _____ _____, preferably early in the _____, using a _____ _____ _____.

6. Parenteral injection of chloroquine is avoided because the drug can cause _____ _____, _____, and _____ _____ when given _____ or _____.

7. Paromomycin may be _____ in large amounts by patients with _____ _____, causing _____ and _____ _____.

8. Diagnosis of amebiasis is made by _____ the _____, as well as by considering the _____ _____.

9. The nurse _____ delivers all _____ _____ saved for amebiasic examination to the _____ because the organisms _____ when the specimen _____.

10. Ingestion of _____ while taking metronidazole may cause a _____ to _____ reaction with symptoms of _____ _____, _____, _____, _____ _____, _____ and _____.

III. Crossword Puzzle

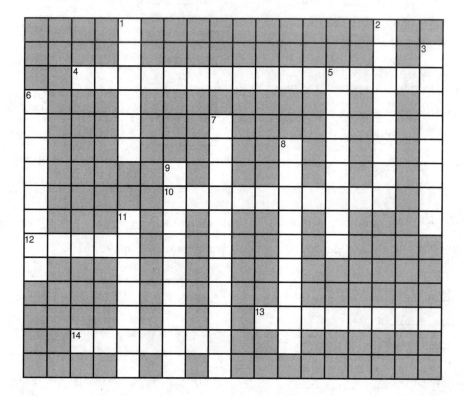

ACROSS CLUES

4. Easy bruising or bleeding.
10. Cells formed as a result of asexual reproduction.
12. One-celled organism found in soil and water.
13. Worms found in the body.
14. The first antimalarial drug.

DOWN CLUES

1. Another name for mebendazole.
2. Helminth infection that is universally common.
3. Organism that lives in or on another organism without contributing to the survival or well-being of the host.
5. Drug used to treat roundworm and pinworm.
6. Combination of sulfadoxine and pyrimethamine.
7. An animal reproductive cell.
8. A type of mosquito that transmits malaria.
9. Invasion of the body by the ameba.
11. An infectious disease transmitted to humans through a bite from an infected mosquito.

IV. Multiple Choice

Circle the letter of the most appropriate answer.

A team conference is held to discuss helminth infections. All members attending are asked to consult reference books before the conference to become familiar with the different types of helminth infections and the drugs used to treat them. Questions 1–4 pertain to topics covered at the conference.

1. When discussing administration of specific anthelmintic drugs, the nurse would be correct to state:
   a. albendazole is given once a day on an empty stomach.
   b. mebendazole should be taken with high-fat food to increase absorption.
   c. pyrantel should not be taken with food, milk, or fruit juice.
   d. thiabendazole is always taken on an empty stomach.

2. A nurse asks what can be done if a patient cannot swallow the anthelmintic mebendazole and refuses to chew the tablet. Another nurse correctly answers that the drug can:

   a. be mixed with food.

   b. only be swallowed whole.

   c. not be chewed.

   d. only be taken with water.

3. A nurse assistant asks how the diagnosis of a helminth infection is made. The nurse correctly answers that a diagnosis is made by:

   a. examination of the blood for antibodies associated with the helminths.

   b. obtaining a careful history of symptoms of a helminth infection.

   c. examination of the stool for ova and the helminths.

   d. endoscopic examination of the sigmoid colon.

4. A nurse asks, "How should I take a specimen from the patient suspected of pinworm infection?" The correct instructions would be:

   a. collect the first stool of the day.

   b. use a cotton swab smeared with stool.

   c. the patient will need a colonoscopy.

   d. use a cellophane tape swab in the anal area.

5. When caring for the patient with a helminth infection, the nurse:

   a. wears gloves and thoroughly washes hands after removing gloves.

   b. instructs the patient to wear gloves when using the bathroom or bedpan.

   c. keeps the patient in bed until the helminth is expelled.

   d. wears a gown, mask, shoe coverings, and gloves.

6. A patient asks about the use of antimalarial drugs used for the prevention of malaria. The nurse would describe the treatment regimen as:

   a. begin treatment 6 weeks before expected exposure and continue for 2 weeks after leaving infected area.

   b. begin taking the drug every day for 2 weeks before exposure and continue for 6 weeks.

   c. take the drug every 3 days for 21 days.

   d. take the drug once a week on the same day each week.

7. When a patient has amebiasis, the nurse carries out:

   a. strict isolation.   c. reverse isolation.

   b. stool precautions.   d. respiratory isolation.

8. When obtaining a stool specimen for amebiasis, the nurse immediately takes the specimen to the laboratory because the:

   a. amebas die when the stool cools.

   b. specimen must be examined within 48 hours.

   c. specimen must be immediately refrigerated.

   d. amebas undergo changes in warm temperature.

9. The nurse instructs food handlers who are to undergo treatment for amebiasis to:

   a. wear gloves while at work.

   b. handle only nonperishable food.

   c. wear a mask when handling fresh food.

   d. not return to work until stools are negative for ameba.

10. What two anthelmintic drugs have exhibited embryotoxic effects and are contraindicated during pregnancy?

    a. Chloroquine and pyrantel

    b. Thiabendazole and albendazole

    c. Pyrantel and mebendazole

    d. Albendazole and mebendazole

11. The physician has ordered the first dose of quinine for your patient, to be administered IV. As the nurse, you would know:

    a. quinine must be administered at a very fast rate.

    b. quinine does not require any further dilution.

    c. the patient must be monitored for respiratory distress.

    d. the drug is nonirritating to the vein.

12. The nurse is educating a patient who will be taking chloroquine in high dose for an extended period. It is important for the patient to know:

    a. frequent renal function tests are required.

    b. frequent ophthalmic examinations are necessary.

    c. liver function tests are required after treatment.

    d. the drug must be taken with antacids containing aluminum.

V. Dosage Problems

Solve the following dosage calculations.

1. The physician has ordered chloroquine hydrochloride for a patient experiencing an acute malaria attack. The dose ordered is 1 gram, PO, initially, followed 6 hours later with a 500-mg dose. The dosing schedule is to be repeated on days 2 and 3. Chloroquine is available as Aralen, 200-mg and 500-mg tablets.

    a. How many tablets will be administered for the first dose? _____

    b. How many milligrams are to be administered daily? _____

    c. How many tablets will be administered for the complete 3-day regimen? _____

2. A patient diagnosed with hydatid disease has been prescribed a treatment regimen of albendazole. The dose ordered is 400 mg, PO, BID, with meals for 38 days followed by 14 days with no albendazole; repeating for a total of three cycles. Albendazole (Albenza) is available in 200-mg tablets.

    a. How many tablets will be taken for each dose? _____

    b. How many milligrams of medication will the patient take each day? _____

    c. How many tablets will the patient need for each cycle of the medication regimen? _____

    d. How many days will have elapsed at the end of the last 14-day drug-free period of the medication regimen? _____

    e. Approximately how many months of drug therapy will the patient undergo? _____

3. A patient receiving ciprofloxacin for a gram-negative infection has developed pseudomembranous colitis. The physician orders metronidazole (Flagyl) for the antibiotic-associated infection. The dose ordered is 2 grams per day for 7 days, PO Flagyl is available in 250-mg and 500-mg tablets.

    a. How many 500-mg tablets would the nurse administer at each dose? _____

    b. For a 7-day treatment regimen, the patient would need how many tablets? _____

4. A 12-year-old and his mother are diagnosed with roundworm infection. The physician has ordered pyrantel pamoate for both patients. The instructions from the physician are: 5 mg per pound of body weight, PO, single dose. The 12-year-old weighs 72 pounds and the mother weighs 144 pounds. Pyrantel is available in 180-mg capsules.

    a. How many milligrams of pyrantel will be given to the 12-year-old? _____

    b. How many milligrams will the mother receive? _____

    c. How many capsules will each patient receive? _____

VI. Critical Thinking

1. A patient is admitted to your unit with severe diarrhea. The physician orders stool samples and stool cultures for microscopic examination for ova and parasites. In addition to a history of the patient's symptoms and a drug and allergy history, discuss what other questions you would ask this patient.

2. A couple planning to do missionary work is going to a country where malaria is prevalent. Their estimated stay in the country is 2 to 3 years. The physician has prescribed hydroxychloroquine (Plaquenil) to be taken weekly. Discuss what additional information and instructions you would give these patients.

3. A patient diagnosed with amebic dysentery is prescribed the combination of metronidazole and iodoquinol. Discuss the drug-specific teaching points that must be covered by the nurse for both of these drugs. Also discuss what the nurse must include in the assessment of this patient, and why.

CHAPTER 17

Nonnarcotic Analgesics: Salicylates and Nonsalicylates

I. Matching

Match each term in Column A with the correct statement or definition in Column B.

COLUMN A

_____ 1. aggregation

_____ 2. antipyretic

_____ 3. pain

_____ 4. salicylism

_____ 5. asterixis

_____ 6. analgesic

_____ 7. NSAID

_____ 8. salicylates

_____ 9. pancytopenia

_____ 10. aspirin

_____ 11. chronic

_____ 12. Reye's syndrome

_____ 13. prostaglandins

_____ 14. tinnitus

_____ 15. acute

COLUMN B

A. Involuntary jerking movements, especially of the hands.

B. Fatty acid derivatives found in almost every tissue of the body.

C. Clumping.

D. Type of pain that is short in duration and can be mild or severe.

E. Nonsteroidal anti-inflammatory drug.

F. Type of drug used to treat elevated body temperature.

G. Has a greater anti-inflammatory effect than the other salicylates.

H. Usually occurs with repeated large doses of a salicylate.

I. A life-threatening condition characterized by vomiting and lethargy progressing to coma.

J. A reduction in all cellular components of the blood.

K. Ringing sound in the ear.

L. Defined as an unpleasant sensory and emotional experience.

M. Type of pain lasting longer than 6 months and can be mild or severe.

N. Aspirin and related drugs.

O. Type of drug used to relieve pain.

II. Fill in the Blanks

1. List two examples of NSAIDs discussed in this chapter. Include the generic as well as the trade name.

   a) _____ _____

   b) _____

2. Side effects of the nonnarcotic analgesics include:

   a) _____

   b) _____

   c) _____

   d) _____

   e) _____

   f) _____

3. Foods that naturally contain salicylate and may increase the risk of adverse reactions when salicylates are administered include:

   a) _____

   b) _____

   c) _____

d) _____

e) _____

f) _____

4. _____ may increase the risk of bleeding during heparin administration.

5. _____ has analgesic and antipyretic activity but does not possess _____ action.

6. List 10 of the symptoms of salicylism:

a) _____

b) _____

c) _____

d) _____

e) _____

f) _____

g) _____

h) _____

i) _____

j) _____

7. List the signs and symptoms of acetaminophen toxicity:

a) _____

b) _____

c) _____

d) _____

e) _____

f) _____

g) _____

h) _____

i) _____

j) _____

k) _____

l) _____

8. Pain is _____ and the patient's report of pain should always be taken _____.

9. The _____ analgesics are a group of _____ used to relieve _____ without the possibility of causing _____ _____.

10. Loss of _____ through the gastrointestinal tract occurs with _____ use.

III. Multiple Choice

Circle the letter of the most appropriate answer.

1. A nurse asks how aspirin prolongs bleeding time. The most correct response is that aspirin prolongs bleeding time by:
   a. interfering with the manufacture of prothrombin.
   b. inhibiting the aggregation of platelets.
   c. a direct action on the liver.
   d. increasing the manufacture of platelets.

2. At a team conference, the nurse explains that acetaminophen has:
   a. analgesic and antipyretic activity.
   b. analgesic activity only.
   c. analgesic and anti-inflammatory activity.
   d. analgesic, antipyretic, and anti-inflammatory activity.

3. Salicylism may occur with salicylate overdose. Which of the following signs would alert the nurse to the possibility of mild salicylism?
   a. Nausea, vomiting, constipation
   b. Insomnia, anxiety, headache
   c. Dizziness, tinnitus, difficulty hearing
   d. Mental confusion, dyspnea, heartburn

4. When doing discharge teaching, the nurse informs the patient that prolonged salicylate use can cause:

   a. an increase in the ability of the blood to clot.

   b. an increase in the number of platelets.

   c. a loss of blood through the gastrointestinal tract.

   d. a decrease in the number of white blood cells.

5. At a team conference, the nurse explains that salicylates, especially aspirin, may be responsible for the development of:

   a. Reye's syndrome in children with influenza or chickenpox.

   b. liver disorders.

   c. intestinal polyps in older adults.

   d. pancreatitis.

6. A patient being seen in the clinic tells the nurse, "I take Tylenol every day." The nurse should explain the adverse reactions that may occur with the use of acetaminophen, and also tell the patient that these reactions usually occur:

   a. in those with inflammatory conditions.

   b. with chronic use or when exceeding the recommended dosage.

   c. when the drug is combined with an antacid.

   d. if the patient is also taking an anticoagulant.

7. Which of the following statements by the patient would indicate to the nurse that the patient is developing an adverse reaction to salicylates?

   a. "My pain is decreasing."

   b. "My eyes are swollen each morning when I awaken."

   c. "My feet and legs are swollen at the end of the day."

   d. "The color of my stools is very dark, almost black."

8. Which of the following items of information will the nurse be certain to include in a teaching plan for the patient taking a nonsteroidal anti-inflammatory drug?

   a. These drugs can cause extreme confusion and should be used with caution.

   b. Relief from pain and inflammation should occur immediately after the first dose.

   c. Avoid the use of aspirin or other salicylates when taking these drugs

   d. If gastrointestinal upset occurs, take this drug on an empty stomach.

9. As a nurse, you are responsible for helping the patient manage pain. The nurse must always remember that:

   a. patients will often be overmedicated for pain.

   b. chronic pain will not be helped with medication.

   c. acute pain is of short duration and rarely needs medication.

   d. pain is subjective and patients' report of pain should be taken seriously.

10. A patient who is on anticoagulation therapy asks why the physician told her to use acetaminophen in place of aspirin for pain. You would be correct in stating:

    a. aspirin will cause your blood to clot easily.

    b. aspirin is known to cause Reye's syndrome in adults.

    c. acetaminophen is an effective pain reliever without the side effects of aspirin.

    d. aspirin and acetaminophen can be taken concurrently.

IV. Crossword Puzzle

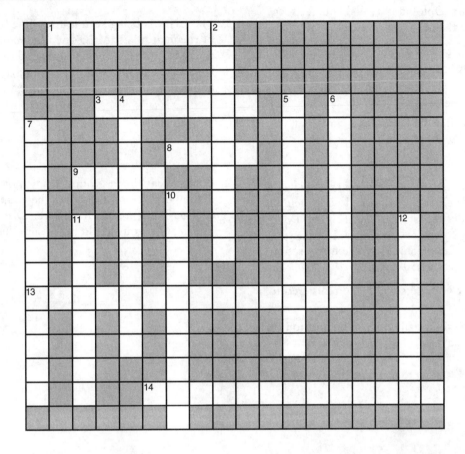

ACROSS CLUES

1. Ringing sound in the ear.
3. Has a greater anti-inflammatory effect than the other salicylates.
8. Life-threatening syndrome seen in children with influenza or chickenpox who take aspirin.
9. Defined as an unpleasant sensory and emotional experience.
13. Fatty acid derivatives found in almost every tissue of the body.
14. Major drug classified as a nonsalicylate.

DOWN CLUES

2. Another word for salicylate toxicity.
4. Aspirin and related drugs.
5. Clumping of platelets.
6. Involuntary jerking movements, especially of the hands.
7. A reduction of all cellular components of the blood.
10. Drugs used to relieve pain.
11. Drug used to treat acetaminophen overdosage.
12. Yellow discoloration of the skin.

V. Dosage Problems

Solve the following dosage calculations.

1. The physician has ordered Tylenol liquid, 1000 mg, PO, every 6 hours. The available acetaminophen is in dosage strength of 500 mg/15 mL. According to the label, acetaminophen dosage should not exceed 4 grams per day.

   a) How many milliliters of acetaminophen liquid would the nurse administer every 6 hours?
   _____

   b) How many milligrams of acetaminophen will be administered in each 24-hour period?
   _____

   c) Will this dose exceed the recommended daily dose? _____

2. The physician's order reads, diflunisal (Dolobid), 1000 mg, PO, initially follow by 750 mg, PO, every 12 hours. Dolobid is available in 250-mg and 500-mg tablets.

   a) How many tablets will be administered at the initial dose? _____

   b) How many tablets will be administered at each 12-hour dose? _____

   c) During the first 24 hours, how many milligrams of Dolobid will be administered? _____

3. The physician has ordered sodium thiosalicylate (Rexolate) for a patient diagnosed with rheumatic fever. The order reads: Rexolate, 150 mg, IM, every 6 hours for 3 days. Day 4, Rexolate, 100 mg, IM, BID. Rexolate is available for injection in a dose strength of 50 mg/mL.

   a) How many milliliters will be administered for each of the 150-mg doses? _____

   b) What is the total daily dose of medication for the first 3 days? _____

VI. Critical Thinking

1. Ms. Clark is being seen in the clinic for treatment of rheumatoid arthritis. The physician has prescribed Naproxen for her pain and discomfort. Discuss the information you will give Ms. Clark about detecting possible gastrointestinal bleeding.

2. You are teaching a group of new mothers about the importance of using over-the-counter drugs cautiously for treatment of fever. Discuss what information you should make sure they receive.

CHAPTER 18

Nonnarcotic Analgesics: Nonsteroidal Anti-inflammatory Drugs (NSAIDs)

I. Matching

Match each term in Column A with the correct statement or definition in Column B.

COLUMN A

_____ 1. cyclooxygenase-1

_____ 2. cyclooxygenase-2

_____ 3. NSAID

_____ 4. dysmenorrhea

_____ 5. intestinal ulcerations

COLUMN B

A. Nonsteroidal anti-inflammatory drug.

B. Enzyme that helps to maintain the stomach lining.

C. An adverse reaction associated with use of NSAIDs.

D. Enzyme that triggers pain and inflammation.

E. A condition treated with NSAIDs.

II. Multiple Choice

Circle the letter of the most appropriate answer.

1. A patient asks, "What exactly are NSAIDs?" You would be correct in replying:
   a. "They are drugs in the salicylate group."
   b. "They are another type of nonnarcotic analgesic."
   c. "These drugs contain steroids."
   d. "These drugs have only antipyretic properties."

2. Your patient has been prescribed an NSAID and is also taking monopril for treatment of high blood pressure. As his nurse, you would carefully monitor for:
   a. increased urine output.
   b. increased blood pressure.
   c. decreased blood pressure.
   d. decreased hepatic function.

3. Ms. Brown is being seen in the clinic today for complaints of arthritic-type pain. The physician has prescribed Celecoxib. You tell her the adverse reactions that may occur include:
   a. dyspepsia, diarrhea.
   b. dyspepsia, somnolence.
   c. dyspepsia, insomnia.
   d. headache, hemoptysis.

4. When assessing a patient who is taking a diuretic medication, it is important to ask about over-the-counter (OTC) drugs because:
   a. OTC drugs are less likely to interact with the diuretic.
   b. these drugs are not likely to impair renal function.
   c. there is a decreased effect of diuretics when administered with ibuprofen.
   d. naproxen increases the effect of diuretics when used together.

5. When an NSAID is prescribed for treatment of rheumatoid arthritis or osteoarthritis in an elderly patient over a long period, there is an increased probability of:
   a. the patient developing an addiction to the drug.
   b. the development of gastrointestinal bleeding.
   c. increased clotting of the blood.
   d. fewer adverse reactions occurring.

III. Fill in the Blanks

1. List the four commonly used NSAIDs discussed in this chapter. Include the generic and trade names.

    a) _____ _____

    b) _____ _____

    c) _____ _____

    d) _____ _____

2. The NSAIDs are so named because they do not belong to the _____ group of drugs.

3. The NSAIDs have _____,

    _____, and _____ effects.

4. The NSAIDs are used for the following conditions:

    a. _____
    _____
    _____ .

    b. _____
    _____
    _____ .

    c. _____
    _____
    _____ .

    d. _____
    _____
    _____ .

5. Adverse reactions to the NSAIDs may affect the special senses. The nurse should know to monitor

    for _____, _____,
    _____, _____,
    _____, _____,
    _____.

IV. Critical Thinking

1. Discuss why it is important to determine if a patient has a history of gastrointestinal bleeding or peptic ulcer before administration of the NSAIDs.

2. During treatment with an NSAID, your patient complains of increasing pain. Discuss how you would address this situation. Describe any assessment you might complete.

3. Educating patients about their medications is an effective way to ensure compliance with treatment regimens. Describe a teaching plan for the patient who has been prescribed an NSAID.

V. Dosage Problems

Solve the following dosage calculations.

1. A patient has been prescribed naproxen suspension, 500 mg, PO, BID. The available dose strength is 125 mg/5 mL. How many milliliters must be administered to give the ordered dose?

    _____

2. A pediatric patient who weighs 38 kg is to receive naproxen suspension, 7.5 mL, BID. The dose strength is the same as in question 1. How many milligrams of naproxen will be administered at each dose? _____

3. The physician has ordered ibuprofen for your 15-year-old patient who has been diagnosed with mild juvenile arthritis. The order is for ibuprofen, 20 mg/kg per day, PO, in four divided doses. The ibuprofen is available in dose strength of 100 mg/5 mL, and the patient weighs 50 kg.

   a) How many milligrams of medication will be administered at each dose? _____

   b) How many milliliters of medication will be administered at each dose? _____

VI. Crossword Puzzle

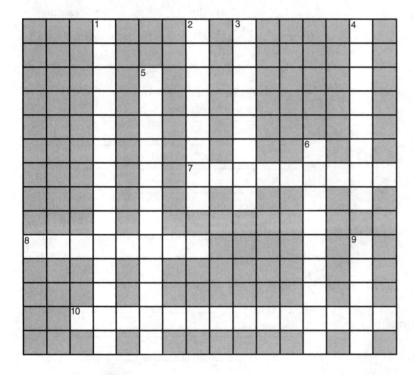

ACROSS CLUES

7. Advil.
8. Administration of this drug can cause dyspepsia and diarrhea.
10. A type of arthritis that is treated with NSAIDs.

DOWN CLUES

1. Enzyme that triggers pain and inflammation.
2. An adverse reaction that can occur with the administration of NSAIDs.
3. An adverse reaction that may occur with the use of NSAIDs.
4. Naprosyn.
5. A condition treated with NSAIDs.
6. Vioxx.
9. Nonsteroidal anti-inflammatory drug.

CHAPTER 19

Narcotic Analgesics

I. Matching

Match each term in Column A with the correct statement or definition in Column B.

COLUMN A

_____ 1. opioid analgesic

_____ 2. narcotic antagonists

_____ 3. PCA

_____ 4. morphine

_____ 5. partial agonist

_____ 6. narcotic analgesic

_____ 7. agonist-antagonist

_____ 8. epidural

_____ 9. antitussive

_____ 10. agonist

COLUMN B

A. Controlled substances used to treat moderate to severe pain.

B. Binds to a receptor and causes a response.

C. Narcotic analgesic obtained from the opium plant.

D. Binds to a receptor, but the response is limited.

E. Allows patients to administer their own analgesic by means of an IV pump system.

F. Catheter is placed in the epidural space of spinal cord.

G. Suppresses the cough reflex.

H. Drugs that counteract the effects of the narcotic analgesics.

I. Have properties of both the agonists and antagonists.

J. Considered the prototype or "model" narcotic.

II. Fill in the Blanks

1. Narcotic antagonists compete with the _____ at the _____ sites and are used to _____ the depressant effects of the _____ _____.

2. List the drugs obtained from raw opium.

   a) _____

   b) _____

   c) _____

   d) _____

3. Synthetic _____ are those man-made _____ with properties and actions similar to the _____ _____.

4. Examples of synthetic narcotic analgesics are:

   a) _____

   b) _____

   c) _____

   d) _____

5. The ability of a narcotic analgesic to relieve pain depends on the:

   a) _____

   b) _____

   c) _____

   d) _____

   e) _____

   f) _____

6. Narcotic analgesics may be used preoperatively to _____ _____ and _____ the patient.

7. List the two opioids used in treatment and management of opioid dependence:

   a) _____

   b) _____

8. A major hazard of narcotic administration is

   _____ _____ with a

   _____ in the _____

   _____ and _____ .

9. Immediately before preparing a narcotic analgesic for administration, the nurse assesses the patient's:

   a) _____

   b) _____

   c) _____

10. What three physiologic changes in the patient would signal the nurse to withhold the narcotic analgesic and contact the primary health care provider?

    a. _____
    _____
    _____ .

    b. _____
    _____
    _____ .

    c. _____
    _____
    _____ .

III. Multiple Choice

Circle the letter of the most appropriate answer.

1. When checking a drug reference, the nurse reads that when a drug has agonist properties, it is capable of:

   a. binding to an opioid receptor and causing no response.

   b. binding to an opioid receptor and causing a response.

   c. binding to an opioid receptor with limited response.

   d. binding to an opioid receptor and reversing the antagonist response.

2. At a team conference, the nurse explains that the administration of a narcotic analgesic:

   a. can produce serious or potentially fatal respiratory depression if given too frequently.

   b. requires an assessment of the patient 2 or 3 hours after drug is given.

   c. always leads to the patient developing a chemical dependence on the drug.

   d. orally or transdermally causes the development of tolerance to the drug very quickly.

3. Which of the following changes in the eye will the nurse be alert for after the administration of morphine?

   a. Mydriasis   c. Diplopia

   b. Myopia   d. Miosis

4. The nurse would anticipate that the effect of morphine on respiration would be:

   a. a decrease in rate and depth.

   b. an increase in the rate.

   c. a decrease in the depth.

   d. an increase in the rate and depth.

5. The nurse expects the patient receiving morphine to experience nausea and vomiting because this drug:

   a. has antiemetic properties.

   b. depresses the chemoreceptor trigger zone (CTZ).

   c. stimulates the pituitary gland.

   d. stimulates the CTZ.

6. At a team conference, the nurse explains that although methadone may be given for pain, it is also used:

   a   when the patient is allergic to morphine.

   b. in the detoxification and treatment of narcotic addiction.

   c. to induce emesis after poison ingestion.

   d. to stimulate respirations after anesthesia.

7. The nurse explains to the patient that patient-controlled analgesia:

   a. allow patients to administer their own analgesic.

   b. appears to increase the need for narcotics in those with mild to moderate pain.

   c. is effective only when oral narcotic analgesics are ordered.

   d. decreases the time between doses of the narcotic.

8. The narcotic agonists are contraindicated in patients with:

   a. congestive heart failure.

   b. gout.

   c   head injuries.

   d. myocardial infarction.

9. The nurse is going over the teaching plan with a patient who has been prescribed a narcotic analgesic transdermal system. The instructions would include which of the following?

   a. After 72 hours, remove the patch and apply a new patch to different site.

   b. Use soap and water to cleanse thoroughly the area of application.

   c. Be sure to apply each new patch to the same spot as the old patch.

   d. Apply the patch to any area of the lower torso or legs.

10. The nurse will obtain the patient's blood pressure, pulse, and respiratory rate _____ after the narcotic analgesic is administered IM.

    a. 1 to 2 hours   c. 5 to 10 minutes

    b. 20 to 30 minutes   d. 30 minutes to 1 hour

IV. Dosage Problems

Solve the following dosage calculations.

1. The patient is prescribed oral morphine, 8 mg. The dosage available is 10 mg/mL. How many milliliters would the nurse give? _____

2. The physician has ordered codeine phosphate 20 mg, subcutaneous every 4 hours. The vial states the dose strength is 30 mg/mL. How many milliliters will the nurse administer? _____

3. The physician's order reads, morphine 6 mg, IM, now. The medication is available in dose strength of 8 mg/mL. How many milliliters will the nurse give? _____

4. A postoperative patient has been prescribed Demerol 100 mg, IM, every 3 to 4 hours as needed for pain. The vials of meperidine you have are in dose strength of 75 mg/mL. How many milliliters of medication will you give?

   _____

V. Crossword Puzzle

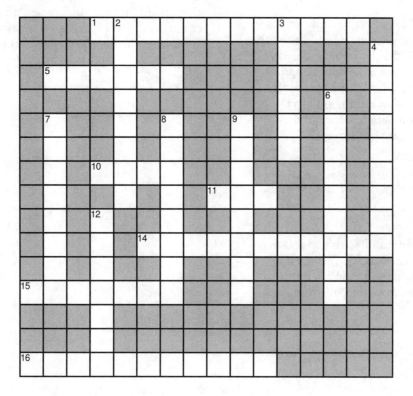

ACROSS CLUES

1. Levorphanol sulfate.
5. Remifentanil hydrochloride.
10. The emotional and sensory perceptions associated with real or potential tissue damage.
11. Abbreviation for patient-controlled analgesia.
13. Suppresses the cough reflex.
14. Meperidine hydrochloride.
15. Substance manufactured in the body that prevents the release of a neurotransmitter from carrying pain impulses to the central nervous system.

DOWN CLUES

2. Route of administration of patient-controlled analgesia.
3. Another word for narcotic.
4. Synthetic narcotic analgesic.
6. Methadone hydrochloride.
7. Prototype or model narcotic.
8. Drug used as an alternative to morphine because patients experience fewer adverse reactions.
9. Type of analgesic used to treat moderate to severe pain.
12. Narcotic used to relieve severe, persistent cough.

VI. Critical Thinking

1. Mr. Adams is a few hours postoperative and is in a considerable amount of pain. He is refusing the meperidine (Demerol) that had been ordered by the physician. Discuss how you would approach this situation to determine why the patient is refusing medication. What information can you give Mr. Adams to help him understand the importance of pain relief after surgery?

2. Undertreatment of pain can be avoided if the nurse has good assessment skills. Discuss the information the nurse must obtain from the patient to meet the needs of the patient in pain.

3. You are to present a program to your fellow nurses about medicating the patient with chronic severe pain. Prepare your presentation using a terminally ill patient with cancer as an example, and discuss the management of his pain.

CHAPTER 20

Narcotic Antagonists

I. Matching

Match each term in Column A with the correct definition or statement in Column B.

COLUMN A

_____ 1. naloxone (Narcan)

_____ 2. respirator

_____ 3. narcotic antagonist

_____ 4. naltrexone (ReVia)

_____ 5. antagonist

COLUMN B

A. Reverses the action of a narcotic.

B. A substance that counteracts the action of something else.

C. Drug given to reverse respiratory depression by narcotic analgesics.

D. Drug used for the treatment of narcotic dependence to block the effects of the opiates.

E. Used for artificial ventilation.

II. Fill in the Blanks

1. A drug that is an antagonist has an _____ for a cell _____, and, by _____ to it, _____ the cell from _____.

2. The two narcotic antagonists in use today are _____ _____ and _____ _____ (list the generic and trade names) .

3. _____ is used primarily to block the _____ effects experienced in _____ dependence.

4. Administration of _____ prevents or _____ the effects of the _____.

5. Naloxone is used for _____ or _____ _____ of _____ _____, including _____ _____.

6. Abrupt reversal of narcotic depression may result in _____, _____, _____, _____, _____ _____ _____, and _____.

7. Patients taking _____ on a scheduled basis will not experience any _____ _____ if they use an _____.

8. The expected outcome for the patient with respiratory _____ is a return to normal _____ _____, _____, and _____.

III. Multiple Choice

Circle the letter of the most appropriate answer.

1. The nurse administering naloxone should continue to monitor vital signs after the patient has shown a response to the drug:

    a every 1 to 2 minutes.

    b. every 5 to 15 minutes.

    c. every 30 to 45 minutes.

    d. once an hour.

2. Your patient has been given naloxone for narcotic depression. As the nurse, you would be aware of the most important nursing task as:

    a. keeping suction equipment available to maintain a patent airway.

    b. maintaining an accurate record of the patient's activities.

    c. maintaining an accurate intake and output record.

    d. monitoring the vital signs at least once every 4 hours.

3. Jane Allen is being treated with naltrexone in the clinic for her narcotic addiction. When completing your assessment, it is important to ask her:

    a. "Have you missed any work lately?"

    b. "Have you had any headaches lately?"

    c. "Do you have identification indicating you are receiving naltrexone?"

    d. "How has your appetite been since you were last here?"

4. A patient is being treated in the emergency department for a suspected overdose of a narcotic analgesic. As a nurse, you would anticipate the treatment to include:

    a methadone.   c. naltrexone.

    b. naloxone.   d. meperidine.

5. Adverse reactions the nurse must monitor for when administering naltrexone would include:

    a. depression.   c. tachycardia.

    b. tremors.   d. increased blood pressure.

6. Andy Parker is being treated with naltrexone for his narcotic addiction. His physician has just prescribed thioridazine for the depression he is expe-

riencing. What will his nurse need to teach him about the concurrent use of these two drugs?

    a. There will be increased anxiety.

    b. He will experience decreased joint pain.

    c. There may be increased lethargy and drowsiness.

    d. Nausea and vomiting should not be a problem anymore.

7. You are monitoring a patient who is receiving morphine by IV drip. Which drug would you expect to be kept at the patient's bedside?

    a. Naloxone   c. Naltrexone

    b. Methadone   d. Fentanyl

8. Mr. James has just been administered naloxone for reversal of narcotic depression. As his nurse, you would know to monitor for the possible reaction of:

    a abdominal cramping.   c. irritability.

    b. depression.   d. tachycardia.

IV. Dosage Problems

Solve the following dosage calculations.

1. A patient is prescribed naloxone for an overdose of morphine. The dosage in the drug guide is 10 mcg/kg and the patient weighs 150 pounds. What dosage would the nurse expect the physician to prescribe for this patient?

    _____

2. Mary Lee has been prescribed naltrexone for treatment of narcotic addiction. The initial dose ordered is: naltrexone, 25 mg, PO, observe 1 hr; if no signs or symptoms observed, complete dose with additional 25 mg, PO. Maintenance dose will be 150 mg every third day. Naltrexone is available in 50-mg tablets.

    a) How many tablets will be administered for the initial dose? _____

    b) How many tablets are needed for each maintenance dose? _____

3. A patient who was given nalbuphine (Nubain) as a preoperative analgesic has developed respiratory depression. The physician has ordered naloxone 1 mg, IV, repeat at 3-minute intervals until desired response. Naloxone is available in an injection dose of 0.4 mg/mL. How many milliliters will be administered in each 3-minute interval? _____

V. Crossword Puzzle

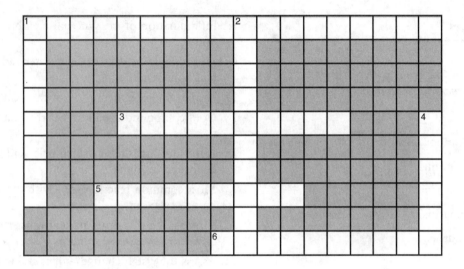

ACROSS CLUES

1. Reverses the action of a narcotic (two words).
3. Used for artificial ventilation.
5. Narcotic used in detoxification of those addicted to narcotics.
6. Adverse reaction the nurse must monitor for when administering naltrexone.

DOWN CLUES

1. Drug used to reverse narcotic-induced respiratory depression.
2. Drug used for the treatment of narcotic dependence to block the effects of the opiates.
4. Naloxone.

VI. Critical Thinking

1. You are asked by your supervisor to present information at a staff meeting on how to promote optimal response in a patient being treated for opioid dependency. Discuss the anxiety issues that may be involved, the nursing responsibilities, and the problems that must be addressed to assist the patient to adhere to his treatment regimen.

2. You are monitoring a patient who is receiving IV morphine. What are the indications that this patient is going into narcotic depression and reparatory depression? If naloxone is ordered, what will you watch for as it is administered?

CHAPTER 21

Drugs That Affect the Musculoskeletal System

I. Matching

Match each term in Column A with the correct definition or statement in Column B.

COLUMN A

_____ 1. thrombocytopenia

_____ 2. auranofin

_____ 3. rheumatoid arthritis

_____ 4. dermatitis

_____ 5. alendronate

_____ 6. drowsiness

_____ 7. cyclobenzaprine

_____ 8. osteoarthritis

_____ 9. Paget's disease

_____ 10. corticosteroids

_____ 11. musculoskeletal

_____ 12. chrysiasis

_____ 13. hydroxychloroquine

_____ 14. gout

_____ 15. synovitis

COLUMN B

A. Pertaining to bone and muscle.

B. A chronic disease characterized by inflammatory changes in the body's connective tissue.

C. A noninflammatory joint disease resulting in degeneration of the articular cartilage and changes in the synovial membrane.

D. Inflammation of the skin.

E. Abnormally low numbers of platelets in the blood.

F. Inflammation of the synovial membrane of the joint.

G. A chronic bone disorder characterized by abnormal bone remodeling.

H. Gray to blue pigmentation of the skin.

I. Gold compound used to treat rheumatoid arthritis.

J. A form of arthritis in which uric acid is deposited in joints.

K. Most common reaction seen with the use of the muscle relaxants.

L. After taking this drug, patient must avoid lying down for at least 30 minutes.

M. Assess for visual changes when giving this drug because irreversible retinal damage may occur.

N. Hormones secreted from the adrenal cortex.

O. Muscle relaxer that appears to have an effect on muscle tone, thus reducing muscle spasms.

II. Fill in the Blanks

1. List the types of drugs, discussed in this chapter, used to treat musculoskeletal disorders.

   a) _____

   b) _____

   c) _____

   d) _____

   e) _____

   f) _____

      1. _____

      2. _____

      3. _____

2. List the gold compounds discussed in this chapter. Include the generic and trade names.

   a) _____ _____

   b) _____ _____

   c) _____ _____

3. List the two most common adverse reactions seen with the gold compounds.

   a) _____

   b) _____

4. Colchicine reduces _____ associated with the deposit of _____ _____ in the _____.

5. List the antigout medications discussed in this chapter. Include the generic and trade names.

   a) _____ _____

   b) _____ _____

   c) _____ _____

   d) _____ _____

6. Serious hypersensitivity reactions that can occur with administration of allopurinal are:

   a) _____

   b) _____

7. List the skeletal muscle relaxants discussed in this chapter. Include generic and trade names.

   a) _____

   b) _____

   c) _____

   d _____

   e) _____

8. Adverse reactions seen with the administration of diazepam would include _____,

   _____, _____,

   _____, _____,

   _____, _____ or

   _____, and _____.

9. Cyclobenzaprine is contraindicated in patients with recent _____

   _____, _____

   _____ disorders, and

   _____.

10. List the bisphosphonates discussed in this chapter. Include generic and trade names.

    a) _____ _____

    b) _____ _____

    c) _____ _____

11. Adverse reactions with the bisphosphonates include _____, _____,

    _____ or _____.

    _____ _____, _____,

    _____, _____ _____,

    _____, and _____ pain.

12. Corticosteroids may be used to treat rheumatic disorders such as _____

    _____, _____

    _____, _____, _____,

    and _____.

13. Hydroxychoroquine is contraindicated in patients with _____,

    _____, and _____ disease.

14. During the assessment of a patient with any type of arthritis, the nurse will include a thorough examination of:

    a) _____

    b) _____

    c) _____

III. Multiple Choice

Circle the letter of the most appropriate answer.

Mr. Morris has rheumatoid arthritis and is prescribed meclofenamate (Meclomen), a nonsteroidal anti-inflammatory drug (NSAID). Questions 1–3 pertain to Mr. Morris' case.

1. Which of the following may indicate a serious adverse reaction to this drug and require withholding the next dose?
   a. Tarry stools
   b. Anorexia
   c. Hypertension
   d. Bradycardia

2. In explaining the difference between the corticosteroids and the NSAIDs to another nurse, you would state that the NSAIDs:
   a. have a greater analgesic activity than corticosteroids.
   b. do not have the antipyretic activity of the corticosteroids.
   c. are related to aspirin, but have no effect on clotting time.
   d. do not possess the adverse reactions associated with the corticosteroids.

3. The physician changes Ms. Morris' medication to aurothioglucose (Solganal), a gold compound. The nurse would include what nursing action in Ms. Morris' plan of care?
   a. Keeping Ms. Morris on complete bed rest
   b. Inspecting Ms. Morris' mouth daily for ulcerations of the mucous membranes
   c. Monitoring Ms. Morris' blood pressure every 4 hours
   d. Withholding fluids from Ms. Morris in the late evening hours

4. When asked to discuss carisoprodal (Soma) at a team conference, the nurse states that the mode of action of this drug may be due to its:
   a. anti-inflammatory actions.
   b. effect on muscle tone.
   c. sedative action.
   d. direct action on skeletal muscles.

5. When a patient is prescribed a corticosteroid long term for treatment of arthritis, alternate-day therapy may be used to:
   a. ensure compliance with the drug regime.
   b. minimize certain undesirable reactions.
   c. create high plasma levels of the drug.
   d. deactivate the feedback mechanism.

6. When allopurinol is used for the treatment of gout, the nurse will:
   a. place patient on complete bed rest.
   b. give the medication after the evening meal.
   c. restrict the intake of fluids in late evening.
   d. encourage increased fluid intake.

7. When the nurse is administering colchicine for an acute attack of gout, the drug will be given every 1 to 2 hours:
   a. for a total of 12 doses.
   b. until pain is relieved or vomiting or diarrhea develops.
   c. until all signs of inflammation in the affected joint decrease.
   d. for the duration of the treatment regimen.

8. You are administering the antigout medication sulfinpyrazone to a patient with gout. The patient complains of stomach distress after the medication is given. Your nursing actions for this patient would include:
   a. notifying the primary health care provider.
   b. withholding the next scheduled dose of the drug.
   c. administering the medication with food or after a meal.
   d. ordering an antidiarrheal for this patient.

9. Patients being treated with the skeletal muscle relaxants are cautioned not to perform tasks requiring concentration or attention because of the:
   a. attention deficit created by the drug.
   b. state of drowsiness that may occur.
   c. feelings of agitation and nervousness.
   d. relaxation of muscle tone and decreased response time.

10. Which of the following is the most important to include in a plan of care for the patient receiving a corticosteroid?

    a. Give the drug with food or milk.

    b. Do not omit doses or suddenly stop taking drug.

    c. Monitor vital signs every 2 to 4 hours.

    d. Force fluids throughout the daytime hours.

11. The nurse is teaching an outpatient about the gold compound the doctor has prescribed. Which of the following reactions should the nurse tell the patient to notify the doctor of?

    a. A metallic taste

    b. Arthralgia pain 2 days after IM injection

    c. Occurrence of chrysiasis

    d. Photosensitivity reaction

12. Patients receiving high-dose, long-term NSAID therapy are assessed for:

    a. ulcerations of the skin.

    b. signs of blood clots in the legs.

    c. evidence of pulmonary complications.

    d. evidence of gastrointestinal bleeding.

13. In teaching a patient with gout about the medications used to treat this condition, the nurse would be sure to include the instruction to:

    a. drink at least 10 glasses of water a day.

    b. take your medications on an empty stomach.

    c. notify the physician if pain is not relieved in a few weeks.

    d. continue to take the drug if diarrhea occurs.

14. Patients taking methotrexate are instructed:

    a. to take the weekly dose close to the same day each week.

    b. to report all adverse reactions to the physician.

    c. that the weekly dose may be switched to a daily dose with no ill effects.

    d. to increase the dose if no therapeutic response in a week.

IV. Crossword Puzzle

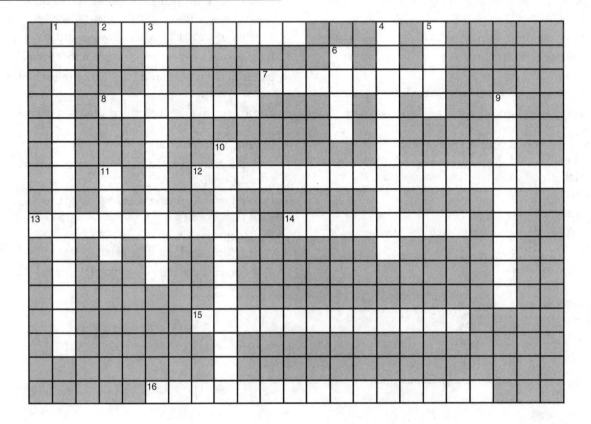

ACROSS CLUES

2. Drug classification used for the treatment of pain.
7. Brand name of allopurinol.
8. Brand name for probenecid.
12. Drugs that work against inflammation.
13. Type of arthritis characterized by inflammatory changes in the body's connective tissue.
14. Ringing in the ears.
15. Pregnancy Category X drug.
16. Pertaining to bone and muscle.

DOWN CLUES

1. Noninflammatory joint disease resulting in degeneration of the articular cartilage.
3. After taking this drug, the patient must avoid lying down for at least 30 minutes.
4. Gray to blue pigmentation of the skin.
5. Brand name for carisoprodol.
6. Compound used to treat active juvenile and adult rheumatoid arthritis not controlled by other drugs.
9. Inflammation of the synovial membrane of the joint.
10. Type of drug used to decrease an elevated temperature.
11. Form of arthritis in which uric acid accumulates in the blood and may be deposited in the joints.

V. Dosage Problems

Solve the following dosage calculations.

1. Betty Jones has been prescribed methotrexate (Rheumatrex) for severe rheumatoid arthritis. The doctor has ordered 7.5 mg, PO, weekly. Rheumatrex is available in 2.5-mg tablets. How many tablets will the nurse instruct Betty to take at each dose? _____

2. A patient with repeated attacks of gout has been prescribed sulfinpyrazone and is to begin prophylactic treatment. The order states: Anturane, 200 mg per day, PO, in two divided doses with milk. Gradually increase dose over 1 week to reach maintenance dose of 600 mg per day, PO, in two divided doses. Anturane is available in 100-mg tablets.

   a) How many tablets will be taken at each dose when medication is first started?_____

   b) How many tablets will be taken at each maintenance dose? _____

   c) What instructions will you give about fluid intake? _____

3. The physician has ordered colchicine, 1.2 mg, PO, every 2 hours until pain is relieved or nausea, vomiting, or diarrhea occurs. Colchicine is available in 0.6-mg tablets. How many tablets will you administer every 2 hours? _____

4. The physician has prescribed predisone (liquid Pred) for a patient who has difficulty swallowing tablets. The order reads, prednisone, 7.5 mg, PO, daily. Liquid Pred is available in syrup with a dose strength of 5 mg/mL.

   a) How many milliliters will be given at each dose? _____

   b) At what time should the daily dose be given? _____

VI. Critical Thinking

1. Develop a teaching plan for a patient who is to be started on a medication regimen using a corticosteroid. Try to be as thorough as possible. Use a Nursing Drug Guide for further reference. (*Note*: Nursing Drug Guides are books with information about all available drugs.)

2. An 84-year-old patient with dementia has been prescribed risedronate daily. What are the nursing actions you should anticipate with this patient? What might be areas of concern that would require discussion with the prescribing physician?

3. Discuss why medication histories are important when the patient has been prescribed methotrexate or penicillamine.

Adrenergic Drugs

I. Matching

Match each term in Column A with the correct definition or statement in Column B.

COLUMN A

_____ 1. sympathetic nervous system

_____ 2. central nervous system

_____ 3. shock

_____ 4. norepinephrine

_____ 5. peripheral nervous system

_____ 6. epinephrine

_____ 7. parasympathetic nervous system

_____ 8. somatic nervous system

_____ 9. neurotransmitters

_____ 10. autonomic nervous system

_____ 11. hypoxia

_____ 12. hypovolemic shock

_____ 13. septic shock

_____ 14. cardiogenic shock

_____ 15. obstructive shock

_____ 16. neurogenic shock

COLUMN B

A. Consists of the brain and the spinal cord, and receives, integrates, and interprets nerve impulses.

B. All nerves outside of the brain and spinal cord.

C. Type of shock resulting from a direct injury to the spinal cord.

D. Concerned with sensation and voluntary movement.

E. Type of shock occurring when obstruction of blood flow results in inadequate tissue perfusion.

F. System controlling blood pressure, heart rate, gastrointestinal activity, and glandular secretions.

G. Shock resulting from circulatory insufficiency associated with overwhelming infection.

H. Regulates the expenditure of energy and is operative when we are stressed or in danger, or during intense emotion or severe illness.

I. Shock resulting from hemorrhage or other large fluid loss.

J. Helps conserve body energy by slowing heart rate, digestion, and other body activities.

K. Chemical substances also called *neurohormones.*

L. Shock resulting from inadequate cardiac output failing to maintain perfusion to vital organs.

M. Neurohormone secreted by the adrenal medulla.

N. Life-threatening condition resulting from an inadequate supply of arterial blood flow and oxygen to cells and tissues.

O. Neurohormone secreted mainly at nerve endings of sympathetic nerve fiber.

P. Decreased oxygen reaching the cells.

II. Labeling

Label the parts of the nervous system.

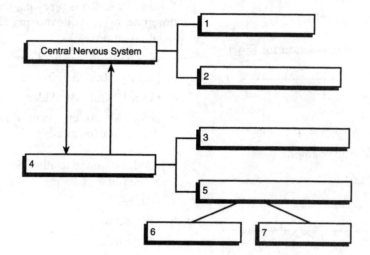

III. Fill in the Blanks

1. The primary effects of the adrenergic drugs
   occur on the _____, the _____ _____,
   and the _____ _____, such as the
   _____.

2. Adrenergic drugs mimic the activity of the
   _____ _____
   _____ .

3. List three synthetic adrenergic drugs. Include the
   generic and trade names.

   a) _____ _____

   b) _____ _____

   c) _____

4. The adrenergic drugs are important in
   _____ and _____ of
   patients in _____.

5. List the responses that are produced in the
   peripheral nervous system by the adrenergic
   drugs.

   a) _____ .

   b) _____ .

   c) _____ .

   d) _____ .

6. Adrenergic drugs are used to improve
   _____ status during shock, by
   improving _____ contractility and
   _____ heart _____, which
   results in _____ cardiac
   _____.

7. Some of the more common adverse reactions seen
   with the adrenergic drugs would include
   _____ _____ such as
   _____ and _____,
   _____, _____,
   _____, _____, and
   _____ blood pressure.

8. Although adrenergic drugs are potentially dangerous, proper _____ and _____ before, during, and after _____ will _____ the occurrence of any serious problems.

9. Initial _____ intervention for shock is aimed at supporting the _____ with _____.

10. List three of the more potent vasopressors. Include the generic and trade names.

   a) _____ _____
   b) _____ _____
   c) _____ _____

IV. Multiple Choice

Circle the letter of the most appropriate answer.

Mr. Alden is in shock, and the physician has ordered norepinephrine, a potent vasopressor, to be given IV. Questions 1–4 concern Mr. Alden's case.

1. The rate of administration of the IV fluid containing norepinephrine is:
   a. maintained at a set rate of infusion.
   b. adjusted according to the patient's blood pressure.
   c. given at a rate not to exceed 5 drops/minute.
   d. discontinued when his blood pressure is 100 systolic.

2. As Mr. Alden's nurse, you would know to monitor his blood pressure every:
   a. 5 to 15 minutes.　　c. hour.
   b. 30 minutes.　　　　d. 2 to 3 hours.

3. Mr. Alden's IV fluid containing norepinephrine extravasates into the subcutaneous tissue surrounding the needle site. Which of the following actions by the nurse would be most correct?
   a. Closely watch the IV for further extravasation.
   b. Continue the IV and notify the physician.

   c. Place warm compress on IV site and notify physician.
   d. Immediately establish a new IV line and discontinue the IV containing norepinephrine.

4. While Mr. Alden is receiving the IV containing norepinephrine, your nursing responsibilities would include:
   a. observing Mr. Alden hourly.
   b. placing Mr. Alden in semi-Fowler's position.
   c. never leaving Mr. Alden unattended.
   d. giving Mr. Alden a central nervous system depressant for anxiety.

5. When dobutamine is administered with phenytoin, the nurse is aware of the increased risk for:
   a. seizures.
   b. arrhythmias.
   c. tachycardia.
   d. hypertension.

6. A nurse assistant asks the nurse to explain the autonomic nervous system. The nurse begins by explaining that the autonomic nervous system consists of:
   a. the brain and spinal cord.
   b. the somatic and peripheral nervous systems.
   c. the sympathetic and parasympathetic nervous systems.
   d. all the nerves concerned with voluntary movement.

7. Epinephrine coadministered with propranolol may cause:
   a. heart failure.
   b. rigidity and tremor.
   c. excessive hypertension.
   d. extreme confusion.

8. When discussing the voluntary part of the somatic nervous system, the nurse explains that it is concerned with:
   a. voluntary movement of skeletal muscles.
   b. the gastrointestinal system and the digestion of food.
   c. voluntary movement of the smooth muscles.
   d. heart rate and respiratory rate.

9. Which are the more common adverse reactions the nurse would expect with the administration of adrenergic drugs?

   a. Bradycardia, hypotension, bronchial constriction

   b. Increase in appetite, nervousness, drowsiness

   c. Nausea, vomiting, hypotension

   d. Cardiac arrhythmias, increased blood pressure, headache

10. The nurse would question giving the patient epinephrine if the patient is suffering from:

    a. glaucoma.   c. diabetes.

    b. gout.   d. arthritis.

11. When midodrine is being administered, the nurse should know that the patient should be:

    a. on bed rest.   c. on a high-fat diet.

    b. out of bed.   d. limiting fluids.

12. The patient beginning treatment with midodrine should be told:

    a. to take the drug at bedtime.

    b. to lie down after taking the midodrine.

    c. to sleep with the head of the bed elevated.

    d. she will experience urinary frequency.

V. Dosage Problems

Solve the following dosage calculations.

1. A patient being treated in the emergency department for respiratory distress, caused by bronchial asthma, is to be given epinephrine. The physician has ordered 1.5 mg, subcutaneous. The drug is available in dose strength of 5 mg/1 mL. The nurse would administer how many milliliters of medication subcutaneously? _____

2. The physician has ordered ephedrine sulfate for a patient's acute asthma attack. The order reads: Ephedrine, 12.5 mg, SC. Dosage available is 50 mg/mL. How many milliliters will be given?

   _____

3. The physician has ordered phenylephrine hydrochloride, 4 mg, IM. The drug is available as 10 mg/mL. The nurse will administer how many milliliters? _____

4. The physician has ordered midodrine, starting dose 2.5 mg, PO, TID, Day 2, dose #1 and #2, 5 mg, PO, dose #3, 7.5 mg, PO. Day 3 and on, 7.5 mg, PO, TID. The dosage available is tablets, 5 mg.

   a) How many tablets will be given at each dose on day 1? _____

   b) How many tablets will be given at dose #1 and dose #2 on day 2? _____

   c) How many tablets will be given at each dose from day 3 on? _____

VI. Crossword Puzzle

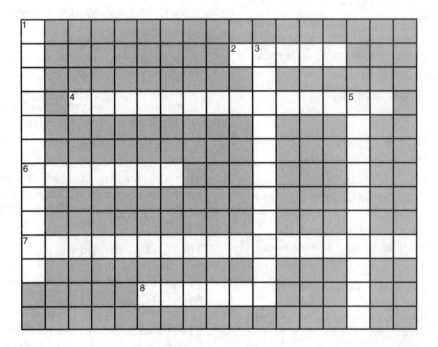

ACROSS CLUES

2. Life-threatening condition resulting from an inadequate supply of arterial blood flow and oxygen to cells and tissues.
4. Neurohormone secreted mainly at nerve endings of sympathetic nerve fibers.
6. Decreased oxygen reaching the cells.
7. Chemical substances also called *neurohormones*.
8. Type of shock resulting from circulatory insufficiency associated with overwhelming infection.

DOWN CLUES

1. Neurohormone secreted by the adrenal medulla.
3. Type of shock resulting from hemorrhage or other large fluid loss.
5. Type of shock resulting from a direct injury to the spinal cord.

VII. Critical Thinking

1. Your nursing supervisor has asked you to prepare a presentation for the staff meeting. You have decided to discuss the sympathetic and parasympathetic nervous systems. Discuss some everyday situations that could be used to demonstrate the actions of these two systems.

2. You are caring for a patient who is being prescribed midodrine. Discuss how you would explain the actions of this drug and the patient teaching that will be needed.

CHAPTER 23

Adrenergic Blocking Drugs

I. Matching

Match each term in Column A with the correct definition or statement in Column B.

COLUMN A

_____ 1. glaucoma

_____ 2. pheochromocytoma

_____ 3. α-adrenergic blocking drugs

_____ 4. β-adrenergic blocking drugs

_____ 5. cardiac arrhythmias

_____ 6. orthostatic hypotension

_____ 7. α/β-adrenergic blocking drugs

_____ 8. first-dose effect

_____ 9. postural hypotension

_____ 10. antiadrenergic drugs

_____ 11. phentolamine

_____ 12. β-adrenergic receptors

COLUMN B

A. Are found mainly in the heart.

B. Abnormal rhythm of the heart.

C. Drug used to treat or prevent tissue damage caused by extravasation of norepinephrine or dopamine.

D. A tumor of the adrenal gland that produces excessive amounts of epinephrine and norepinephrine.

E. A narrowing or blockage of the drainage channels between the anterior and posterior chambers of the eye creating increased intraocular pressure in the eye.

F. Inhibit the release of norepinephrine from certain adrenergic nerve endings in the peripheral nervous system.

G. Produce greatest effect on receptors of adrenergic nerves that control the vascular system.

H. A feeling of light-headedness and dizziness when suddenly changing from a lying to a sitting or standing position, or from a sitting to a standing position.

I. Act on both α and β nerve fibers.

J. Produce an effect primarily on the β-receptors of the heart.

K. Occurs when position is shifted or changed after standing in one place for a long time.

L. Occurs with the first few doses of the drug. Patient may experience marked hypotension, syncope, and sudden loss of consciousness.

II. Labeling

Label the following figure to correctly illustrate the actions of the beta-adrenergic blocking drugs.

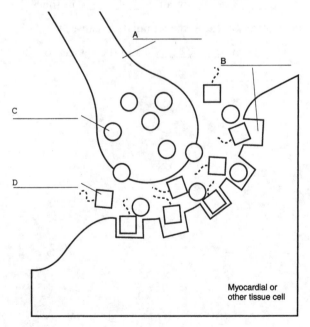

Myocardial or other tissue cell

III. Fill in the Blanks

1. List the four types of adrenergic drugs.

   a) _____

   b) _____

   c) _____

   d) _____

2. Alpha-adrenergic blocking drugs produce their greatest effect on the _____ of the adrenergic nerves that control the _____ _____.

3. Beta-adrenergic blocking drugs produce their greatest effect on the _____ of the _____.

4. Administration of an α-adrenergic blocking drug may result in the adverse reactions of _____, _____ _____, _____ _____, _____, and _____.

5. Stimulation of _____ of the _____ results in an _____ in the heart rate. Blocking the stimulation causes the heart rate to _____ and the vessels to _____.

6. Beta-adrenergic blocking ophthalmic drugs _____ the production of _____ _____ in the _____ _____ of the eye, to relieve the _____ _____ of _____.

7. Beta-adrenergic blocking drugs are used mainly in the treatment of _____ and certain _____ _____.

8. More serious adverse reactions that may be seen with the β-adrenergic blocking drugs can include symptoms of _____ _____ _____, which are _____, _____ _____, and _____ _____.

9. Some of the adverse reactions observed with the administration of β-adrenergic blocking drugs include _____ _____, _____, _____, _____, _____, _____, _____, _____, and _____.

10. The nurse should withhold the _____ _____ drug propranolol (Inderal) if the patient has a heart rate of less than _____ beats per minute and notify the _____.

IV. Crossword Puzzle

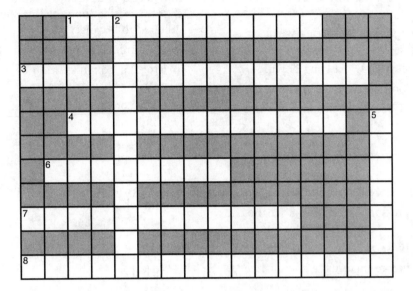

ACROSS CLUES

1. Beta-adrenergic drug that should be withheld if patient's heart rate is less than 60 bpm.
3. Effect occurring with the first dose of a drug (three words).
4. Adverse reaction observed with the administration of β-adrenergic blocking drugs.
6. Hypotension characterized by light-headedness and dizziness when suddenly standing from a lying or sitting position.
7. Drug used to treat or prevent tissue damage caused by extravasation of norepinephrine or dopamine.
8. A tumor of the adrenal gland that produces excessive amounts of epinephrine and norepinephrine.

DOWN CLUES

2. Hypotension produced by shifting or changing position after standing in one place for long periods.
5. Symptom of congestive heart failure.

V. Multiple Choice

Circle the letter of the most appropriate answer.

Mr. Hartsel has hypertension and his physician has decided to prescribe a β-adrenergic blocking agent. Questions 1–4 pertain to Mr. Hartsel's case.

1. Before giving Mr. Hartsel the first dose of his medication, the most important physical assessment performed by the nurse would be:
   a. weighing him.
   b. obtaining blood for laboratory tests.
   c. taking a past medical history.
   d. taking his blood pressure in both arms.

2. Mr. Hartsel complains of dizziness; his pulse is now 58 beats per minute and his blood pressure is significantly decreased. His next dose of the drug is due now. The most appropriate action for the nurse to take is to:
   a. give the next dose of medication and call the physician.
   b. withhold the next dose of medication and notify the physician.
   c. advise Mr. Hartsel to ambulate to raise his blood pressure.
   d. ask Mr. Hartsel to let you know if the dizziness gets worse.

3. After several days of therapy, Mr. Hartsel experiences postural hypotension, which the nurse explains is:

   a. a drop in blood pressure occurring when changing position.

   b. hypotension occurring when lying down.

   c. a decrease in blood pressure when sitting.

   d. hypotension that occurs when standing for a long time.

4. When giving Mr. Hartsel his medication, the nurse should:

   a. take his blood pressure before the drug is given.

   b. take his blood pressure 10 minutes after the drug is given.

   c. take his apical pulse after administration.

   d. have him void before the drug is administered.

5. Ms. Slominski developed life-threatening cardiac arrhythmias and is receiving IV propranolol (Inderal). The nurse is aware that while receiving this drug, Ms. Slominski will require:

   a. monitoring of her heart rate and blood pressure every 1 to 2 hours.

   b. a private room, an electrocardiogram every hour, and mechanical ventilation.

   c. constant medical supervision, and frequent monitoring of blood pressure and respiratory rate.

   d. mechanical ventilation.

6. Ms. Slominski's condition has been stabilized and she is being transferred to the intensive care unit. As her nurse, you would know that Ms. Slominski will be receiving:

   a. hourly supervision.

   b. cardiac monitoring.

   c. mechanical ventilation.

   d. an adrenergic drug.

7. Patient teaching is very important for the patient receiving the β-adrenergic blocking drugs. The nurse should make sure the patient knows to report to the physician immediately:

   a. any dental work he or she is to have done.

   b. any drowsiness, dizziness, or light-headedness.

   c. any over-the-counter vitamins he or she is taking.

   d. weight gain, difficulty breathing, or edema of the extremities.

8. The nurse instructs the patient receiving the β-adrenergic drug timolol (Timoptic) for glaucoma that the instillation schedule should be strictly adhered to because:

   a. the intraocular pressure can decrease.

   b. irregular administration of medication decreases ocular pressure.

   c. ocular pressure can increase and lead to blindness.

   d. regular instillation of drops helps increase ocular pressure.

9. The physician has asked the nurse to teach a patient who is being discharged how to take his blood pressure. The nurse's instructions should include:

   a. take the blood pressure at a different time each day.

   b. take the blood pressure in a different arm each day.

   c. make sure you are in a different position each time you check your blood pressure.

   d. make sure you use the same arm each time you check your blood pressure.

10. A patient just admitted to your unit is diagnosed with hypertension due to pheochromocytoma. During your initial assessment, the patient tells you he also has coronary artery disease. The physician has ordered the drug phentolamine (Regitime). As this patient's nurse, you would:

    a. give the drug ordered by the physician.

    b. hold the medication and talk to the physician.

    c. ask your supervisor to give the drug.

    d. call the pharmacist and ask for a different drug.

VI. Dosage Problems

Solve the following dosage calculations.

1. The physician has prescribed clonidine (Catapres), 0.3 mg, PO, BID. You have available Catapres tablets in dosage strength of 0.2 mg/tablet.

   a) How many tablets will the nurse give at each dose? _____

   b) What will be the total daily dosage for this patient? _____

2. The physician's order reads: Metoprolol (Lopressor), 100 mg, PO, now. The drug is available in dosage strength of 50-mg tablets.

   a) How many tablets will the nurse give?

   _____

   b) How often will the drug be administered?

   _____

3. A patient is on a maintenance dose of propranolol SR, 320 mg, PO, daily. The drug is available in sustained-release form as 160-mg capsules. How many capsules should she take daily? _____

4. A patient has been prescribed carvedilol for hypertension. The initial week of treatment, the physician orders 6.25 mg, PO, BID. The second week, the dose is to be increased to 12.5 mg, PO, BID. The drug is available in a dose strength of 6.25-mg tablets.

   a) How many tablets will be administered for each dose, starting week 2? _____

   a) What is the total daily milligram dosage during week 1? _____

   b) What is the total daily milligram dosage, starting week 2? _____

   c) Using a Nursing Drug Guide, find out what is the maximum dose for hypertension.

   _____

VII. Critical Thinking

1. Ms. Marshal has just been diagnosed with glaucoma. The primary health care provider has prescribed timolol (Timoptic) drops. Discuss in detail the patient teaching that is needed for this patient.

2. John Thomas, an 88-year-old patient diagnosed with cardiac arrhythmias, is being released from the hospital. His physician has prescribed propranolol (Inderal). Mr. Thomas has difficulty hearing and poor vision. He will be living with his son when he leaves the hospital. Discuss the problems his nurse will have to address in his patient teaching in regard to his medication and its adverse reactions.

CHAPTER 24

Cholinergic Drugs

I. Matching

Match each term in Column A with the correct definition or statement in Column B.

COLUMN A

_____ 1. direct-acting cholinergics

_____ 2. parasympathomimetic drug

_____ 3. myasthenia gravis

_____ 4. acetylcholinesterase (AChE)

_____ 5. indirect-acting cholinergics

_____ 6. acetylcholine (ACh)

_____ 7. cholinergic crisis

_____ 8. miosis

_____ 9. micturition

_____ 10. glaucoma

COLUMN B

A. Inhibit the release of AChE, prolonging the activity of ACh.

B. Constriction of the iris.

C. Cholinergic drugs that act like ACh.

D. Disorder of increased pressure within the eye caused by an obstruction of the outflow of aqueous humor through the canal of Schlemm.

E. A disease that involves rapid fatigue of skeletal muscles due to the lack of ACh released at the nerve endings of parasympathetic nerve fibers.

F. Voiding of urine.

G. Drug that mimics the activity of the parasympathetic nervous system.

H. Neurotransmitter responsible for the transmission of nerve impulses to effector cells of the parasympathetic nervous system.

I. Neurotransmitter that inactivates and destroys ACh.

J. Cholinergic drug toxicity.

II. Fill in the Blanks

1. List the symptoms that characterize cholinergic crisis.

a) _____

b) _____

c) _____

d) _____

e) _____

f) _____

2. List the signs of cholinergic drug underdosage.

a) _____

b) _____

c) _____

3. List three responsibilities of the parasympathetic nervous system that help conserve body energy.

a) _____

b) _____

c) _____

4. List the major uses of the cholinergic drugs.

Treatment of:

a) _____

b) _____

c) _____

5. List two drugs used to treat glaucoma. Include the generic and trade name for the second one.

a) _____

b) _____

List the two adverse reactions seen with the administration of these drugs.

c) _____

d) _____

6. List two drugs used to treat myasthenia gravis. Include the generic and trade names.

a) _____ _____

b) _____ _____

7. List three drugs used to treat urinary retention. Include the generic and trade names.

a) _____ _____

b) _____ _____

c) _____ _____

III. Multiple Choice

Circle the letter of the most appropriate answer.

Mr. Stanford, age 43, has been diagnosed as having glaucoma. Questions 1–6 pertain to Mr. Stanford's case.

1. For initial therapy, the physician orders pilocarpine eye drops. One adverse reaction that the nurse tells Mr. Stanford to expect with the use of this drug is:
   a. temporary loss of visual acuity.
   b. occasional urinary retention.
   c. salivation and sweating.
   d. extreme muscle weakness.

2. Before instilling the eye drops, the nurse should check the label of the bottle to see if the drug is:
   a. for topical use.
   b. sterile.
   c. for ophthalmic use.
   d. for glaucoma.

3. Unless the physician orders otherwise, the nurse instills eye drops into the:
   a. outer corner (canthus) of the eye.
   b. lower conjunctival sac of the eye.
   c. upper conjunctival sac of the eye.
   d. inner corner (canthus) of the eye.

4. When the nurse administers eye drops, the hand holding the dropper is supported against the patient's:
   a. opposite cheek.   c. lower jaw.
   b. nose.   d. forehead.

5. Mr. Stanford is learning to self-administer his eye drops. It is the nurse's responsibility to:
   a. allow the patient to document administration of the drug.
   b. observe return demonstration of the patient's technique for administration of the drug.
   c. continue to administer the drops until the patient goes home.
   d. allow Mr. Stanford to administer eye drops to another patient for practice.

6. Mr. Stanford is not able to self-administer his eye drops. The physician has prescribed a pilocarpine ocular system. The nurse instructs the patient that the system disk is normally changed every:
   a. 4 hours.   c. 7 days.
   b. day.   d. month.

Ms. Martin has been diagnosed as having myasthenia gravis and is started on drug therapy with ambenonium (Mytelase). Questions 7–11 pertain to Ms. Martin's case.

7. During early drug therapy, it will be important for the nurse to assess Ms. Martin for:
   a. the effects of the drug on her cardiovascular system.
   b. muscle contractions.
   c. dilation of the pupils of her eyes.
   d. her response to the drug.

8. It is important for the nurse to reassess Ms. Martin before each dose of medication is administered because:
   a. a decrease in symptoms may require dosage adjustment.
   b. an increase in symptoms of the disease will necessitate decreasing the dosage of the drug.
   c. symptoms of drooling or drooping eyelids indicate dosage needs to be decreased.
   d. rapid muscular fatigue and difficulty breathing indicate cholinergic overdosage.

9. The dose of a cholinergic drug for myasthenia gravis may be difficult to regulate, and signs of overdose may occur. When monitoring Ms. Martin for signs of overdose, the nurse must be alert for:

   a. muscle rigidity, clenching of the jaw.

   b. muscle weakness, abdominal tenderness.

   c. drop in blood pressure, diarrhea.

   d. headache, double vision.

10. If Ms. Martin experiences effects of under-dosage of her medication, the nurse will most likely observe:

    a. abdominal rigidity.

    b. drooping of the eyelids.

    c. clenching of the jaw.

    d. anorexia and vomiting.

11. If Ms. Martin has a drug overdose and an anti-dote is needed, which one of the following drugs would the nurse anticipate having available?

    a. Morphine   c. Atropine

    b. Pilocarpine   d. Phenobarbital

IV. Dosage Problems

Solve the following dosage calculations.

1. Harold Moss, a 38-year-old, is being treated with ambenonium (Mytelase). His optimum dose has been determined to be 15 mg, QID. The Mytelase is available in 10-mg tablets.

   a) How many tablets will Mr. Moss take at each dose? _____

   b) What is the total daily milligram dose for Mr. Moss? _____

2. A hospitalized patient has developed urinary retention. The physician has ordered bethanecol, 2.5 mg, SC, at 30-minute intervals for four doses. The bethanecol is available in vials of 5 mg/mL.

   a) How many milliliters are to be given at each dose? _____

   b) How many vials of bethanecol will be needed for the four doses? _____

3. The physician has ordered neostigmine methylsulfate, 0.25 mg, IM. The drug is available as Prostigmin, 0.5 mg/1 mL of 1:2000 solution. How many milliliters of medication will be used for the 0.25-mg dose? _____

V. Crossword Puzzle

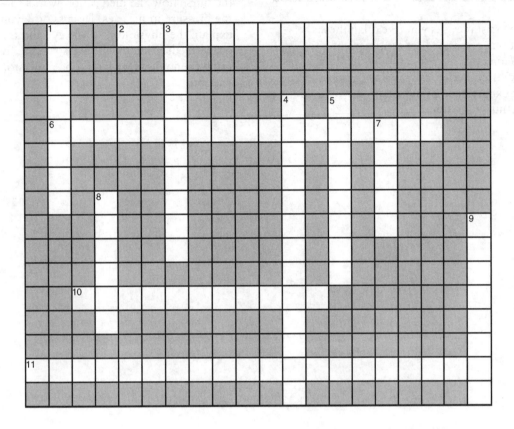

ACROSS CLUES

2. A disease that involves rapid fatigue of the skeletal muscles due to the lack of ACh (two words).
6. Cholinergic drug toxicity (two words).
10. Voiding.
11. Neurotransmitter that inactivates and destroys ACh.

DOWN CLUES

1. A disorder of increased pressure within the eye.
3. Drug used to treat myasthenia gravis.
4. Neurohormone abbreviated as ACh.
5. Sign of facial muscle weakness.
7. The pilocarpine ocular system is changed every _____ days.
8. Treatment of glaucoma with a cholinergic agent produces _____.
9. To check for urinary retention, the nurse _____ the bladder.

VI. Critical Thinking

1. A nurse assistant asks you to explain how the medications prescribed for treatment of myasthenia gravis work and why the dosage has to be adjusted periodically. Using pyridostigmine as your example, what information would you give the nurse assistant?

2. A patient newly diagnosed with glaucoma asks the nurse how the medication works to reduce the pressure in his eyes. Discuss how you would explain the physiology of the eye and the effects of the medication on the eye structure. Be sure to use terminology that would be understood by the patient.

CHAPTER 25

Cholinergic Blocking Drugs

I. Matching

Match each term in Column A with the correct definition or statement in Column B.

COLUMN A

_____ 1. mydriasis

_____ 2. photophobia

_____ 3. cholinergic blocking drugs

_____ 4. cycloplegia

_____ 5. drug idiosyncrasy

COLUMN B

A. Block the action of acetylcholine in the parasympathetic nervous system.

B. An unexpected or unusual drug effect.

C. Paralysis of accommodation or inability to focus the eye.

D. Aversion to bright light.

E. Dilation of the pupil.

II. Multiple Choice

Circle the letter of the most appropriate answer.

Mr. Baker has a peptic ulcer. He is currently being treated with the cholinergic blocking drug clidinium (Quorzan). Questions 1 and 2 pertain to Mr. Baker's case.

1. Mr. Baker complains of constipation. Knowing the adverse reactions associated with cholinergic blocking drugs, the nurse should:

   a. consider this complaint to be unusual and notify the physician.

   b. encourage Mr. Baker to increase fluid intake to 2000 mL daily.

   c. ignore Mr. Baker's complaint because constipation is temporary.

   d. place Mr. Baker on a high-carbohydrate diet.

2. Mr. Baker's ulcer has begun to bleed and he is scheduled for surgery. Part of his preoperative medication regimen is the cholinergic blocking agent glycopyrrolate (Robinul). After giving the drug, what information or instructions should the nurse give to the patient?

   a. "A severe dry mouth will occur; this is normal."

   b. "You can remain out of bed until you get sleepy."

   c. "In about 30 minutes, go to the bathroom and urinate."

   d. "You will not feel any effects as a result of this drug."

3. When reviewing a patient's chart for preoperative orders, the nurse would expect a cholinergic blocking drug such as atropine to be given before surgery to:

   a. inhibit the action of the anesthesia.

   b. reduce secretions of the upper respiratory tract.

   c. inhibit the action of the preoperative narcotic.

   d. increase gastric motility.

4. A patient administered atropine before surgery will experience the adverse reaction of an extremely dry mouth. The nurse would also expect the patient to experience:

   a. diarrhea.

   b. urinary frequency.

   c. constriction of the pupils.

   d. drowsiness.

5. Because of the effect of the cholinergic blocking drugs on intestinal motility, the nurse must monitor patients taking these drugs for a long time for the development of:

 a. gastric irritation due to increased secretions.

 b. diarrhea.

 c. constipation.

 d. heartburn.

6. The nurse must be aware that administering cholinergic blocking drugs to elderly patients during the hot summer months may result in:

 a. an increase in sweating.

 b. heat prostration.

 c. decreased heart rate.

 d. intolerance to air conditioning.

7. The nurse would anticipate atropine being administered for the condition of:

 a. third-degree heart block.

 b. severe tachycardia.

 c. angina.

 d. hypertensive crisis.

8. When the patient is given atropine for the cardiac problem in question 7, the nurse would expect the patient to be:

 a. transferred to a private room.

 b. placed in a supine position.

 c. started on intravenous fluids.

 d. placed on a cardiac monitor.

9. If a patient is experiencing photophobia as a result of administration of a cholinergic blocking drug, the nurse would most likely place the patient:

 a. in a quiet room, away from the nurse's station.

 b. close to the nurse's station.

 c. in a semidarkened room.

 d. in a brightly lighted area.

10. Anticholinergic drugs are contraindicated in patients with:

 a. glaucoma.   c. bradycardia.

 b. gout.   d. diabetes.

III. Fill in the Blanks

1. The nurse would offer what suggestions to the patient experiencing dry mouth caused by the anticholinergic drugs?

 a) _____

 b) _____

 c) _____

 d) _____

 e) _____

 f) _____

 g) _____

 h) _____

2. The nurse should contact the primary health care provider if the elderly patient taking a cholinergic blocking drug experiences _____, _____, _____ _____, _____, or _____ _____.

3. The anesthesiologist must be _____ if the _____ medications are given _____.

4. The parasympathomimetic drugs may affect the following organs and structures of the body:

 a) _____

 b) _____

 c) _____

 d) _____

 e) _____

5. The cholinergic blocking drug _____ _____ is used only to treat peptic ulcer.

6. Cholinergic blocking drugs may cause the adverse reaction of heat exhaustion, which is characterized by:

a) _____

b) _____

c) _____

d) _____

e) _____

7. The effects of atropine may be increased when administered with (include the generic and trade names for the first three):

a) _____ _____

b) _____ _____

c) _____ _____

d) _____

e) _____

IV. Crossword Puzzle

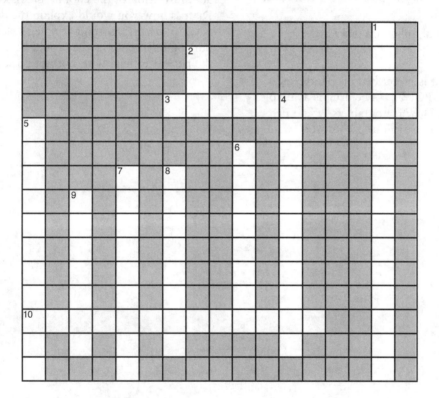

ACROSS CLUES

3. Paralysis of accommodation.
10. An unexpected or unusual drug effect.

DOWN CLUES

1. Another word for cholinergic blocking drugs.
2. Anticholinergic drugs cause the mucous membranes of the mouth to become _____.
4. Aversion to bright light.
5. Anticholinergic drug that may cause an idiosyncratic reaction of excitement, delirium, and restlessness.

6. Anticholinergic drugs are contraindicated in patients with this condition.
7. Dilation of the pupil.
8. Anticholinergic commonly used as a preoperative medication.
9. Cholinergic blocking drugs' action on acetylcholine.

V. Dosage Problems

Solve the following dosage calculations.

1. The physician's order reads: Atropine, 0.6 mg, SC, 30 minutes before surgery. Atropine is available in dose strength of 1 mg/mL. How many milliliters will be administered? _____

2. The physician's order reads: Flavoxate, 200 mg, PO, QID. The drug Urispas is available in 100-mg tablets.

   a) How many tablets will be given for each dose?
   _____

   b) What is the total milligram daily dose?
   _____

3. A geriatric patient is prescribed propantheline bromide, 7.5 mg, PO, TID. The drug is available in 15-mg tablets. How many tablets would be administered to the patient at each dose?

   _____

VI. Critical Thinking

1. An 84-year-old patient is to have a scopolamine patch applied to prevent motion sickness. What does the nurse need to discuss with this patient's caregiver with respect to the adverse reactions that may occur with this drug?

2. You are asked to lead a team conference on the administration of the cholinergic blocking drugs. Discuss how you would explain the difference between mydriasis and cycloplegia. Identify nursing interventions that could be used to help the patient to deal with both of these problems.

CHAPTER 26

Sedatives and Hypnotics

I. Matching

Match each term in Column A with the correct definition or statement in Column B.

COLUMN A

_____ 1. valerian

_____ 2. hypnotic

_____ 3. NREM

_____ 4. sedative

_____ 5. melatonin

_____ 6. soporifics

_____ 7. REM

_____ 8. ataxia

_____ 9. detoxified

_____ 10. barbiturates

COLUMN B

A Dietary supplement used for treating insomnia.

B. A drug that induces sleep.

C. Drugs that have little or no analgesic action.

D. Drug that produces a relaxing, calming effect.

E. Stage of sleep when dreams occur.

F. Make nontoxic or not harmful.

G. Herb used for its sedative effects.

H. Stage of sleep occurring early in the sleep cycle.

I. Unsteady gait.

J. Another term used to identify the hypnotics.

II. Fill in the Blanks

1. Sedatives make the patient _____, but usually do not produce _____.

2. Hypnotics allow the patient to _____ _____ and _____ _____.

3. Sedatives are given during _____ hours and hypnotics are given at _____.

4. List the groups of barbiturates and how long their action lasts.

   a) _____ _____

   b) _____ _____

   c) _____ _____

   d) _____ _____

5. Sedatives and hypnotics have an _____ effect when administered with _____, _____, _____ _____, _____, or _____.

6. Assessment of the patient receiving a _____ or _____ drug depends on the _____ for administration and whether the drug is given _____ or as _____.

7. Barbiturates, when given in the presence of pain, may cause _____, _____, and _____.

8. Patients who have been taking a _____ or _____ for several weeks should be gradually _____ from the drug to prevent _____ symptoms.

III. Multiple Choice

Circle the letter of the most appropriate answer.

Ms. Brown, age 54, is admitted for diagnostic tests. Her blood pressure, pulse, and respiratory rate are 144/78, 86, and 14, respectively. She had a breast biopsy under general anesthesia late this afternoon and will be discharged from the hospital tomorrow morning and readmitted in 1 week for a mastectomy. Questions 1–3 pertain to Ms. Brown's case.

1. Ms. Brown tells you that she is feeling uncomfortable and she is afraid she won't be able to sleep. She asks if she can have a "sleeping pill." In assessing Ms. Brown, the nurse determines:

    a. the sleeping pill should be left at the bedside in case Ms. Brown can't sleep.

    b. Ms. Brown's discomfort is really pain and a hypnotic has no analgesic effect.

    c. a hypnotic will be the best drug for relief of Ms. Brown's pain.

    d. Ms. Brown received a narcotic analgesic 30 minutes earlier and must wait 4 hours for a hypnotic.

2. Ms. Brown's analgesic was administered at 7:00 P.M. The nurse can plan on administering a hypnotic, if it is needed, at:

    a. 9:00 P.M.   c. 8:00 P.M.

    b. 7:30 P.M.   d. 11:00 P.M.

3. After administration of a hypnotic to Ms. Brown, the nurse assesses the results of the drug in:

    a. 15 minutes.   c. 1 to 2 hours.

    b. 30 minutes.   d. 4 hours.

4. Which of the following would the nurse consider as a contraindication to administering a hypnotic?

    a. A pulse rate of 74   c. Mild anxiety

    b. Nervousness   d. Respiratory rate of 9

5. An article in a nursing journal states that barbiturates reduce the amount of time spent in the REM stage of sleep. When checking a reference, the nurse finds that the REM stage is the:

    a. time just before waking.

    b. the first stage of sleep.

    c. the dreaming stage of sleep.

    d. stage before falling asleep.

6. Further reading about the REM stage of sleep reveals that:

    a. being deprived of the REM stage may result in development of a psychosis.

    b. a long REM stage can result in an increase in respiration.

    c. it is best if the REM stage is eliminated from sleep.

    d. tachycardia during the REM stage is harmful.

7. While checking a pharmacology reference in preparation for a team conference, the nurse finds that the barbiturates and nonbarbiturates are detoxified by the:

    a. spleen.   c. liver.

    b. kidneys.   d. stomach.

8. A nurse working in the emergency department is asked by the physician to administer a sedative-type drug to a patient. The nurse knows that this type of drug is given to:

    a. help the patient sleep.

    b. treat anxiety and apprehension.

    c. treat psychosis.

    d. prevent a psychosis.

9. After the administration of a hypnotic, the nurse instructs the patient to:

    a. wait 30 minutes, then go to the bathroom.

    b. drink extra fluids before becoming sleepy.

    c. sit in a chair until the drug takes effect.

    d. remain in bed and call for assistance if needed.

10. The physician has ordered propiomazine (Largon), 20 mg, IM, as a preoperative medication for Mr. Jackson. The nurse knows the injection must be administered into the:

    a. deltoid muscle.

    b. trapezius muscle.

    c. gluteus maximus muscle.

    d. forearm.

11. A new nurse asks why the physicians sometimes order hypnotics PRN for sleep when patients are first admitted to the hospital. You would be correct in answering:

   a. "Patients will need the hypnotic to sleep if they are in pain."

   b. "Helping the patient sleep is an important part of management of the illness."

   c. "Patients need a hypnotic to relieve their anxiety and calm them down."

   d. "Hypnotics are ordered only for the geriatric patients."

IV. Crossword Puzzle

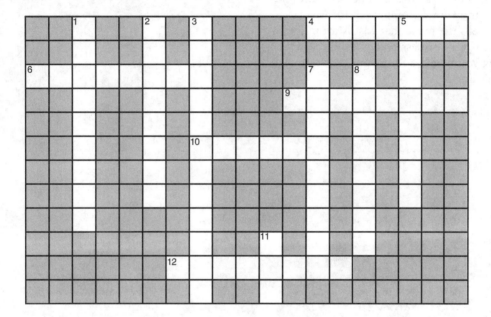

ACROSS CLUES

4. Example of a benzodiazepine used as a sedative.
6. Drug that induces sleep.
9. Drug that produces a relaxing, calming effect.
10. Unsteady gait.
12. Individuals taking a sedative or hypnotic are discouraged from eating foods containing this ingredient.

DOWN CLUES

1. Another name for hypnotic.
2. Make nontoxic or harmless.
3. Example of a short-acting barbiturate.
5. Effect that occurs when alcohol and a sedative are taken together.
7. Dietary supplement used for treating insomnia.
8. Herb used for its sedative effects.
11. Dreaming occurs in this stage of sleep.

V. Dosage Problems

1. The physician's order reads: Phenobarbital, grain 1, PO, HS. The drug is available as phenobarbital, 60-mg tablets. How many tablets will the nurse administer? _____

2. Mary Baker is having difficulty sleeping. The physician has ordered temazepam (Restoril), 30 mg, PO, HS, PRN. The Restoril is available in 15-mg capsules. How many capsules should be given to Ms. Baker? _____

3. The physician's order reads: Phenobarbital, gr iss, IM, stat. Phenobarbital sodium is available in 1-milliliter vials, which contain 120 mg of the drug. How many milliliters of the solution would you administer to give the ordered dose? _____

4. The physician's order reads: Secobarbital (Seconal) sodium, 90 mg, IM, HS, PRN. Seconal sodium is available in a dose strength of 50 mg/mL. How many milliliters will be administered for the ordered dose? _____

VI. Critical Thinking

1. Ms. Martin, an 87-year-old patient, is in the orthopedic unit after surgery to repair a fractured hip. Her daughter is staying with her at night and she asks the nurse for a sleeping pill for Ms. Martin. She tells the nurse that Ms. Martin goes to sleep, but is very restless and awakens easily. Discuss how you would address this situation as Ms. Martin's nurse.

2. Mr. Adams has been admitted to the hospital with complaints of chest pain. He is scheduled for tests tomorrow to rule out myocardial infarction. The physician has written an order for Restoril, 15 mg, HS, PRN. Mr. Adams is refusing the Restoril because he doesn't want to "get hooked" on sleeping pills. Discuss what you would tell Mr. Adams about his need for this medication and about developing dependence for these types of drugs.

CHAPTER 27

Central Nervous System Stimulants

I. Matching

Match each term in Column A with the correct definition or statement in Column B.

COLUMN A

_____ 1. psychological dependence

_____ 2. narcolepsy

_____ 3. doxapram

_____ 4. attention deficit disorder

_____ 5. analeptics

_____ 6. modafinil

_____ 7. exogenous obesity

_____ 8. anorexiants

_____ 9. amphetamines

COLUMN B

A. Drugs that stimulate the respiratory center of the central nervous system (CNS).

B. Occurs with long-term use of the amphetamines.

C. Drugs used to suppress the appetite.

D. Disorder causing an uncontrollable desire to sleep during normal waking hours.

E. An analeptic used to treat narcolepsy.

F. Sympathomimetic drugs that stimulate the CNS.

G. Used to treat drug-induced respiratory depression.

H. Obesity due to a persistent calorie intake that is greater than needed by the body.

I. Children with this disorder exhibit short attention span, hyperactivity, impulsiveness, and emotional lability.

II. Fill in the Blanks

1. List the three types of nervous system stimulants.

    a) _____

    b) _____

    c) _____

2. List the analeptics (include the generic and trade name for the first one).

    a) _____ _____

    b) _____

    c) _____

3. Caffeine has mild _____ activity and also results in _____ stimulation, dilation of _____ and _____ blood vessels, constriction of _____ blood vessels, and _____ muscle stimulation.

4. Amphetamines and anorexiants should not be given _____ or _____ 14 days after administration of _____ _____ _____, because the patient may develop _____ _____ and _____ _____.

5. When CNS stimulants are prescribed for respiratory depression, nursing assessment should include the _____ of _____ and any pattern to the _____ _____, such as _____ respirations or alternating _____ and _____ respirations.

6. When amphetamines are prescribed for any reason, the nurse _____ the patient and takes the _____ _____, _____ and _____ _____ before starting _____ _____.

7. After administration of an analeptic, the nurse carefully monitors _____ _____ and _____ until _____ return to normal.

III. Crossword Puzzle

ACROSS CLUES

1. Abbreviation for attention deficit disorder.
6. Disorder manifested by an uncontrollable desire to sleep during normal waking hours.
7. Type of obesity due to a caloric intake greater than needed by the body.

DOWN CLUES

1. CNS stimulants with a high abuse potential.
2. Drugs used to suppress the appetite.
3. Example of an anorexiant.
4. Drugs that stimulate the respiratory center of the CNS.
5. Example of an analeptic.
6. Brand name for caffeine and sodium benzoate.

IV. Multiple Choice

Circle the letter of the most appropriate answer.

1. A nurse assessing a patient receiving doxapram postanesthesia will know that administration of an analeptic can cause adverse reactions that necessitate keeping a _____ at the bedside.
   a. bedside commode   c. portable x-ray
   b. suction machine   d. chest tube tray

2. When discussing the use of amphetamines as anorexiants at a team conference, the nurse correctly states that these drugs:
   a. are of value only for patients more than 40 pounds overweight.
   b. slow fat and carbohydrate metabolism.
   c. cannot be used for weight reduction for more than 6 months.
   d. have a high abuse and addiction potential.

3. When asked by another nurse how doxapram (Dorram) increases the depth of respirations, the nurse is correct in stating:
   a. by direct stimulation of the cerebellum.
   b. by stimulating chemoreceptors in the carotid artery and aorta.
   c. by increasing nerve activity in the upper spinal cord.
   d. by indirect stimulation of the spinal cord's basal ganglia.

4. Before administering an analeptic, the nurse notes and records the patient's:

   a. weight and blood pressure.

   b. ability to understand why the drug is being given.

   c. respiratory rate, depth, and character.

   d. pulse and temperature.

5. When discussing weight loss with a patient who wants to lose weight by taking a nonprescription diet aid, the nurse states that these drugs:

   a. have limited appetite-suppressing ability.

   b. can be addicting when used longer than 6 months.

   c. have abuse potential and should be avoided.

   d. are superior to the anorexiants.

6. Ongoing assessment of the child receiving a CNS stimulant for attention deficit disorder will include:

   a. monitoring the child's behavior once a month.

   b. asking the teacher to monitor the child once a month.

   c. checking the child's nightly dosing schedule.

   d. writing a daily summary of the child's behavior.

7. After administration of doxapram for postanesthesia respiratory depression, the patient is closely observed until the respiratory rate is:

   a. between 6 and 10 breaths per minute.

   b. 10 breaths per minute or below.

   c. normal.

   d. above 24 breaths per minute.

8. Ms. Black, age 72, is receiving a CNS stimulant. The nurse closely observes this patient for:

   a. somnolence.

   b. mental confusion.

   c. depression.

   d. increased appetite.

V. Dosage Problems

1. A patient undergoing an appendectomy is to receive doxapram postanesthesia to stimulate his respirations. The physician's order is for doxapram, 5 mg/minute, IV. How many milligrams of doxapram will be administered the first 5 minutes? _____

2. Phendimetrazine titrate is ordered, 105 mg, PO, daily, in A.M. The drug is available in 35-mg capsules. How many capsules will be administered for each dose? _____

3. An 11-year-old pediatric patient is in the third week of treatment with methylphenidate (Ritalin SR). His daily dosage has been increased to 30 mg daily. The drug is available in 10-mg and 20-mg sustained-release tablets. How many tablets will be administered at each dose?

   _____

VI. Critical Thinking

1. After a month of treatment with pemoline for attention deficit disorder, a 9-year-old is to be reassessed to determine if treatment with the medication should continue. Discuss what information and observed behaviors would indicate that the pemoline should be discontinued.

2. A patient with possible narcolepsy is being seen in the clinic. He states that he falls asleep several times a day and he has been using a nonprescription tablet form of caffeine to help him stay awake. As a nurse, discuss the information you can give him about narcolepsy and the over-the-counter caffeine he has been taking.

CHAPTER 28

Anticonvulsants

I. Matching

Match each term in Column A with the correct definition or statement in Column B.

COLUMN A

_____ 1. absence seizures

_____ 2. anticonvulsants

_____ 3. ataxia

_____ 4. convulsion

_____ 5. epilepsy

_____ 6. gingival hyperplasia

_____ 7. jacksonian seizure

_____ 8. myoclonic seizures

_____ 9. nystagmus

_____ 10. pancytopenia

_____ 11. psychomotor seizures

_____ 12. seizure

_____ 13. status epilepticus

_____ 14. tonic-clonic seizure

COLUMN B

A. Periodic attack of disturbed cerebral function.

B. Abnormal disturbance in the electrical activity in one or more areas of the brain.

C. A focal seizure that begins with an uncontrolled stiffening or jerking in one part of the body such as finger, mouth, hand, or foot and that may progress to a generalized seizure.

D. A seizure where the most common motor symptom is drawing or jerking of the mouth and face.

E. Seizure that includes alternate contraction (tonic phase) and relaxation (clonic phase) of muscles, a loss of consciousness, and abnormal behavior.

F. Seizures that involve sudden, forceful contractions involving the musculature of the trunk, neck, and extremities.

G. Seizures characterized by a brief loss of consciousness during which physical activity ceases.

H. May be defined as a permanent, recurrent seizure disorder.

I. Drugs used for the management of convulsant disorders.

J. An emergency situation characterized by continual seizure activity with no interruptions.

K. Constant, involuntary movement of the eyeball.

L. An overgrowth of the gum tissue.

M. Loss of control of voluntary movements, especially gait.

N. Decrease in the cellular components of the blood.

II. Fill in the Blanks

1. Anticonvulsant drugs possess the ability to _____ abnormal _____ _____ in the central nervous system, resulting in an _____ of _____ activity.

2. Patients being treated with anticonvulsants may find their _____ of medication may have to be _____ or _____ during the _____ period of _____.

3. List the five types of drugs used as anticonvulsants.

   a) _____

   b) _____

   c) _____

   d) _____

   e) _____

4. With phenobarbital administration, _____ rather than _____ may occur in some patients.

5. The adverse reactions seen with the benzodiazpines include _____, _____, _____, or _____.

6. _____ is the most commonly prescribed anticonvulsant.

7. List the hematologic changes that may be seen with the oxazolidinediones.

a) _____

b) _____

c) _____

d) _____

8. When the hydantoins are administered with the _____ there may be an _____ in the _____ blood level.

9. List the laboratory and diagnostic tests that may be ordered initially for a patient experiencing seizures.

a) _____

b) _____

c) _____

d) _____

e) _____

10. An anticonvulsant drug must never be _____ discontinued or have its _____ omitted.

III. Multiple Choice

Circle the letter of the most appropriate answer.

Mr. Collins, age 25, has recently been diagnosed with epilepsy and has been prescribed phenytoin (Dilantin) to control his seizures. Questions 1 and 2 pertain to Mr. Collins' case.

1. When teaching Mr. Collins about the adverse reactions that he may experience while taking phenytoin, the nurse informs him that the most common adverse reactions are related to the:
   a. gastrointestinal system.
   b. hepatic system.
   c. central nervous system.
   d. reproductive system.

2. The nurse informs Mr. Collins of the need to see his dentist frequently because the hydantoins may cause:
   a. cavities.   c. oral tumors.
   b. staining of the teeth.   d. gingival hyperplasia.

3. For optimum anticonvulsant effect, phenytoin blood plasma levels should be between:
   a. 10 and 20 mcg/mL.   c. 25 and 30 mcg/mL.
   b. 2.5 and 7.5 mcg/mL.   d. 35 and 50 mcg/mL.

4. A patient receiving succinimide must be monitored for overdosage. The nurse would report immediately the symptom of:
   a. rapid, shallow respirations.
   b. hyperactive reflexes.
   c. slight elevation of blood pressure.
   d. slow, shallow respirations.

5. A patient receiving an anticonvulsant states that the medication is causing nausea. It is important for the nurse to determine if the patient:
   a. should decrease the dosage.
   b. drinks extra water during the day.
   c. takes the drug with food.
   d. takes the drug in the morning.

6. Which of the following reported adverse reactions would alert the nurse to the possibility that a patient taking a hydantoin may be developing drug toxicity?

   a. Slurred speech, lethargy, nausea

   b. Diarrhea, blurred vision, rash

   c. Constipation, urinary retention, pruritus

   d. Hyperactivity, insomnia, double vision

7. In planning discharge teaching for a patient receiving an anticonvulsant, which of the following would be most correct for the nurse to include in the discharge instructions? The abrupt withdrawal of an anticonvulsant can result in:

   a. having to use another drug because the first drug would no longer be effective.

   b. a decreased response to any of the anticonvulsants.

   c. having to restart the drug at a higher dose.

   d. status epilepticus.

8. At a team conference, the nurse explains to the staff that until seizures are controlled in patients receiving anticonvulsants:

   a. some activities may need to be limited.

   b. the patient must be hospitalized.

   c. the patient will require two anticonvulsants given together.

   d. the only activity to be avoided is driving a car.

9. The nurse correctly administers IV phenobarbital when the drug is given:

   a. within 30 minutes of preparation.

   b. at no more than 5 mg per minute.

   c. in combination with diazepam.

   d. at a rate of 80 mg per minute.

10. The nurse correctly administers valproic acid (Depakene) when the drug is:

    a. taken on an empty stomach.

    b. sprinkled on a small amount of food and swallowed immediately.

    c. chewed thoroughly.

    d. placed under the tongue.

11. Trimethadione, valproic acid, and phenytoin are classified as pregnancy category:

    a. B.   c. D.

    b. C.   d. X.

12. When anticonvulsants are administered with other central nervous system (CNS) depressant drugs:

    a. a decreased CNS depressant effect may occur.

    b. an additive CNS depressant effect may occur.

    c. a hypertensive crisis may occur.

    d. there is increased risk for toxicity of the anticonvulsants.

IV. Crossword Puzzle

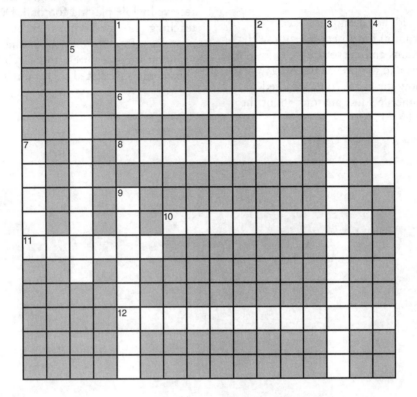

ACROSS CLUES

1. Drug most often prescribed for status epilepticus.
6. Example of a succinimide.
8. Overgrowth of gum tissue is called _____ hyperplasia.
10. Constant involuntary movement of the eyeball.
11. Relaxation phase of a generalized seizure.
12. Decrease in all the cellular components of the blood.

DOWN CLUES

2. Loss of control of voluntary movements.
3. Drugs used for the management of convulsant disorders.
4. Type of seizure where brief loss of consciousness occurs and physical activity ceases.
5. Another term for seizure.
7. Contraction phase of a generalized seizure.
9. A permanent recurrent seizure disorder.

V. Dosage Problems

Solve the following dosage calculations.

1. The physician orders Dilantin, 100 mg, via gastrostomy tube, TID. Available dose strength is 125 mg per 5 mL of solution. How many milliliters will be administered at each dose?

_____

2. The physician orders phenobarbital, gr ss, PO, TID. You have phenobarbital tablets, 30 mg on hand. How many tablets will be administered?

_____

3. The physician orders phenobarbital elixir, 45 mg, PO, TID. Available dose is 20 mg/5 mL. How many milliliters will be given at each dose?

_____

4. The physician orders clonazepam, 0.25 mg, PO, BID and HS. Drug available is clonazepam, 0.5 mg, scored tablets. How many tablets will be administered at each dose? _____

VI. Critical Thinking

1. Melinda, a 6-year-old, has been prescribed ethosuximide (Zarontin) for absence seizures. Her mother is very anxious and nervous about Melinda's diagnosis and the prescribed drug therapy. Discuss how the nurse could proceed to help Melinda's mother feel less anxious about the drug Melinda will be taking.

2. Tommy, age 15, is prescribed phenobarbital for a convulsive disorder that began after a head injury received while playing football. Develop a teaching plan for Tommy and his parents that includes information about his medication, how to monitor his seizures, and special considerations related to Tommy's age.

CHAPTER 29

Antiparkinsonism Drugs

I. Matching

Match each term in Column A with the correct definition or statement in Column B.

COLUMN A

_____ 1. blood-brain barrier

_____ 2. choreiform movements

_____ 3. dystonic movements

_____ 4. on-off phenomenon

_____ 5. Parkinson's disease

_____ 6. parkinsonism

_____ 7. achalasia

_____ 8. ataxia

COLUMN B

A. Degenerative disorder of the central nervous system.

B. Term referring to the symptoms of Parkinson's disease.

C. A meshwork of tightly packed cells in the walls of the brain's capillaries that screen out certain substances.

D. Muscular spasms most often affecting the tongue, jaw, eyes, and neck.

E. Failure of the muscles of the lower esophagus to relax, causing difficulty swallowing.

F. Condition where the patient alternates between improved clinical status and loss of therapeutic effect.

G. Involuntary muscular twitching of the limbs or facial muscles.

H. Lack of muscular coordination.

II. Fill in the Blanks

1. _____ disease is characterized by fine _____ and _____ of some muscle groups and _____ of others.

2. The symptoms of _____ are caused by a _____ of dopamine in the _____.

3. The most serious and frequent adverse reactions seen with levodopa include:

   a) _____ _____

   b) _____ _____

4. Foods high in _____ or _____ preparations _____ the effect of levodopa.

5. _____, a COMT inhibitor, is associated with _____ damage and _____ failure.

6. Important data to include in the health history of the patient with Parkinson's disease are:

   a) _____

   b) _____

   c) _____

   d) _____

III. Multiple Choice

Circle the letter of the most appropriate answer.

Ms. Johnson, age 72, has had Parkinson's disease for 10 years. Questions 1–5 pertain to Ms. Johnson's case.

1. Ms. Johnson has been taking an anticholinergic antiparkinsonism drug. Adverse reactions the nurse would observe most frequently with this type of drug include:
   a. constipation, urinary frequency, loss of peripheral vision.
   b. nausea, hypotension, muscle spasms.
   c. diarrhea, hypertension, bradycardia.
   d. dry mouth, blurred vision, dizziness.

2. The physician has decided to discontinue Ms. Johnson's present drug and start her on levodopa. Which of the following would be the most serious and frequent adverse reactions the nurse would expect to observe in patients receiving levodopa?
   a. Tachycardia, hypotension
   b. Choreiform and dystonic movements
   c. Excessive salivation and convulsions
   d. Dry mouth and urinary retention

3. If Ms. Johnson complains of nausea, the nurse would administer levodopa:
   a. with food.
   b. on an empty stomach.
   c. with orange juice.
   d. dissolved in 4 ounces of water.

4. The nurse is alert for a less frequent, but serious adverse reaction that Ms. Johnson may develop to levodopa, which is:
   a. mental changes, such as depression and psychotic episodes.
   b. cardiac arrhythmias, such as ventricular tachycardia.
   c. gastrointestinal upset, such as constipation.
   d. CNS reactions, such as a decrease in tremors.

5. The nurse must monitor Ms. Johnson closely for adverse reactions because:
   a. the patient's cognitive abilities are decreasing and her judgment is becoming impaired.
   b. the drug she is taking causes extreme sedation.

   c. of the possibility of an anaphylactic reaction occurring.
   d. some patients with parkinsonism communicate poorly and are unable to tell the nurse that problems are occurring.

6. Which of the following signs and symptoms of Parkinson's disease would the nurse note during the assessment?
   a. Excessive or abnormal hair loss
   b. Hypertension
   c. Masklike facial expression
   d. Dysuria

7. Carbidopa (Lodosyn) is prescribed for a patient with parkinsonism. In teaching the patient about the drug, the nurse explains that carbidopa:
   a. is the most potent antiparkinsonism drug.
   b. must be given with levodopa (Larodopa).
   c. is more toxic than levodopa (Larodopa).
   d. is given to patients with advanced parkinsonism.

8. Ms. Jones is prescribed selegiline (Eldepryl) for parkinsonism. The nurse explains to Ms. Jones that selegiline is usually used for those:
   a. with a mild form of parkinsonism.
   b. taking an anticholinergic antiparkinsonism drug.
   c. requiring special diets.
   d. not responding to therapy with carbidopa and levodopa.

9. Tolcapone (Tasmar) is a newer antiparkinsonism drug used only when patients do not respond to other therapies. This drug is associated with serious and possibly fatal:
   a. liver failure.
   b. psychotic episodes.
   c. tardive dyskinesia.
   d. suicidal tendencies.

10. The COMT inhibitors are classified as pregnancy category:
    a. X.   c. C.
    b. B.   d. D.

IV. Dosage Problems

Solve the following dosage calculations.

1. Ms. Jones' physician has ordered carbidopa-levodopa 25-100, 2 tablets, PO, TID. The label on the medication reads, Sinemet, 25-100, 100 tablets. Each tablet contains 25 mg carbidopa and 100 mg levodopa.

   a) How many tablets are given at each dose? _____

   b) How many milligrams of each drug are being administered at each dose? _____

   c) What is the total daily dosage of each drug? _____

2. The physician's order reads: Diphenhydramine HCL, 25 mg, PO, QID. The drug available is diphenhydramine hydrochloride elixir in a dosage strength of 12.5 mg/5 mL. How many milliliters would be administered to give the prescribed dose of diphenhydramine? _____

3. Amantadine, 100 mg, PO, BID is ordered. The drug available is Symmetrel syrup, 50 mg/5 mL. How many milliliters are administered for the ordered dose? _____

4. The physician's order reads: Bromocriptine mesylate, 12.5 mg, PO, BID. The drug is available in 5-mg capsules and 2.5-mg tablets. Which form of the drug would you give, capsules or tablets, and how many? _____

V. Crossword Puzzle

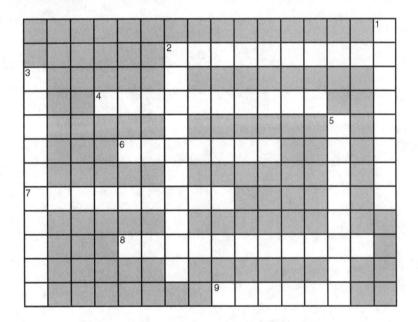

ACROSS CLUES

2. Vitamin to avoid while taking levodopa.
4. Involuntary muscular movements, such as twitching of the limbs or facial muscles.
6. Meat to avoid while taking levodopa.
7. Failure of the muscles of the lower esophagus to relax, causing difficulty swallowing.
8. Generic name for Cogentin.
9. Lack of muscular coordination.

DOWN CLUES

1. Generic name for Larodopa.
2. Another name for paralysis agitans.
3. Generic name for Symmetrel.
5. Movements consisting of spasms affecting the tongue, jaw, eyes, and neck.

VI. Critical Thinking

1. Mr. Martin has had Parkinson's disease for 4 years and, despite treatment with Sinemet, his functional ability continues to decline. His physician prescribes a tricyclic antidepressant. Mr. Martin returns to the clinic 3 weeks later complaining of constipation and difficulty voiding. Discuss your assessment of Mr. Martin and how you could determine if his symptoms are related to his medications. What would you suggest for Mr. Martin to do?

2. Ms. Moore, a patient with Parkinson's disease, has carbidopa-levodopa (Sinemet) 25-100 ordered TID. The pharmacy department has just delivered your patient's medication, which you administer. On returning to the medication cart, you discover the Sinemet that you have just administered was Sinemet 25-250. What would be your response to this situation and how could you prevent it from occurring again?

CHAPTER 30

Antianxiety Drugs

I. Matching

*Match each term in Column A with the correct
definition or statement in Column B.*

COLUMN A

_____ 1. antianxiety drugs

_____ 2. anxiety

_____ 3. anxiolytics

_____ 4. benzodiazepine withdrawal

_____ 5. psychotherapeutic drug

_____ 6. psychotropic drug

_____ 7. tolerance

_____ 8. psychomotor agitation

COLUMN B

A. Drug used to treat disorders of the mind.

B. Drugs used to treat anxiety.

C. Another term used to refer to the psychotropic
drugs.

D. A feeling of apprehension, worry, or uneasiness
that may or may not be based on reality.

E. A term that refers to the anxiety drugs.

F. Increasingly larger doses needed to obtain the
desired effect.

G. Extreme restlessness.

H. A condition that may occur when antianxiety
drugs are abruptly discontinued after 3 to 4
months of therapy.

II. Fill in the Blanks

1. List the symptoms of benzodiazepine withdrawal.

   a) _____

   b) _____

   c) _____

   d) _____

      1. _____

      2. _____

      3. _____

      4. _____

2. List the three types of psychotherapeutic drugs
   used to treat mental illness.

   a) _____

   b) _____

   c) _____

3. Antianxiety drugs include:

   a) _____

   b) _____

4. Long-term treatment with the _____
   drugs may result in _____ _____ and
   _____ _____ _____.

5. Ingestion of _____ with the antianxiety
   drugs can cause _____ and _____.

6. Preadministration assessment _____
   starting therapy with the _____ drugs
   would include complete _____
   _____ with _____ status and
   _____ level.

7. List the physiologic manifestations of anxiety that the nurse may observe during assessment of the patient.

   a) _____

   b) _____

   c)_ _____

   d) _____

   e) _____

8. Benzodiazepine toxicity causes _____, _____ _____, and _____.

9. Flumazenil (Romazicon) is an _____ for benzodiazepine _____ and acts within _____ to _____ minutes after _____ administration.

10. When _____ an antianxiety drug in patients who have used these drugs for _____ periods, the _____ will prescribe a _____ of _____ gradually over _____ to _____ weeks to _____ the possibility of _____ symptoms.

III. Multiple Choice

Circle the lett er of the most appropriate answer.

1. Mr. Ames is receiving chlordiazepoxide (Librium) for treatment of anxiety. Which adverse reaction would the nurse monitor for?
   a. Nausea and vomiting
   b. Diarrhea and abdominal cramping
   c. Ataxia and dysuria
   d. Drowsiness and sedation

2. The nurse should inform a patient being prescribed lorazepam (Ativan) that long-term use of this drug may result in:
   a. insomnia.
   b. physical dependence.
   c. increased anxiety.
   d. idiosyncratic reaction.

3. Ms. Betts has been prescribed oxazepam (Serax) for her anxiety. While she is taking this medication, the nurse will:
   a. monitor her lab tests for plasma concentration levels on a weekly basis.
   b. inform Ms. Betts to expect cardiac arrhythmias.
   c. inform Ms. Betts that some adverse reactions may diminish as therapy continues.
   d. advise Ms. Betts to avoid foods containing tyramine.

4. The nurse administering the benzodiazepines must be aware that the classification of these drugs by the Controlled Substance Act places them in Category:
   a. I.   c. III.
   b. II.   d. IV.

5. Mr. Smith, 78-year-old patient, has been prescribed buspirone (BuSpar) for anxiety. The nurse tells the patient that this drug is a safe choice for older adults with anxiety because it does not:
   a. cause excessive sedation.
   b. increase nervousness.
   c. cause dry mouth and problems swallowing.
   d. cause episodes of postural hypotension.

6. Common adverse reactions seen during initial therapy with the antianxiety drugs would include:
   a. dystonia.
   b. sedation.
   c. ataxia.
   d. urinary retention.

7. Abruptly discontinuing the antianxiety drugs can result in withdrawal symptoms occurring within:
   a. the first 8 hours after discontinuing the drug.
   b. 30 minutes after the first missed dose.
   c. 2 to 3 days after stopping the drug.
   d. 7 to 10 days after discontinuing the drug.

8. Symptoms of withdrawal from antianxiety drugs include:
   a. irritability and tremors.
   b. bradycardia and hypotension.
   c. occipital headache and hypertension.
   d. sedation and lethargy.

IV. Drug Matching

Match the generic name with the trade name.

COLUMN A	COLUMN B
_____ 1. clorazepate	A. Ativan
_____ 2. lorazepam	B. Equanil
_____ 3. chlordiazepoxide	C. Serax
_____ 4. diazepam	D. Valium
_____ 5. oxazepam	E. Librium
_____ 6. alprazolam	F. Tranxene
_____ 7. hydroxyzine	G. Atarax
_____ 8. meprobamate	H. Xanax

V. Crossword Puzzle

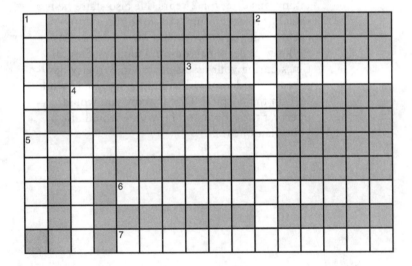

ACROSS CLUES

3. Antianxiety agent that increases the risk of digitalis toxicity when administered with digitalis.
5. Another name for antianxiety drugs.
6. Hydroxyzine produces its effect by acting on which area of the body?
7. A term referring to drugs used to treat disorders of the mind.

DOWN CLUES

1. Condition that may develop when antianxiety drugs are used for periods longer than 2 weeks.
2. What action do the antianxiety agents have on the CNS?
4. Feeling of apprehension or uneasiness that may not be based on reality.

VI. Dosage Problems

Solve the following dosage calculations.

1. The physician orders Xanax, 0.25 mg, PO, BID. Drug available: alprazolam, 0.5-mg tablets. How many tablets will the nurse give? _____

2. The physician orders Ativan, 2 mg, IM, q 4 hours, PRN, agitation. Drug available: lorazepam, 4 mg/mL. How many milliliters will the nurse administer? _____

3. The physician orders Valium, 7.5 mg, IM, stat. Drug available: diazepam, 5 mg/mL. How many milliliters will the nurse need for the ordered dose? _____

4. The physician orders Vistaril, 75 mg, IM, stat. Drug available: hydroxyzine, 25 mg/mL. How many milliliters will be administered? _____

VII. Critical Thinking

1. Mary Burns, a recently divorced 35-year-old, is seen in the clinic today complaining of anxiety and inability to sleep at night. The primary care provider writes Ms. Burns a prescription for diazepam (Valium), 5 mg, three times daily and also for triazelam (Halcion), 0.25 mg, at night for sleep when needed. As Ms. Burns' nurse, you are responsible for developing a teaching plan for her. Consider what additional information from the patient might be helpful. Discuss your plan.

2. Adam Berkeley is admitted to your unit for elective surgery. While completing your assessment, Mr. Berkeley states that he has been taking alprazolam (Xanax), 1 mg, three times a day and at night to help him sleep. He has been taking this drug for 2 years. He also states he is a social drinker, consuming two to three drinks each evening after work and on weekends. Mr. Berkeley appears nervous and anxious. Several times during your assessment, Mr. Berkeley has asked if the doctor will continue his Xanax while he is in the hospital. Discuss how you would interpret these data and how they would affect your plan of care.

CHAPTER 31

Antidepressant Drugs

I. Matching

Match each term in Column A with the correct definition or statement in Column B.

COLUMN A

_____ 1. dysphoric

_____ 2. monoamine oxidase

_____ 3. depression

_____ 4. priapism

_____ 5. orthostatic hypotension

_____ 6. SSRIs

_____ 7. hypertensive crisis

_____ 8. tricyclic

COLUMN B

A. Characterized by feelings of intense sadness, help-lessness, worthlessness, and impaired functioning.

B. Extreme or exaggerated sadness, anxiety, or unhappiness.

C. A significant drop in blood pressure when going from lying to standing.

D. A complex enzyme system that is responsible for breaking down amines.

E. Extremely high blood pressure.

F. Type of antidepressant drug contraindicated in patients scheduled to have a myelogram.

G. Type of antidepressant drug used cautiously in patients with diabetes mellitus.

H. A persistent erection of the penis.

II. Fill in the Blanks

1. List the symptoms of depression.

   a) _____

   b) _____

   c) _____

   d) _____

   e) _____

   f) _____

   g) _____

   h) _____

   i) _____

   j) _____

2. List the different types of antidepressant drugs.

   a) _____

   b) _____

   c) _____

   d) _____

3. List the selective serotonin reuptake inhibitors. Include the generic and trade names.

   a) _____ _____

   b) _____ _____

   c) _____ _____

   d) _____ _____

4. The most common adverse reactions seen with the TCAs are _____ and _____ .

5. _____ hypotension is seen with both the _____ and the _____ .

6. A serious _____ _____ associated with the use of MAOIs is _____ _____ , which may occur when _____ containing _____ are eaten.

7. List the symptoms of hypertensive crisis.

   a) _____

   b) _____

   c) _____

   d) _____

   e) _____

   f) _____

   g) _____

   h) _____

   i) _____

8. There is a _____ _____ of fluoxetine in patients who _____ _____ during administration of the drug.

III. Multiple Choice

Circle the letter of the most appropriate answer.

Ms. Lyons has had varying degrees of depression for the past 7 years. She has recently been admitted to the psychiatric unit for reevaluation of her depression and therapy. Questions 1–4 pertain to Ms. Lyons' case.

1. Ms. Lyons has been seen by a psychiatrist and prescribed nortriptyline (Pamelor), a tricyclic antidepressant. The nurse would expect Ms. Lyons to experience a decrease in depression:
   a. within 24 hours of the first dose.
   b. within 2 to 3 weeks.
   c. within 1 week.
   d. after 6 weeks of continuous treatment.

2. Which of the following adverse reactions would the nurse expect to observe in Ms. Lyons?
   a. Constipation and abdominal cramps
   b. Bradycardia and double vision
   c. Sedation and dry mouth
   d. Polyuria and hypotension

3. The nurse will monitor Ms. Lyons closely because:
   a. an adjustment in drug dosage may be required.
   b. tricyclic antidepressants are rarely effective.
   c. an anaphylactic reaction may occur.
   d. nortriptyline can cause a hypertensive crisis.

4. The nurse will include which of the following facts in the discharge teaching for Ms. Lyons?
   a. Tricyclic antidepressants are physically addicting; do not take for longer than 8 weeks.
   b. Decrease the dose if drowsiness is severe.
   c. Increase the dose by 1 tablet if severe depression occurs.
   d. Do not drink alcoholic beverages unless the physician approves use.

5. Which of the following is a common adverse reaction that the nurse would expect to observe in the patient receiving the antidepressant amitriptyline hydrochloride (Elavil)?
   a. Hyperglycemia   c. Diarrhea
   b. Dry mouth   d. Insomnia

6. Which of the following would indicate to the nurse that the patient receiving fluoxetine (Prozac) is experiencing a therapeutic effect of the drug?
   a. The patient has an increase in anxiety.
   b. A decrease in hallucinations occurred within 24 hours of the first dose.
   c. The patient has a decrease in depression over a period of several weeks.
   d. The patient develops signs of tardive dyskinesia.

7. At a team conference, the nurse states that the monoamine oxidase inhibitors are used for the treatment of:
   a. depression.
   b. anxiety.
   c. nervousness.
   d. restlessness.

8. The nurse instructs the patient taking a monoamine oxidase inhibitor that prohibited foods would include:
   a. apples.
   b. peaches.
   c. bananas.
   d. strawberries.

9. A patient taking phenelzine (Nardil) is complaining of a severe headache. The nurse should:
   a. ask the physician to prescribe an analgesic.
   b. check the patient's temperature and encourage the patient to increase fluid intake.
   c. check the patient's blood pressure and notify the physician immediately.
   d. monitor the patient at regular intervals for the next several hours.

10. The nurse caring for a patient who is taking tranylcypromine (Pronate) must monitor for hypertensive crisis. One of the earliest symptoms is:
    a. sedation.
    b. arrhythmias.
    c. occipital headache
    d. anorexia.

11. A physician has written an order for imipramine (Tofranil). On reviewing the medical history of the patient, you find she was taking phenelzine and had discontinued it a week earlier. As the nurse, you would know the MAOIs must be discontinued _____ before starting the tricyclics.
    a. at least 2 weeks
    b. at least 1 month
    c. 5 days
    d. at least 1 week

12. A nurse would know that patients taking the MAOIs require strict dietary control because foods should not be eaten that contain:
    a. fat.
    b. cholesterol.
    c. purine.
    d. tyramine.

IV. Crossword Puzzle

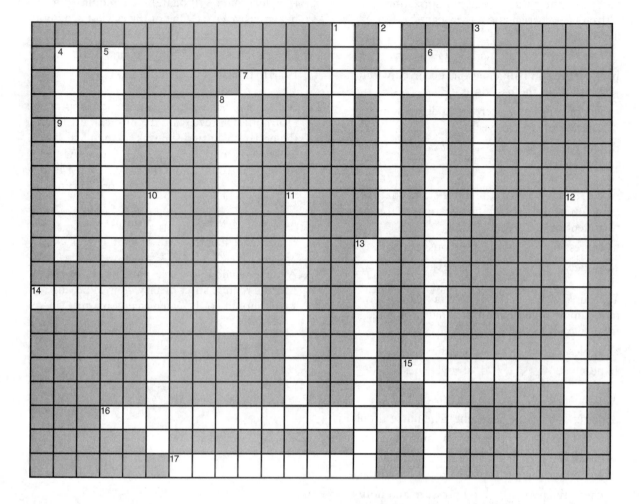

ACROSS CLUES

7. Generic name for Elavil.
9. Generic name for Ludiomil.
14. Generic name for Zoloft.
15. Type of antidepressant drug contraindicated in patients scheduled to have a myelogram.
16. A complex enzyme system that is responsible for breaking down amines (two words).
17. Generic name for Desyrel.

DOWN CLUES

1. Type of antidepressant drug used cautiously in patients with diabetes mellitus.
2. Generic name for Wellbutrin.
3. A persistent erection of the penis.
4. Trade name for trimipramine.
5. Extreme or exaggerated sadness, anxiety, or unhappiness.
6. Extremely high blood pressure (two words).
8. Generic name for Prozac.

10. Generic name for Effexor.
11. Generic name for Paxil.
12. Characterized by feelings of intense sadness, helplessness, worthlessness, and impaired function.
13. Generic name for Tofranil.

V. Dosage Problems

Solve the following dosage calculations.

1. The physician orders Prozac, 20 mg, PO, qd. Prozac is available in 10-mg capsules. How many capsules will be taken at each dose? _____

2. The physician has ordered fluoxetine, 40 mg, PO, qd. The Prozac available is liquid in a dosage strength of 20 mg/5 mL. How many milliliters will be needed for the ordered dose of Prozac? _____

3. Venlafaxine, 75 mg is ordered. The drug is available in 37.5-mg tablets. The nurse would administer how many tablets? _____

4. A patient is prescribed 300 mg of bupropion daily. How many tablets would the nurse need to have on hand if the drug is available in 75-mg tablets? _____

VI. Critical Thinking

1. Michael, a 15-year-old, has been prescribed bupropion (Wellbutrin) for depression. You are preparing a patient teaching plan for Michael and his parents. Discuss important points that must be covered in your teaching.

2. Jane, a 17-year-old, was admitted to your psychiatric unit after a suicide attempt. When you approach her with her morning dose of her antidepressant, she is lying on her bed in a fetal position. She opens her eyes when you call her name. Jane tells you just to leave her medication on the bedside table and she will take it at breakfast. Discuss how you would respond to Jane's request without disrupting the therapeutic relationship you have established with her.

CHAPTER 32

Antipsychotic Drugs

I. Matching

Match each term in Column A with the correct definition or statement in Column B.

COLUMN A

_____ 1. akathisia

_____ 2. antipsychotic drugs

_____ 3. bipolar disorder

_____ 4. delusion

_____ 5. dystonia

_____ 6. extrapyramidal effects

_____ 7. hallucination

_____ 8. neuroleptic drugs

_____ 9. neuroleptic malignant syndrome

_____ 10. photophobia

_____ 11. photosensitivity

_____ 12. psychotic disorder

_____ 13. tardive dyskinesia

_____ 14. flattened affect

_____ 15. anhedonia

COLUMN B

A. Characterized by extreme personality disorganization and the loss of contact with reality.

B. False beliefs that cannot be changed with reason.

C. A false perception having no basis in reality.

D. Drugs given to patients with a psychotic disorder.

E. Another term used to refer to antipsychotic drugs.

F. A psychiatric disorder characterized by severe mood swings from extreme hyperactivity to depression.

G. Absence of emotional response to any situation or condition.

H. Intolerance to light.

I. Abnormal muscle movements resulting from the use of antipsychotic drugs.

J. Extreme restlessness and increased motor activity.

K. Facial grimacing and twisting of the neck into unnatural positions.

L. Finding no pleasure in activities that are normally pleasurable.

M. Abnormal response or sensitivity when exposed to light.

N. Syndrome consisting of potentially irreversible, involuntary dyskinetic movements.

O. Characterized by a combination of extrapyramidal effects, hyperthermia, and autonomic disturbance.

II. Fill in the Blanks

1. The most common adverse reactions that may occur with lithium carbonate include _____, _____, _____, _____, and _____.

2. The _____ of lithium is _____ according to _____ levels and _____ response to the drug.

3. Adverse reactions that indicate bone marrow suppression would include _____, _____, _____ _____, _____, _____ _____ _____, and _____ _____.

4. Signs of lithium toxicity would include _____, _____, _____, _____, _____ _____, and lack of _____.

III. Multiple Choice

Circle the letter of the most appropriate answer.

Mr. Howard has been diagnosed with a bipolar disorder and is being started on drug therapy using lithium. Questions 1–4 pertain to Mr. Howard's case.

1. Because of the possibility of toxicity associated with high plasma levels of lithium, the nurse would anticipate the physician ordering hematological testing of Mr. Howard's:
   a. hepatic functioning.
   b. renal functioning.
   c. serum lithium levels.
   d. immune status.

2. Patient teaching for Mr. Howard would include information on recognizing the symptoms of lithium toxicity. These symptoms would include:
   a. nausea, vomiting, diarrhea.
   b. constipation and abdominal cramps.
   c. stupor, oliguria, hypertension.
   d. dry mouth, blurred vision, difficulty swallowing.

3. The nurse would question Mr. Howard about his type of work and activities he is involved with in his daily life because:
   a. lithium is contraindicated in patients who must operate machinery.
   b. lithium is used cautiously in patients exposed to situations that cause profuse sweating.
   c. lithium is contraindicated in patients who are constantly exposed to the elements of weather.
   d. lithium is used cautiously in patients involved in activities requiring mental alertness.

4. During an ongoing assessment of Mr. Howard, the nurse would note in the patient record symptoms that may indicate that Mr. Howard is experiencing a manic episode. These symptoms would include:
   a. direct eye contact and smiling.
   b. animated speech with appropriate answers.
   c. indirect eye contact and bizarre delusions.
   d. direct eye contact and spontaneous laughter.

5. The nurse explains to the family that when higher doses of some antipsychotic drugs are administered, the physician may prescribe _____ to reduce the possibility of the occurrence of parkinson-like symptoms.
   a. cortisone
   b. an NSAID
   c. epinephrine
   d. an antiparkinsonism drug

6. Ms. Clark's drug therapy includes an antipsychotic drug and an antiparkinsonism drug to treat the extrapyramidal effects she may experience. The nurse would know that Ms. Clark must be monitored closely for symptoms of:
   a. hypertensive crisis.
   b. tardive dyskinesia.
   c. narcolepsy.
   d. increased heart rate.

7. In Mr. Ross' patient record, the nurse finds that clozapine was discontinued 1 week ago. The nurse is now aware that the patient's current symptoms may indicate:
   a. bone marrow suppression.
   b. tardive dyskinesia.
   c. a bacterial infection.
   d. a viral infection.

8. Ms. Edwards has been prescribed haloperidol (Haldol). The drug is available in tablet and liquid concentrate form. The patient states she has difficulty swallowing pills, but can swallow liquids. Patient teaching for the liquid Haldol would include:
   a. mix the medication with apple juice.
   b. protect the medication from light.
   c. keep the medication refrigerated.
   d. do not mix the medication with pudding.

9. Which drug would be contraindicated for a patient with Parkinson's disease?
   a. Donepezil   c. Tacrine
   b. Lithium   d. Haloperidol

10. The nurse would avoid administering lithium with:
   a. highly salted foods.
   b. meals or immediately after meals.
   c. large amounts of water.
   d. an antacid.

IV. Crossword Puzzle

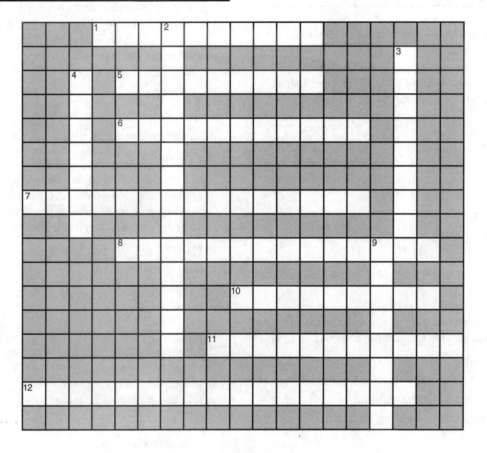

ACROSS CLUES

1. Disease characterized by a progressive deterioration of mental, physical, and cognitive abilities.
5. False beliefs that cannot be changed with reason.
6. Another word for antipsychotic drugs.
7. Absence of emotional response to any situation or condition. (Two words)
8. Effects of the antipsychotic drugs characterized by abnormal muscle movements.
10. Extreme restlessness and increased motor activity.
11. Intolerance to light.
12. Syndrome consisting of potentially irreversible, involuntary dyskinetic movements. (Two words)

DOWN CLUES

2. False perceptions having no basis in reality.
3. Finding no pleasure in activities that are normally pleasurable.
4. A psychiatric disorder characterized by severe mood swings of extreme hyperactivity to depression.
9. Facial grimacing and twisting of the neck into unnatural positions.

V. Dosage Problems

Solve the following dosage calculations.

1. The physician's order reads: Chlorpromazine, 75 mg, PO, BID. Available drug: Thorazine, 25-mg tablets. The patient will receive how many tablets at each dose? _____

2. The physician has ordered lithium carbonate, 600 mg, PO, HS. The label on the bottle reads: Lithium Citrate syrup. Each 5-mL container contains lithium carbonate 300 mg.

   a. How many milliliters are needed to administer the ordered dose? _____

   b. How many containers of the drug will you need to prepare each dose? _____

3. The physician has written an order for Haldol, 10 mg, PO, BID. The drug you have on hand is haloperidol concentrate labeled 2 mg/mL. The nurse will administer how many milliliters of the day? _____

4. A patient has been prescribed Trilafon, 24 mg, PO, BID. The pharmacy has sent a container whose label reads: Perphenazine concentrate, 16 mg/5 mL. How many milliliters of the medication will be administered? _____

5. The physician's order reads: Thorazine concentrate, 150 mg, PO, BID. Available drug: chlorpromazine concentrate, 100 mg/mL. How many milliliters will be administered? _____

VI. Critical Thinking

1. A patient, 37 years old and homeless, has been admitted to the hospital with pneumonia. His patient record shows that he has been diagnosed and treated for schizophrenia and alcohol abuse for the last 15 years. When you enter his room to administer his prescribed antipsychotic medication and his antibiotic, he swears at you and tells you to leave the room because he has no plans to take that poison. Discuss how you would respond to this patient if you were his nurse and identify how you might convince him to take his medication.

2. You are the nurse assigned to care for Charles Grey, hospitalized 2 weeks ago and started on perphenazine (Trilafon) to treat acute psychotic symptoms. During your assessment, Charles appears restless, unable to sit still, and uncoordinated. You also observe that he has developed a fine hand tremor. How would you interpret this collective information and how would you respond as Mr. Grey's nurse?

CHAPTER 33

Cholinesterase Inhibitors

I. Matching

Match the term in Column A with the correct definition or statement in Column B.

COLUMN A

_____ 1. acetylcholine

_____ 2. alanine aminotransferase

_____ 3. Alzheimer's disease

_____ 4. dementia

_____ 5. ginkgo

_____ 6. ginseng

COLUMN B

A. Herb taken to improve memory and brain function.

B. A progressive deterioration of mental, physical, and cognitive abilities from which there is no recovery.

C. Herb taken to improve energy and mental performance.

D. A natural chemical in the brain required for memory and thinking.

E. Decrease in cognitive functioning.

F. An enzyme found predominantly in the liver.

II. Fill in the Blanks

1. Drugs used to treat Alzheimer's disease do not _____ the disease, but are aimed at _____ the _____.

2. Examples of the cholinesterase inhibitors include (*list the generic and trade names*):

   a) _____ _____

   b) _____ _____

   c) _____ _____

   d) _____ _____

3. The cholinesterase inhibitors act to _____ the level of _____ in the _____ by inhibiting its _____.

4. In the patient with Alzheimer's disease, _____ ability and _____ ability is assessed _____ and _____ therapy.

5. The nurse assesses the patient with AD for:

   a) _____

   b) _____

   c) _____

   d) _____

   e) _____

   f) _____

III. Multiple Choice

Circle the letter of the most appropriate answer.

1. Ms. Gilbert, a 61-year-old patient with Alzheimer's-type dementia, is being treated with tacrine. Her oldest daughter Rose has assumed the caregiver role for Ms. Gilbert. Ms. Gilbert's nurse would teach Rose to monitor for indications of liver damage. The symptoms would include:
   a. loss of appetite.
   b. jaundice.
   c. tachycardia.
   d. lethargy.

2. Mr. Tolbert has been prescribed donepezil (Aricept) for his Alzheimer's symptoms. When teaching the patient about his medication, the nurse would be correct to state:
   a. take this drug at bedtime.
   b. this drug will cure Alzheimer's.
   c. this drug is taken twice daily.
   d. take this drug with breakfast.

3. A patient being treated with the drug rivastigmine (Exelon) has begun to experience episodes of nausea and vomiting. As this patient's nurse, you would notify the physician and:
   a. encourage the patient to take the drug on an empty stomach.
   b. expect the drug to be discontinued and restarted with a smaller dose.
   c. tell the patient that this is the drug of first choice for treating Alzheimer's disease.
   d. suggest the patient take the drug every other day until nausea and vomiting stop.

4. The nurse caring for a patient being treated with tacrine will expect periodic monitoring of:
   a. renal function.
   b. complete blood counts.
   c. liver function.
   d. cardiac enzymes.

5. Ms. Bell is at the clinic for her regular checkup. During your assessment, you question the patient about her medications. Ms. Bell states she takes only one drug, Aricept, and she always takes it just before going to bed. As a nurse, you would know that Ms. Bell:
   a. should be taking the drug Aricept three times a day.
   b. is taking her medication appropriately.
   c. should take her medication with breakfast.
   d. should be having plasma levels of ALT checked.

6. Mary Brown has brought her father to the clinic because she doesn't think his medicine is working. Mary's father has recently been diagnosed with Alzheimer's-type dementia and has been prescribed galantamine. Mary wants to know when her father will get well. You would be correct in explaining to Mary that:
   a. if the drug doesn't work in a week, the doctor will probably change it.
   b. her father will be able to take the drug only for 30 days.
   c. she should increase the dose of the drug daily until improvement occurs.
   d. the drug is not going to cure the Alzheimer's disease, but symptoms may improve.

7. A patient is receiving tacrine and bethanechol. The nurse would expect to see:
   a. an adverse reaction.
   b. antagonist effects.
   c. a synergistic effect.
   d. an agonist effect.

8. At a team conference on caring for patients with Alzheimer's disease, a new nurse asks if there are any natural herbal therapies for treating Alzheimer's. You tell her that there are two herbs that are said to improve memory and mental function. These are:
   a. ginger and garlic.
   b. gotu kola and goldenseal.
   c. guayusa and goldenrod.
   d. ginkgo and ginseng.

IV. Crossword Puzzle

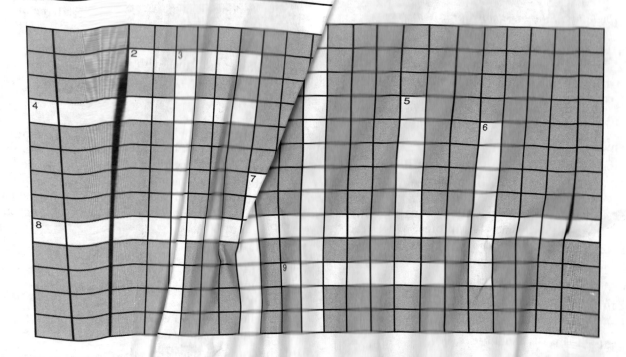

ACROSS CLUES

2. Trade name for tade.
4. Decrease in cognit function.
8. An enzyme found dominantly in the liver.
9. Herb taken to imve energy and mental performance.

DOWN CLUES

1. A natural chemi in the brain required for memory and thing.
3. Herb taken to rove memory and brain function (two vds).
5. Trade name for vastigmine tartrate.
6. Trade name for onepezil.
7. Trade name for galantamine hydrobromide.

V. Dosage Problems

Solve the follow dosage calculations.

1. A patien has been receiving Aricept 5-mg tablets at bedtime for 6 weeks. The physician has decided to increase the dosage of Aricept to 10 mg, PO, qd, HS. Aricept is available in 5-mg tablets. How many tablets will the patient take with the new dosage? _____

2. Ms. Brown has been diagnosed with Alzheimer's-type dementia and started on therapy with Exelon. The physician has written orders for the administration schedule to be used for this drug. The orders are Exelon, 1.5 mg, PO, BID for 2 weeks, increase dose to 3 mg, PO, BID for 2 weeks, increase dose to 4.5 mg, PO, BID for 2 weeks, increase dose to 6 mg, PO, BID. The pharmacy has sent the nursing home rivastigmine in liquid form with a dosage strength of 2 mg/2mL.

   a) How many milliliters of drug will be given for each dose for the first 2 weeks? _____

   b) How many milliliters will be administered for the 4.5-mg doses? _____

3. The physician has prescribed galantamine (Reminyl), 32 mg, PO, qd, in 2 divided doses. Galantamine is available in 4-mg tablets.

   a) How many milligrams will be given at each dose? _____

   b) How many tablets will be administered for each dose? _____

VI. Critical Thinking

1. Beth Martin is caring for her father, who has been diagnosed with early-stage Alzheimer's disease. Beth's father has been demonstrating increasing signs of forgetfulness and confusion for the last few weeks. At their regular monthly visit to the clinic, Beth asks you for suggestions on how to get her father to take his medicine without the usual arguments and questions. Discuss suggestions you could make and also what information you can give Beth on the progression of Alzheimer's disease that might help her to understand her father's actions more fully.

2. A patient has been receiving donepezil for treatment of Alzheimer's disease. The therapy is in its third month. When the patient returns for a follow-up visit, you are expected to complete an assessment to determine if there has been any therapeutic effect from the medication. Discuss what you would look for specifically and what questions you could ask to assist in making your determination.

CHAPTER 34

Antiemetic and Antivertigo Drugs

I. Matching

Match each term in Column A with the correct definition or statement in Column B.

COLUMN A

_____ 1. Ménière's

_____ 2. ondansetron

_____ 3. antiemetic

_____ 4. CTZ

_____ 5. antivertigo

_____ 6. Anzemet

_____ 7. nausea

_____ 8. vertigo

_____ 9. vestibular neuritis

_____ 10. vomiting

COLUMN B

A. Drug administered orally 1 hour before chemotherapy to prevent nausea and vomiting.

B. Disease of the ear causing dizziness and other symptoms.

C. A drug that can be given intravenously 30 minutes before administration of antineoplastic drugs.

D. Forceful expulsion of gastric contents through the mouth.

E. Drug used to treat or prevent nausea.

F. A feeling of spinning or rotation-type motion.

G. Drug used to prevent or treat vertigo.

H. Inflammation of the vestibular nerve.

I. A group of nerve fibers located on the surface of the fourth ventricle of the brain and known as the chemoreceptor trigger zone.

J. Unpleasant gastric sensation usually preceding vomiting.

II. Fill in the Blanks

1. Vertigo is usually accompanied by _____, _____, and _____.

2. Dronabinol is a derivative of the active substance found in _____ and is a second-line _____ used after _____ with other _____ have failed.

3. Antivertigo drugs are essentially _____ because they have _____ or _____ _____ properties.

4. Thiethylperazine is classified as a Pregnancy Category _____ drug and is _____ during pregnancy.

5. _____ decrease absorption of the _____.

6. Preadministration _____ for the patient with nausea and vomiting should include the _____ of times the patient has _____ and approximate amount of _____ lost.

7. The nurse notifies the _____ if the drug _____ to _____ or _____ symptoms.

8. The nurse instructs the patient to take buclizine by placing the _____ in the _____ and allowing it to _____ or to _____ or _____ the _____ whole.

9. List examples of antiemeics used to treat chemotherapy induce nausea and vomiting (*include generic and trade names*).

   a) _____ _____

   b) _____ _____

   c) _____ _____

   d) _____ _____

   e) _____ _____

10. The nurse must immediately report symptoms of dehydration, which include:

   a) _____

   b) _____

   c) _____

   d) _____

   e) _____

III. Multiple Choice

Circle the letter of the most appropriate answer.

1. When asked by a patient why the physician has prescribed an antivertigo drug for her motion sickness, the nurse would respond that the antivertigo drugs:
   a. depress the gastric reflex, as well as relieve vertigo.
   b. relieve nausea by stimulating the CTZ.
   c. have direct or indirect antiemetic properties.
   d. stimulate the vestibular nerves and the CTZ.

2. After administration of an antiemetic, the nurse advises the patient to:
   a. request assistance if drowsiness occurs.
   b. drink plenty of fluid to prevent dehydration.
   c. lie flat in bed to prevent vomiting.
   d. take nothing by mouth until nausea subsides.

3. A patient asks the nurse what to do if the scopolamine patch she has applied falls off in 1 or 2 days. The nurse would instruct the patient to:
   a. leave the patch off because it has probably dispensed enough medication.
   b. discard the used disk and apply a new disk behind the opposite ear.
   c. reapply the old disk behind the same ear using tape to reattach.
   d. apply a new disk behind the same ear used for the old disk.

4. When vomiting is severe, the patient is observed for signs and symptoms of dehydration, which include:
   a. absence of bowel sounds, increase urine output.
   b. distended abdomen, decreased respiratory rate.
   c. diarrhea, anxiety, rash.
   d. poor skin turgor, dry mucous membranes.

5. If vomiting is severe, the blood pressure, pulse, and respiratory rate are monitored:
   a. every 15 minutes.   c. every 12 hours
   b. every 2 to 4 hours.   d. daily.

6. When asked at a team conference why nausea and vomiting occur, the nurse states that one cause is:
   a. inhibition of the vestibular apparatus.
   b. stimulation of the cerebral cortex.
   c. stimulation of the CTZ.
   d. inhibition of the gastric nerve supply.

7. When an antiemetic is used to relieve the nausea and vomiting caused by the administration of an antineoplastic drug, the nurse may be responsible for preparing the antiemetic, which is given:
   a. along with the antineoplastic drug.
   b. 30 minutes before administering the antineoplastic drug.
   c. 10 minutes before administering the antineoplastic drug.
   d. at least 24 hours before the chemotherapy treatment.

8. A patient being prescribed buclizine for motion sickness would be instructed by the nurse:

   a. that one dose is usually effective.

   b. to place the drug behind both ears.

   c. to start taking the drug 1 week before traveling.

   d. to wait until nausea occurs, then take the drug.

9. A nurse reviewing the Summary Drug Table for this chapter will find that the adverse reactions to monitor for meclizine would include:

   a. somnolence. c. headache.

   b. restlessness. d. diarrhea.

10. Which of these drugs could mask the symptoms of ototoxicity when administered with other ototoxic drugs?

    a. Scopolamine c. Dimenhydrinate

    b. Promethazine d. Dolasetron

IV. Crossword Puzzle

ACROSS CLUES

2. Drug that can be given intravenously 30 minutes before administration of antineoplastic drugs to prevent nausea.
6. Classified as a Pregnancy Category X drug.
8. Drug administered orally 1 hour before chemotherapy to prevent nausea and vomiting.
11. Action of antiemetics on the chemoreceptor trigger zone.
12. Trade name for ondansetron hydrochloride.
13. Generic name for Phenergran.

16. Trade name for dronabinol.
17. A derivative of the active substance found in marijuana.

DOWN CLUES

1. Inflammation of the vestibular nerve (two words).
3. Trade name for chlorpromazine hydrochloride.
5. Drug type used to prevent dizziness.
7. Drug type used to prevent vomiting.
9. Abbreviation for chemoreceptor trigger zone.

V. Dosage Problems

Solve the following dosage calculations.

1. The physician's order reads: Thorazine concentrate, 75 mg, PO, qd. Drug available: Chlorpromazine HCl, 100 mg/mL. How many milliliters will be given? _____

2. The physician's order reads: Reglan, 10 mg, PO, TID, 1/2 hour before meals. Drug available: Metoclopramide, 5-mg tablets. How many tablets would be administered before each meal?

   _____

3. The physician's order reads: Phenergan, 12.5 mg, IM, q4h, PRN, nausea. Available drug: Promethazine, 50 mg/mL. How many milliliters will the nurse administer? _____

4. The physician's order reads: Scopolamine grain 1/300, SC, stat. Drug available: Scopolamine hydrobromide injection, 0.4 mg/mL. How many milliliters will be given? _____

5. The physician's order reads: Thorazine, 75 mg, IM, q4h, PRN. Drug available: Chlorpromazine HCL, 25 mg/mL. What will the milliliter dose be?

   _____

VI. Critical Thinking

1. Kelly Compton, a 38-year-old patient, is having elective abdominal surgery. In the past, she has experienced significant postoperative nausea. Her physician has written orders for lorazepam (Ativan), prochlorperaxine (Compazine), and metoclopramide (Reglan) on a PRN basis to treat postoperative nausea and vomiting. Discuss how each antiemetic may work to decrease the postoperative nausea and vomiting and why you think the physician prescribed more than one antiemetic. How would you decide which drug to give?

2. Sally Perkins is being treated in an outpatient chemotherapy unit that operates 24 hours a day. Sally always comes in the late evening to receive her treatment and then stays the night. She receives cisplatin, a very emetogenic chemotherapeutic drug. The following drugs are ordered IV 30 minutes before her treatment: ondansetron (Zofran), metoclopramide (Reglan), and lorazepam (Ativan). Explain why you think Sally's treatment is given in the evening and discuss the rationale for her pretreatment drug orders.

CHAPTER **35**

Anesthetic Drugs

I. Matching

Match each term in Column A with the correct definition or statement in Column B.

COLUMN A

_____ 1. nurse anesthetist

_____ 2. preanesthesia drug

_____ 3. anesthesia

_____ 4. volatile liquids

_____ 5. anesthesiologist

_____ 6. local anesthesia

_____ 7. induction

_____ 8. general anesthesia

_____ 9. local infiltration

_____ 10. topical anesthesia

COLUMN B

A. Begins with administration of an anesthetic drug and lasts until consciousness is lost.

B. Loss of feeling or sensation.

C. A pain-free state in a specific area or region

D. Provision of a pain-free state for the entire body.

E. A physician with special training in administering anesthesia.

F. Application of the anesthetic to the surface of the skin, open area, or mucous membrane; may be applied by a nurse.

G. Injection of a local anesthetic drug into tissues.

H. A nurse with special training who is qualified to administer anesthetics.

I. A drug given before the administration of anes-thesia.

J. Liquids that evaporate on exposure to air.

II. Fill in the Blanks

1. There are two types of anesthesia: _____ anesthesia and _____ anesthesia.

2. In some instances, a _____ anesthetic may be applied by a nurse.

3. The nurse usually gives a _____ drug before the administration of _____ _____.

4. The narcotic or antianxiety drugs are given before surgery to decrease_____ and _____ immediately _____ surgery.

5. Antiemetics are administered before surgery to _____ the _____ of _____ and _____ during the immediate _____ _____ period.

6. Preanesthesia drugs are usually selected by the _____ and may consist of a _____ drug, an _____ drug, and/or a _____.

7. Antianxiety drugs have the ability to _____ the _____ action of the _____ drugs.

8. The choice of drug used for general anesthesia depends on many factors, including:

a) _____

b) _____

c) _____

9. When a nurse first sees the postoperative patient, a priority nursing task will be checking the _____ for patency, assessing the _____ status, and giving _____ as needed.

10. After surgery, the nurse will monitor the patient's _____ _____, _____, and _____ _____ every _____ to _____ minutes until the patient is _____ from the area.

III. Multiple Choice

Circle the letter of the most appropriate answer.

1. A nurse planning the preoperative care for a patient knows the preoperative narcotic drug the physician has ordered is mainly given for the purpose of:
   a. decreasing secretions in the upper respiratory tract.
   b. lessening the incidence of nausea and vomiting.
   c. decreasing anxiety and apprehension before surgery.
   d. providing a pain-free state for the entire body.

2. After the nurse administers the preanesthesia medication, the patient will be instructed to:
   a. sit in a chair for a few minutes and then lie down.
   b. void immediately after the medication is given.
   c. be very quiet and refrain from talking.
   d. remain in bed after the medication is given.

3. When asked at a team conference where the anesthetic agent is injected for spinal anesthesia, the nurse correctly replies "at the level of the _____."
   a. second lumbar vertebra
   b. junction of the thoracic and lumbar vertebrae
   c. in the lower thoracic region
   d. fourth lumbar vertebra

4. John Blake is scheduled for a surgical procedure that requires general anesthesia. He has been fasting (NPO) since midnight and is now asking for a small drink of water. You have already administered his preoperative medications. You explain to Mr. Blake that he must remain NPO because:
   a. some general anesthetics cause nausea and vomiting.
   b. the general anesthetic will work faster with NPO patients.
   c. NPO status helps to reduce the chances of excess blood loss.
   d. IV sedatives may not be as effective if the patient is not fasting.

5. A nurse assistant asks the nurse what the term *neuroleptic-analgesia* means. The nurse correctly replies that this is a type of general anesthesia characterized by:
   a. complete loss of consciousness and decreased respirations.
   b. lack of movement, excitation, increased respiration rate.
   c. quietness, reduced motor activity, profound analgesia.
   d. lack of analgesia, unconsciousness, respiratory depression.

6. A nurse working in the postanesthesia recovery room is aware that the endotracheal tube can be removed:
   a. when swallowing and gag reflexes return.
   b. when the patient is aware of his surroundings.
   c. after the surgeon applies the surgical dressing.
   d. during stage II of the general anesthesia.

7. You are presenting information at a team conference on the importance of administering the preanesthesia drugs at the time ordered by the physician, especially the cholinergic blocking drugs. A new nurse asks what action the cholinergic blocking drugs have. You would be correct to reply that these drugs:
   a. increase the sedative effect of anesthesia.
   b. decrease secretions of the upper respiratory tract.
   c. reduce anxiety and apprehension before surgery.
   d. need to have time to sedate the patient.

8. Fifteen minutes before Mr. Grant's surgery, the laboratory calls to report an abnormal laboratory test. At this time, the nurse:

   a. attaches the report to the laboratory sheet in the chart.

   b. notifies the unit secretary.

   c. contacts the surgeon or anesthesiologist.

   d. calls the laboratory for verification of the test.

9. When reviewing a patient's chart in the postanesthesia recovery room, the nurse notices that the patient was given droperidol (Inapsine) and fentanyl (Sublimaze) for anesthesia. When checking a reference, the nurse reads that the combination of these two drugs is called:

   a. neuroleptic-analgesia.

   b. regional anesthesia.

   c. local infiltration anesthesia.

   d. epidural anesthesia.

10. In the postanesthesia recovery room, the nurse must exercise caution when administering narcotics. Before and after administering narcotics, the nurse must check the patient's:

   a. blood pressure.   c. reflexes.

   b. pulse rate.   d. respiratory rate.

IV. Crossword Puzzle

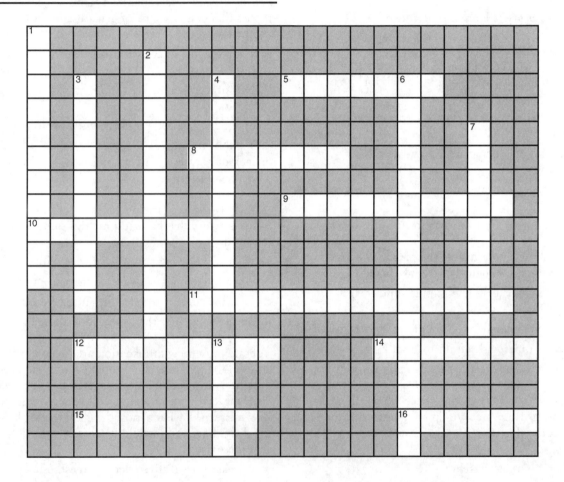

ACROSS CLUES

5. Type of anesthesia that provides a pain-free state for the entire body.
8. Trade name for glycopyrrolate.
9. Loss of feeling.
10. Begins with administration of an anesthetic drug and lasts until consciousness is lost.
11. Cholinergic blocking drug used to dry up secretions of the upper respiratory tract and decrease excessive mucus production during surgery.
12. Generic name for Versed.
14. Type of anesthesia that involves application of the agent to the surface of the skin.

15. Type of anesthesia injected around nerves so that the area supplied by these nerves will not send pain signals to the brain.
16. Type of anesthesia that involves the injection of a local anesthetic into the subarachnoid space of the spinal cord.

DOWN CLUES

1. Generic name for Vistaril.
2. A drug given prior to the administration of anesthesia.
3. Generic name for Demerol.
4. Anesthetic drug sometimes used to control convulsive states.
6. A physician with special training in administering anesthesia.
7. Type of drug used to decrease nausea and vomiting during the immediate postoperative period.
13. Type of anesthesia that provides a pain-free state in a specific area.

V. Dosage Problems

Solve the following dosage calculations.

1. The physician's order reads: Robinul, 200 mcg, IM on call to the OR. Drug available: glycopyrrolate, 0.4 mg/2 mL. How many milliliters will be administered for the dose ordered? _____

2. The physician's order reads: Vistaril, 25 mg, IM on call to OR. Drug available: Hydroxyzine, 50 mg/mL. The nurse will administer how many milliliters? _____

3. The physician's order reads: Versed, 5 mg, IM on call to OR. Drug available: Midazolam, 2 mg/mL, 0.05–0.08 mg/kg. The patient weighs 150 pounds.

   a) What is the patient's weight in kilograms?
   _____

   b) What is the safe dose range for your patient?
   _____

   c) Is the ordered dose within the safe range?
   _____

   d) How many milliliters will the nurse give?
   _____

VI. Critical Thinking

1. Mr. and Mrs. Jackson are in the emergency department with their 6-year-old daughter, who has a small laceration that requires sutures. Mrs. Jackson asks you if her little girl will have to be sedated. Discuss the information you would give the Jacksons about the anesthetic that will probably be used for their daughter.

2. Mr. James is admitted to the postanesthesia recovery room after an exploratory laparotomy. He appears to be in pain and has an order for the narcotic meperidine (Demerol), 75 mg, IM q4h, PRN for pain. Discuss the nursing task that is performed before giving this medication. Analyze the situation to determine what event might raise a question about whether this drug should be given. Give rationales for your answers.

CHAPTER 36

Antihistamines and Decongestants

I. Matching

Match each term in Column A with the correct definition or statement in Column B.

COLUMN A

_____ 1. antihistamine

_____ 2. anticholinergic effects

_____ 3. decongestant

_____ 4. histamine

_____ 5. basophil

_____ 6. rebound nasal congestion

_____ 7. drowsiness

_____ 8. Benadryl

_____ 9. desloratadine

_____ 10. additive sedative

COLUMN B

A. Substance produced by the body in response to injury, which causes dilation of the arterioles and an increased permeability of capillaries and venules.

B. Drugs used to counteract the effects of histamine on body organs and structures.

C. A type of white blood cell.

D. Generic name for Clarinex.

E. Dryness of the mouth, nose, and throat and a thickening of bronchial secretions.

F. Combining antihistamines and alcohol results in an _____ _____ effect.

G. Type of drug that reduces swelling of the nasal passages, resulting in opening of clogged nasal passages and enhancing drainage of the sinuses.

H. Adverse reaction seen with most of the antihistamines.

I. Nasal congestion that occurs as a result of over-use of the topical form of decongestants.

J. Trade name for diphenhydramine.

II. Fill in the Blanks

1. Examples of antihistamines include (*list the generic and trade names*):

   a) _____ _____

   b) _____ _____

   c) _____ _____

   d) _____ _____

   e) _____ _____

   f) _____ _____

2. The respiratory system consists of the _____ and _____ airways, the _____, and the _____ cavity.

3. Histamine acts on the _____ system and the _____ muscle, producing _____ of the arterioles and an _____ permeability of _____ and _____.

4. The body produces histamine and releases it in response to _____, _____ reactions, and _____ reactions.

5. Antihistamines are drugs used to _____ the effects of histamine on _____ _____ and _____.

6. _____ and _____ are _____ reactions seen with the use of many of the antihistamines.

160

Copyright © 2004 by Lippincott Williams & Wilkins. *Study Guide to Accompany Introductory Clinical Pharmacology*, seventh edition, by Bonnie J. Smith and Sally S. Roach.

7. Decongestants are used for the temporary relief of _____ _____ due to the _____ _____, _____ _____, _____, and other _____ allergies.

8. Decongestants are used as adjunctive therapy of _____ _____ infections to _____ congestion around the _____ tube.

9. Hypertensive crisis can result from the use of decongestants with the _____.

10. _____ of the topical form of decongestants can cause _____ nasal congestion.

III. Multiple Choice

Circle the letter of the most appropriate answer.

1. A patient with asthma is being seen in the clinic today with symptoms of seasonal allergies. The nurse knows that antihistamines are not routinely prescribed for patients with lower respiratory disorders because:
   a. the depressant effect may cause a hypotensive crisis.
   b. the drying effects of the drug may cause thickening of bronchial secretions.
   c. paradoxical excitement may occur as a result of stimulation of the CNS.
   d. antihistamines may irritate the bronchi, causing bronchospasm.

2. The nurse would expect the patient to experience fewer cholinergic effects with the administration of:
   a. promethazine.   c. loratadine.
   b. diphenhydramine.   d. hydroxyzine.

3. A patient has received an antihistamine to treat the symptoms of a severe allergic reaction. The nurse must assess the patient at frequent intervals until the symptoms of the reaction appear relieved and for:
   a. 24 hours after the incident.
   b. 12 hours after the incident.
   c. 2 hours after symptoms subside.
   d. 8 hours after symptoms subside.

4. The physician has prescribed an antihistamine for your 82-year-old patient. You would monitor this patient for:
   a. a decreased drug response.
   b. anticholinergic effects.
   c. stimulation of the CNS.
   d. hypertension.

5. Antihistamines may be administered together with a narcotic to achieve:
   a. decreased anticholinergic effects.
   b. decreased blood pressure.
   c. decreased seizure activity.
   d. an increase of the narcotic's sedative effect.

6. A nursing student asks the nurse how decongestants relieve nasal congestion. The nurse would be correct in stating:
   a. they produce localized vasodilation, allowing the sinuses to drain.
   b. they relieve swelling of the nasal passages by vasoconstriction of small blood vessels.
   c. they produce vasodilation, increasing production of nasal secretions.
   d. they thin the secretions, allowing easier passage through swollen nasal passages.

7. At a team conference, the nurse explains that decongestants produce localized:
   a. vasoconstriction.   c. congestion.
   b. vasodilation.   d. inflammation.

8. The nurse explains to the patient taking a decongestant that the drug is prescribed to:
   a. relieve congestion in the lungs.
   b. reduce the viscosity of respiratory secretions.
   c. enhance the drainage of the sinuses.
   d. encourage increased nasal secretions.

9. A patient experiencing rebound nasal congestion asks the nurse what causes this to occur. The nurse correctly states:
   a. the decongestant was not used often enough.
   b. this occurs as a result of overuse of the decongestant.
   c. this always occurs with nasal decongestants.
   d. less frequent use of the decongestant has caused increased mucus production.

10. The antihistamine that needs to be administered
    1 hour before meals or 2 hours after is:

   a. loratadine.

   b. diphenhydramine.

   c. promethazine.

   d. hydroxyzine.

IV. Crossword Puzzle

ACROSS CLUES

1. Type of white blood cell.
4. Generic name for Allegra.
6. Substance produced in the body in response to injury.
7. Body system that provides a mechanism for exchange of oxygen and carbon dioxide in the lungs.
8. Generic name for Claritin.
11. Generic name for Clarinex.
12. Common adverse reaction seen with many antihistamines.

DOWN CLUES

2. Drug classification of gexofenadine.
3. Example of a decongestant.
5. Type of drug that reduces swelling of the nasal passages.
9. Trade name for diphen-hydramine hydrochloride.
10. Trade name for cetirizine.

V. Dosage Problems

Solve the following dosage calculations.

1. The physician's order reads: Vistaril, 25 mg, PO, QID for pruritus. The drug available is hydroxyzine pamoate, oral suspension, 25 mg/5 mL.

   a) How many milliliters will be administered at each dose? _____

   b) What is the total milligram dosage per 24 hours? _____

2. The physician's order reads: Tavist, 1.34 mg, PO, BID. The available drug is clemastine fumarate syrup, 0.67 mg/5 mL.

   a) How many milliliters will be administered at each dose? _____

   b) What will be the total milligram dosage for each 24-hour period? _____

3. An 8-year old patient has been prescribed Polaramine, 1 mg, PO, every 6 hours. The drug available is dexchlorpheniramine maleate syrup, 2 mg/5 mL. The nurse would instruct the parent to give how many milliliters at each dose?

   _____

VI. Critical Thinking

1. You are the nurse on duty at the college health center. Mark, a freshman, comes to the clinic complaining of seasonal pollen allergies that have worsened significantly since his relocation at college. He has been self-treating his symptoms with over-the-counter (OTC) medications that a friend in the dorm gave him. Discuss what questions you might ask Mark about his symptoms and the information he needs for informed use of OTC allergy medication.

2. Mr. Martin, an elderly man with a history of diabetes and hypertension, has a cold. The resident in the emergency department does not know Mr. Martin well and prescribes pseudoephedrine (Sudafed) to relieve nasal congestion. The nurse administers the medication as ordered. Discuss the nurse's responsibility in this situation and the impact this drug will have on Mr. Martin.

CHAPTER 37

Bronchodilators and Antiasthma Drugs

I. Matching

Match each term in Column A with the correct definition or statement in Column B.

COLUMN A

_____1.   prophylaxis

_____2.   asthma

_____3.   leukotrienes

_____4.   extrinsic

_____5.   sympathomimetic

_____6.   intrinsic

_____7.   theophyllinization

_____8.   mixed

_____9.   bronchodilator

_____10. xanthine derivatives

_____11. emphysema

_____12. chronic bronchitis

_____13. COPD

_____14. dyspnea

_____15. mast cell stabilizers

COLUMN B

A. Lung disorder in which the terminal bronchioles or alveoli become enlarged and plugged with mucus.

B. Prevention.

C. Type of asthma caused by both intrinsic and extrinsic factors.

D. Chronic inflammation and possible infection of the bronchi.

E. Type of asthma, also referred to as allergic asthma, occurring in response to an allergen such as pollen, dust, and animal dander.

F. Difficulty breathing.

G. A drug used to relieve bronchospasm associated with respiratory disorders such as bronchial asthma, chronic bronchitis, and emphysema.

H. Chronic obstructive pulmonary disease, a name given collectively to emphysema and chronic bronchitis because obstruction to the airflow is present most of the time.

I. Drug that mimics the sympathetic nervous system, used primarily to treat reversible airway obstruction caused by bronchospasm associated with respiratory conditions and diseases.

J. Drugs that stimulate the central nervous system, resulting in bronchodilation.

K. A respiratory condition characterized by recurrent attacks of dyspnea and wheezing caused by spasmodic constriction of the bronchi.

L. Bronchoconstrictive substances released by the body during the inflammatory process.

M. Drugs that prevent the mast cells in the respiratory tract from releasing substances that cause bronchoconstriction and inflammation.

N. Accomplished by giving the patient a higher initial dose, called a *loading dose*, to bring blood levels to a therapeutic range more quickly.

O. Type of asthma, also known as nonallergic asthma, caused by chronic or recurrent respiratory infections, emotional upset, and exercise.

II. Fill in the Blanks

1. List the two major types of bronchodilators.

   a) _____

   b) _____

2. Use of bronchodilating drug _____ the bronchi and allows _____ air to _____ the lungs, which in turn _____ or _____ relieves _____ _____.

3. Administration of a sympathomimetic bronchodilator may result in the following reactions:

a) _____

b) _____

c) _____

d) _____

e) _____

f) _____

4. List the xanthine derivatives classified as pregnancy category C drugs.

a) _____

b) _____

c) _____

d) _____

5. List the corticosteroids used as antiasthma drugs (*include the generic and trade names*).

a) _____ _____

b) _____ _____

c) _____ _____

d) _____ _____

e) _____ _____

6. Leukotriene receptor antagonists include

_____ _____ and _____ _____

_____. _____ _____ is classified as a

leukotriene formation inhibitor.

7. The leukotriene receptor antagonists inhibit

_____ receptor sites in the _____ tract,

preventing _____ _____ and facilitating

_____.

8. Mast cell stabilizers include (*list the generic and trade names*):

a) _____ _____

b) _____ _____

9. The patient taking theophylline may complain of

_____ because the drug relaxes the lower

_____ _____, allowing _____ reflux.

10. Symptoms associated with serum theophylline levels greater than 35 mcg/mL would include:

a) _____

b) _____

c) _____

d) _____

e) _____

f) _____

III. Multiple Choice

Circle the letter of the most appropriate answer.

1. A patient is receiving albuterol sulfate for treatment of bronchospasm. The nurse would monitor the patient for adverse reactions associated with drugs of this type. These reactions could include:

a. weight gain, bradycardia.

b. anorexia, hypoglycemia.

c. cardiac arrhythmias and insomnia.

d. sedation, nausea, and vomiting.

2. Mr. Moore is being treated with zileuton (Zyflo) as prophylaxis treatment for bronchial asthma. The nurse will anticipate the primary care provider ordering periodic laboratory tests to monitor:

a. hepatic function.

b. respiratory function.

c. cardiac function.

d. gastrointestinal function.

3. A patient with asthma is receiving triamcinolone (Azmacort) as prophylactic therapy in the maintenance treatment of the disease. The nurse must teach the patient to use strict oral hygiene to prevent:

a. hyperplasia of gingival tissue.

b. an unpleasant taste in the mouth.

c. the occurrence of oral candidiasis.

d. gastroesophageal reflux disease.

4. The physician has ordered daily plasma theophylline levels for a patient receiving a sustained-release theophylline preparation. To measure the levels at peak absorption, the blood needs to be obtained:

    a. 5 to 9 hours after morning dose.

    b. 1 to 2 hours after morning dose.

    c. 30 minutes after morning dose.

    d. 12 hours after morning dose.

5. Your patient has been receiving aminophylline for prevention of bronchial asthma. Adverse reactions you could expect from this type of bronchodilator would include:

    a. hypoglycemia, hypothyroidism.

    b. tachycardia, increased respirations.

    c. bradycardia, constriction of bronchi.

    d. drowsiness, lethargy.

6. Which of these drugs, if ordered, would the nurse withhold for a patient experiencing an acute asthma attack?

    a. Epinephrine   c. Terbutaline

    b. Albuterol   d. Salmeterol

7. As a nurse, your would know that formoterol fumarate is administered only by inhalation using:

    a. a nebulizer.

    b. a peak flow meter.

    c. the aerolizer inhaler.

    d. a metered-dose inhaler.

8. A new nurse is having difficulty identifying the sounds that occur in the respiratory tract of the patient experiencing an asthma attack. You explain that when bronchospasm occurs, the lumen of the bronchi decreases and narrows, producing a musical sound with breathing that the nurse documents as:

    a. crackles.   c. rales.

    b. wheezing.   d. rattling.

9. A nurse is teaching a patient about his newly prescribed inhaler. The medication, salmeterol (Serevent), is being used as a preventative for bronchospasm induced by exercise. The nurse stresses the importance of not using the inhaler more often than ordered because of the possibility of _____ occurring.

    a. occipital headache

    b. heart block

    c. paradoxical bronchospasm

    d. narcoleptic episodes

10. Patients prescribed aminophylline must be aware of certain dietary restrictions with bronchodilators of this type. Foods to avoid would include:

    a. green leafy vegetables.   c. citrus fruits.

    b. coffee and colas.   d. fish.

11. The physician has changed an asthma patient's medication to zafirlukast (Accolate). In reviewing the patient record, the nurse finds that the patient also takes warfarin (Coumadin). The nurse wold expect the physician to order laboratory tests to check the:

    a. BUN.   c. H and H.

    b. CBC.   d. PT.

12. An example of a mast cell stabilizer is:

    a. cromolyn.   c. zafirlukast.

    b. zileuton.   d. epinephrine.

13. Patient teaching for the drug cromolyn would include:

    a. mix with any liquid and drink with meals.

    b. mix with milk only and drink after meals.

    c. mix with water and drink 1/2 hour before meals.

    d. open ampule and place contents directly on tongue.

14. A nurse working in the urgent care unit is caring for a patient with symptoms of an acute asthma attack. The symptoms manifested by the attack include:

    a. dyspnea and wheezing.

    b. lethargy and somnolence.

    c. slow, deep respirations.

    d. bradycardia with hypertension.

15. When assessing the patient experiencing an acute asthma attack, the nurse will monitor the patient closely for signs and symptoms of hypoxia, which include:

    a. mental alertness.

    b. restlessness.

    c. pink mucous membranes.

    d. somnolence.

IV. Crossword Puzzle

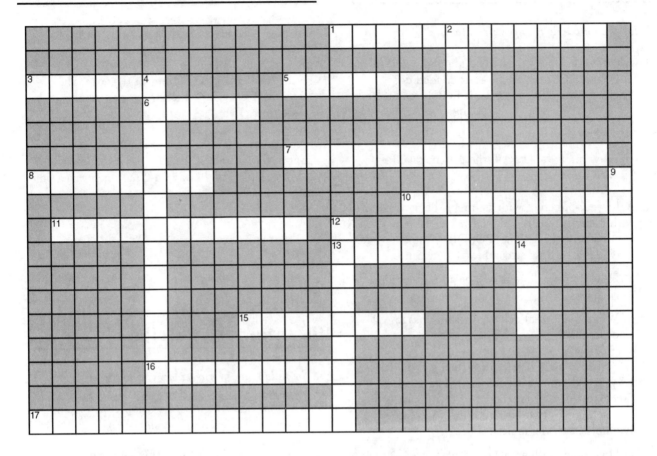

ACROSS CLUES

1. Bronchoconstrictive substances released by the body during the inflammatory process.
3. A respiratory condition characterized by recurrent attacks of dyspnea and wheezing due to constriction of the bronchi.
5. Trade name for budesonide.
6. Type of asthma caused by both intrinsic and extrinsic factors.
7. Generic name for Beclovent.
8. Trade name for triamcinolone.
10. Drug that is contraindicated during acute bronchospasm.
11. Prevention.
13. Type of asthma also known as nonallergic asthma.
15. Generic name for Zyflo.
16. Lung disorder in which the terminal bronchioles or alveoli become enlarged and plugged with mucus.
17. Drug type used to relieve bronchospasm.

DOWN CLUES

2. Example of a sympathomimetic bronchodilator.
4. Example of a xanthine derivative used as a bronchodilator.
9. Generic name for Flonase.
12. Trade name for montelukast sodium.
14. Progressive disorder of the respiratory tract characterized by a decrease in the inspiratory and expiratory capacity of the lung. (abbreviation)

V. Dosage Problems

Solve the following dosage calculations.

1. A patient has been prescribed aminophylline, 1600 mg, PO, each day in four divided doses. The aminophylline is available in 200-mg tablets.

   a) How many milligrams will be administered for each dose? _____

   b) How many tablets will the patient take for each dose? _____

2. A 13-year-old child with asthma is being treated with metaproterenol (Alupent). The dose ordered for this patient is 20 mg, PO, QID. Alupent syrup is available in dose strength of 10 mg/5 mL.

   a) How many milliliters will be administered at each dose? _____

   b) What is the total daily milligram dosage ordered? _____

3. Prophylaxis treatment of bronchial asthma for a 15-year-old patient includes zafirlukast (Accolate). The ordered dose of zafirlukast is 40 mg each day in two divided doses. Accolate is available in 20-mg tablets.

   a) How many milligrams of accolate are taken at each dose? _____

   b) How many tablets will the patient take each dose? _____

4. A patient is taking a low-dose corticosteroid as part of his asthma therapy: triamcinolone, 10 mg, PO, each day before 9:00 AM. The medication is available in syrup form, 4 mg/5 mL. How many milliliters of the syrup must be administered for the ordered dose? _____

VI. Critical Thinking

1. Grace, a 12-year-old middle school student, was recently diagnosed with asthma. She uses two inhalers four times a day, in addition to using a rescue inhaler during periods of dyspnea. She is also taking peak flow measurements. As the school nurse, you are responsible for overseeing Grace's care while she is in school. School regulations usually require that all medication be kept in the nurse's office. Discuss what impact this regulation might have if Grace experiences an asthma attack.

VII. Internet Exercise

Use the following Internet addresses to locate information on any current clinical trials being conducted for new treatments of asthma. Be prepared for classroom discussion of this subject.

http://www.mayoclinic.com/index.cfm
http://www.treatments-for-asthma.com/
http://www.nih.gov/
http://www.healthfinder.gov/
http://health.nih.gov/

CHAPTER 38

Antitussives, Mucolytics, and Expectorants

I. Matching

Match each term in Column A with the correct definition or statement in Column B.

COLUMN A

_____ 1. antitussive

_____ 2. acetylcysteine

_____ 3. mucolytic

_____ 4. guaifenesin

_____ 5. nonproductive cough

_____ 6. expectorant

_____ 7. coughing

_____ 8. viscosity

_____ 9. benzonatate

_____ 10. productive cough

COLUMN B

A. Cough that expels secretions from the lower repiratory tract.

B. A dry, hacking cough that produces no secretions.

C. A drug used to relieve a nonproductive cough.

D. The forceful expulsion of air from the lungs.

E. A drug that loosens respiratory secretions.

F. A drug that aids in raising thick, tenacious mucus from the respiratory passages by increasing production of sputum.

G. A mucolytic drug used as adjunct treatment of acetaminophen overdosage.

H. Thickness.

I. Example of an expectorant.

J. Example of a peripherally acting antitussive.

II. Fill in the Blanks

1. List the two types of antitussives used to treat coughs.

   a) _____

   b) _____

2. Terpin hydrate is classified as both a _____ and an _____.

3. The centrally acting antitussives _____ the _____ _____ located in the _____.

4. Depression of the cough _____ can cause a _____ of _____ in the lungs.

5. Acetylcysteine is an example of a _____ drug.

6. Expectorants _____ the production of _____ secretions, which in turn appears to _____ the _____ of the mucus.

III. Multiple Choice

Circle the letter of the most appropriate answer.

1. A patient's wife asks why the medication her husband is receiving isn't stopping his cough. The nurse explains that the patient's medication is a mucolytic and its action is to:

   a. increase the production of respiratory secretions.

   b. reduce the viscosity of respiratory secretions.

   c. depress the cough center in the brain.

   d. anesthetize the stretch receptors in the respiratory passages.

2. A nurse asks why an antitussive cannot be used for every type of cough. The team leader responds that an antitussive is most appropriate for treatment of a:

   a. productive cough.

   b. nonbacterial upper respiratory infection.

   c. nonproductive cough.

   d. bacterial upper respiratory infection.

3. A new nurse asks what danger may be associated with depression of the cough reflex. The team leader correctly answers that, on occasion, an antitussive may:

   a. cause a pooling of secretions in the lungs.

   b. result in an increase in the respiratory rate.

   c. decrease the viscosity of respiratory secretions.

   d. result in a decrease in the respiratory rate.

4. The team leader asks the new nurse what nurses should do when a patient has a productive cough. The nurse would be correct in stating that the nurse should:

   a. keep the patient seated in a chair most of the day.

   b. keep the patient lying flat in bed.

   c. document in the patient record the number of coughing episodes.

   d. observe and record the appearance and amount of the sputum.

5. If an antitussive is prescribed for use at home, the nurse can advise the patient to:

   a. limit fluid intake until the cough is relieved.

   b. not exceed the recommended dose.

   c. add extra carbohydrates to the diet.

   d. remain in bed until the cough is relieved.

6. When acetylcysteine (Mucomyst) is administered to a patient by nebulization, the nurse will expect to see a(n):

   a. increase in the amount of sputum.

   b. increase in the viscosity of the sputum.

   c. decrease in the viscosity of the sputum.

   d. decrease in the amount of sputum.

7. After administration of guaifenesin (Hytuss) to a patient, the nurse will expect to see a(n):

   a. increase in the viscosity of mucus.

   b. increase in mucus production and a decrease in the viscosity of the mucus.

   c. decrease in mucus production.

   d. decrease in mucus production and an increase in the viscosity of the mucus.

8. Discharge instructions for the patient who will be using a drug nebulizer at home should include:

   a. a list of companies for the patient to contact about equipment.

   b. instructions to clean the equipment at least monthly.

   c. instructions to relax in a reclining position during the treatment.

   d. instructions to observe for misting as evidence of proper equipment function.

9. The nurse is completing an assessment of a client who is visiting the clinic with an upper respiratory infection that is causing a nonproductive cough. The patient states, "I can't sleep because of this cough." The nurse determines that the appropriate nursing diagnosis for this patient would be:

   a. Ineffective Airway Clearance related to cough.

   b. Disturbed Sleep Pattern related to coughing at night.

   c. Ineffective Breathing Pattern related to thick sputum.

   d. Disturbed Sleep Pattern related to medication regimen.

10. You are caring for a patient who is postoperative from eye surgery. The patient has started to exhibit a nonproductive cough. The physician is in the process of writing orders for this patient. The nurse asks the physician to write an order for:

    a. a nonnarcotic antitussive.

    b. a mucolytic.

    c. an expectorant.

    d. an antitussive with codeine.

IV. Crossword Puzzle

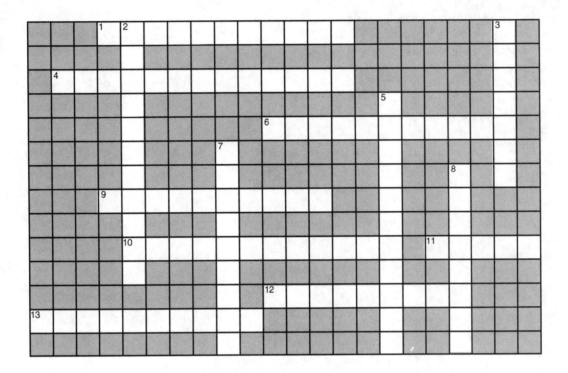

ACROSS CLUES

1. Example of a peripherally acting antitussive.
4. A dry, hacking cough that produces no secretions.
6. Drug used to relieve coughing.
9. A cough that produces secretions from the lower respiratory tract.
10. Acetylcysteine is administered by _____.
11. Forceful expulsion of air from the lungs.
12. Thickness.
13. Trade name for guaifenesin.

DOWN CLUES

2. Drug that aids in raising mucus from the respiratory passages.
3. What action do some antitussives have on the cough center?
5. Example of an expectorant.
7. Drug that loosens respiratory secretions.
8. Trade name for acetylcysteine.

V. Dosage Problems

Solve the following dosage calculations.

1. The physician's order reads: guaifenesin, 300 mg, PO, q4h. Available drug: Robitussin liquid, 200 mg/5 mL. How many milliliters of medication will be administered at each dose? _____

2. The physician's order reads: dextromethorphan, 60 mg, PO, BID. Available drug: dextromethorphan sustained action liquid, 30 mg/5 mL. How many milliliters will be given at each dose? _____

3. The physician's order reads: benzonatate, 200 mg, PO, TID. Available drug: Tessalon Perles, 100-mg capsules. How many capsules will the patient take with each dose? _____

VI. Critical Thinking

1. Your next-door neighbor knows you are a nurse and is always asking you for medical advice. Today she has asked you to recommend a cough medicine for her. She tells you she has a low-grade fever and a dry, hacking cough. Discuss how you should address your neighbor's questions about her health problems and the advice you could give her about over-the-counter cough products.

CHAPTER 39

Cardiotonics and Miscellaneous Inotropic Drugs

I. Matching

Match each term in Column A with the correct definition or statement in Column B.

COLUMN A

_____ 1. atrial fibrillation

_____ 2. cardiac glycosides

_____ 3. cardiac output

_____ 4. Digibind

_____ 5. digitalis toxicity

_____ 6. digitalization

_____ 7. heart failure

_____ 8. hypokalemia

_____ 9. left ventricular failure

_____ 10. neurohormonal activity

_____ 11. positive inotropic action

_____ 12. right ventricular failure

_____ 13. digoxin

_____ 14. bigeminy

_____ 15. trigeminy

COLUMN B

A. The most commonly used cardiotonic drug.

B. Drug administered when digoxin overdosage occurs.

C. Toxicity that occurs from the cumulative effect of digitalis.

D. Drugs used to increase the efficiency and improve contraction of the heart.

E. A condition in which the heart cannot pump enough blood to meet the tissue needs of the body.

F. Leads to pulmonary symptoms such as dyspnea and moist cough.

G. The amount of blood leaving the left ventricle with each contraction.

H. Drug action that causes an increase in the force of the contraction of the muscle of the heart.

I. A cardiac arrhythmia characterized by rapid contractions of the atrial myocardium resulting in an irregular and often rapid ventricular rate.

J. Leads to neck vein distention, peripheral edema, weight gain, and hepatic engorgement.

K. Series of doses given until the drug begins to exert a full therapeutic effect.

L. Low serum potassium levels.

M. Two heartbeats followed by a pause.

N. Three heartbeats followed by a pause.

O. Secretion of neurohormones is increased, which results in increased heart rate and vasoconstriction.

II. Fill in the Blanks

1. List the most common symptoms associated with left ventricular failure.

   a) _____

   b) _____

   c) _____

   d) _____

2. List the most common symptoms associated with right ventricular failure.

   a) _____

   b) _____

   c) _____

   d) _____

   e) _____

   f) _____

3. _____ _____ _____ is the most

   common form of _____ _____ and results

   in _____ cardiac output and _____

   ejection fraction.

4. Diastolic heart failure occurs as the _____ do

   not _____ adequately becoming _____

   and unable to _____ during diastole.

5. List the two types of drugs that have become the treatment of choice for heart failure over the last several years.

   a) _____

   b) _____

6. _____ _____ is the most commonly used

   cardiotonic drug.

7. Miscellaneous drugs with _____ inotropic action, such as _____ and _____, are nonglycosides used in the _____ management of heart failure.

8. List the two actions of digitalis.

   a) _____

   b) _____

9. Uses of the cardiotonics include:

   a) _____

   b) _____

10. List five contraindications to the use of the cardiotonics.

    a) _____

    b) _____

    c) _____

    d) _____

    e) _____

III. Multiple Choice

Circle the letter of the most appropriate answer.

Mr. Martin is admitted to the hospital with heart failure. His physician orders digoxin, 0.25 mg, IV, q8h for 24 hours, followed by digoxin, 0.125 mg, PO, daily. Questions 1–5 pertain to Mr. Martin's case.

1. Mrs. Martin asks the nurse to explain the term *loading dose*, stating that the doctor has used the term when discussing her husband's care. The nurse would be correct in stating:

   a. that is something that you must ask the doctor.

   b. the first dose you receive is the loading dose.

   c. loading dose is the manner by which the doctor calculates the amount of drug you need.

   d. loading dose is a series of doses of the medication given until the drug begins to exert a full therapeutic effect.

2. Three days after beginning digoxin therapy, Mr. Martin develops nausea and complains of blurred vision. What action should the nurse take?

   a. Keep the patient on bed rest until nausea subsides.

   b. Request an order for an antiemetic.

   c. Contact the physician immediately.

   d. Monitor the patient closely for the next 24 hours.

3. Mr. Martin's serum digoxin level is 2.1 ng/mL. The nurse anticipates that the physician will:

   a. change the medication to a different cardiotonic.

   b. discontinue the order for the digoxin.

   c. discontinue the use of the cardiac monitor.

   d. increase the dosage of the drug digoxin.

4. The nurse is reviewing Mr. Martin's laboratory reports. Which condition is most likely to increase the possibility of Mr. Martin developing digitalis toxicity?

   a. Hypomagnesemia   c. Hypocalcemia

   b. Hyperkalemia   d. Hypercalcemia

5. Which of the following points would the nurse include when providing discharge teaching for Mr. Martin?

   a. Vision changes are common and clear with continued use of your medications.

   b. Take this drug with an antacid to enhance the absorption.

   c. Take this drug at the same time every day.

   d. Discontinue the drug when you can walk 1 mile each day.

6. During an assessment of the patient with right ventricular dysfunction, the nurse would expect to find:

   a. restlessness.

   b. swollen ankles and legs.

   c. orthopnea.

   d. wheezing.

7. A patient is to receive a loading dose of digoxin of 0.25 mg IV. The nurse is aware that the first dose of the loading dose will be:

   a. 0.25 mg.   c. 0.05 mg.

   b. 0.025 mg.   d. 0.125 mg.

8. Mr. King has finished his loading dose of digoxin and the nurse is preparing his maintenance dose. With digoxin maintenance dosing, the nurse will know to observe for signs of digitalis toxicity:

   a. one to two times a day.

   b. every 3 or 4 hours.

   c. every other day.

   d. four or five times a day.

9. Cardiotonic drugs may be administered orally, intravenously, and intramuscularly. Which method of administration is not recommended for these drugs?

   a. Crushing the tablets

   b. Slow IV

   c. Intramuscular

   d. Mixing the drugs with food

10. Ms. Moore has been taking digoxin for 2 months and she is in the clinic today for her weekly visit to have her serum digoxin level checked. The lab slip shows her digoxin level to be 1.1 ng/mL. The nurse would recognize this laboratory value to be:

    a. indicative of toxicity.

    b. less than the therapeutic level.

    c. requiring a dose of Digibind.

    d. at the therapeutic level.

11. A patient is being discharged from the hospital with a prescription for digoxin. The nurse knows it is imperative that the patient demonstrate proficiency in the task of taking his:

    a. blood pressure.   c. temperature.

    b. radial pulse.   d. respiratory rate.

12. Before administering a cardiotonic, the nurse knows to check the patient's apical pulse by counting for:

    a. 10 seconds and multiplying by six.

    b. 30 seconds and multiplying by two.

    c. 1 full minute.

    d. 15 seconds and multiplying by four.

IV. Crossword Puzzle

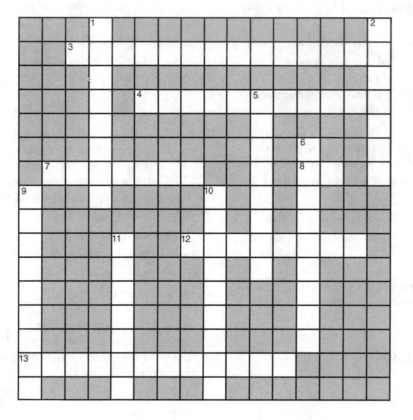

ACROSS CLUES

3. A series of doses of digitalis given until the drug begins to exert a full therapeutic effect.
4. Low serum potassium levels.
7. Trade name for digoxin.
8. Route used when administering amrinone (abbreviation).
12. Drug administered when digoxin overdose occurs.
13. Drugs used to increase the efficiency of heart muscle contraction.

DOWN CLUES

1. Two heartbeats followed by a pause.
2. Type of drug that may decrease plasma digitalis levels.
5. Symptom of digitalis toxicity.
6. Most commonly used miscellaneous inotropic drug.
9. Class of drug that increases the risks of toxicity when taken with a digitalis glycoside.
10. Three heartbeats followed by a pause.
11. The most commonly used cardiotonic drug.

V. Dosage Problems

Solve the following dosage calculations.

1. The physician's order reads: Digoxin, 125 mcg, PO, OD. Available drug: Lanoxin Elixir, 50 mcg/mL. How many milliliters will be administered? _____

2. The physician's order reads: Digoxin 0.125 mg, IV, first dose of loading dose followed in 8 hours with 0.125 mg, IV, second dose of loading dose. Available drug: 0.5 mg/2 mL solution, digoxin. How many milliliters will be administered for each dose of the loading dose of digoxin?

   _____

3. The physician's order reads: Digoxin, 100 mcg, IM, qd. Available drug: Digoxin injection, 0.5 mg/2 mL. How many milliliters will be administered each day? _____

VI. Critical Thinking

1. You have just started your 12-hour shift with five patients assigned to your care. As you are making your rounds and completing the patient assessment on your last patient, Paul Moore, you find Mr. Moore with vital signs of 120/94, 110, 34 and labored. Mr. Moore's respiratory assessment reveals coarse ronchi and wheezing bilaterally. His urine output has been less than 30 cc per hour, and on weighing him you find he has a weight gain of 10 pounds over the last 2 days. You place Mr. Moore in a high Fowler's position and notify his physician of your assessment findings. After examining Mr. Moore, the physician orders digoxin, 0.25 mg, IV, STAT; repeat in 4 hours; then give 0.125 mg qd. Discuss Mr. Moore's symptoms and give the rationale for the physician's order.

2. Discuss the physiology of the electrical conduction system of the heart and how the system responds to compensate for the effects of heart failure. Explain what happens when the cardiotonics are administered to the patient with heart failure; include the effects of these drugs on the heart, kidneys, and other vital organs.

CHAPTER 40

Antiarrhythmic Drugs

I. Matching

Match each term in Column A with the correct definition or statement in Column B.

COLUMN A

_____ 1. action potential

_____ 2. blockade effect

_____ 3. electrocardiogram (ECG)

_____ 4. amiodarone

_____ 5. arrhythmia

_____ 6. depolarization

_____ 7. refractory period

_____ 8. half-life

_____ 9. proarrhythmic effect

_____ 10. diastole

COLUMN B

A. A disturbance or irregularity in the heart rate, rhythm, or both that requires administration of one of the antiarrhythmic drugs.

B. Provides a record of the electrical activity of the heart.

C. An electrical impulse that passes from cell to cell in the myocardium, stimulating the fibers to shorten and causing muscular contraction (systole).

D. The relaxation phase that occurs after systole.

E. Period between the transmission of nerve impulses along a nerve fiber.

F. Blocking the effect of the neurohormones that increase heart rate.

G. Effect that can occur when antiarrhythmics are used to treat an existing arrhythmia and new arrhythmias are created or existing arrhythmias are worsened.

H. Pregnancy Category D drug.

I. Time required for the blood level of a drug to decrease by 50%.

J. Movement of cellular ions; positive ions move from outside into the cell, and negative ions move from inside the cell to outside.

II. Fill in the Blanks

1. List the cardiac arrhythmias identified in this chapter.

   a) _____

   b) _____

   c) _____

   d) _____

   e) _____

   f) _____

   g) _____

2. An arrhythmia that results from heartbeats originating in the ventricles instead of the SA node and causes the ventricles to contract before the atria is identified as a _____

   _____ _____.

3. _____ _____ is the rapid contraction of the atria at a rate too rapid for the ventricles to pump efficiently.

4. _____ _____ is a rapid heartbeat with a rate of more than 100 beats per minute, usually originating in the ventricles.

5. An ECG provides a graphical record of the

   _____ _____ of the _____.

6. The goal of antiarrhythmic drug therapy is to

   restore _____ _____ _____

   and to prevent _____ _____

   _____.

7. List the general adverse reactions common to
   most antiarrhythmic drugs.

   a) _____

   b) _____

   c) _____

   d) _____

   e) _____

8. Two antiarrhythmic drugs contraindicated in
   patients with myasthenia gravis are:

   a) _____

   b) _____

9. When monitoring a patient receiving lidocaine
   for treatment of arrhythmias, the nurse must
   observe the patient closely for:

   a) _____

   b) _____

   c) _____

   d) _____

   e) _____

   f) _____

10. Monitoring for signs and symptoms of
    agranulocytosis is important when
    administering:

    a) _____

    b) _____

    c) _____

    d) _____

    e) _____

III. Multiple Choice

Circle the letter of the most appropriate answer.

Mr. Tate, age 56 years, is admitted to the hospital
with a possible myocardial infarction. He has
developed a cardiac arrhythmia and his physician
orders an antiarrhythmic drug. Questions 1–4
pertain to Mr. Tate's case.

1. While Mr. Tate is being treated with an antiarrhythmic, the nurse should:

   a. assess blood pressure, apical and radial
      pulses, and respiratory rate every 1 to 4
      hours.

   b. restrict fluids during the evening hours.

   c. encourage Mr. Tate to eat a high-calorie diet
      to increase his energy level.

   d. monitor Mr. Tate's blood glucose level for
      hyperglycemia.

2. Mr. Tate is given disopyramide (Norpace) and
   has been experiencing a dry mouth. To relieve
   his discomfort, the nurse may:

   a. suggest he have his family bring in ice cream.

   b. offer him frequent sips of water.

   c. suggest he drink less water so as not to
      stimulate his thirst.

   d. offer him coffee between meals.

3. Which one of the following pulse rates would
   indicate to the nurse that the physician needs to
   be notified?

   a. Pulse rate above 60 beats per minute

   b. Pulse rate above 80 beats per minute

   c. Rate does not remain between 60 and 70
      beats per minute

   d. Rate above 120 or below 60 beats per minute

4. Mr. Tate will be taking disopyramide (Norpace)
   when he is discharged home. The nurse will
   need to teach Mr. Tate and his family to:

   a. monitor his pulse rate.

   b. measure his own intake and output.

   c. monitor and measure his respiratory rate.

   d. avoid all forms of physical exercise.

5. During the administration of quinidine, the nurse must monitor for signs of cinchonism, which include:

   a. tingling in the hands and feet, insomnia, rash.

   b. edema, lung congestion, abdominal pain.

   c. ringing in the ears, headache, dizziness.

   d. occipital headache, hypertension, rash.

6. The initial preadministration assessment the nurse performs before initiating therapy for a patient who is to receive an antiarrhythmic drug would include:

   a. a baseline blood pressure, pulse, and respiratory rate.

   b. keeping the patient NPO except for other medications.

   c. monitoring blood glucose levels before each meal.

   d. ordering an electroencephalogram and electrocardiogram.

7. Patients who are being treated with quinidine have periodic laboratory tests to determine if the plasma levels of quinidine are within the therapeutic range, which is:

   a. 1 to 1.9 mcg/mL.   c. 8 to 8.9 mcg/mL.

   b. 2 to 6 mcg/mL.   d. 0.5 to 1.9 mcg/mL.

8. During the initial treatment with bretylium, the nurse observes an increase in arrhythmias and an elevation of blood pressure. The nurse must be aware that this situation is:

   a. life-threatening and must be reported to the physician immediately.

   b. a sign that the dosage administered is too large and should be discontinued immediately.

   c. a transient increase in arrhythmias and hypertension that occurs within 1 hour of initial therapy with bretylium.

   d. an indication that the dosage should be increased and notify the physician immediately.

9. When lidocaine is being administered intravenously for life-threatening arrhythmias, the nurse must monitor the blood pressure and respiratory rate every:

   a. 6 to 10 minutes.

   b. 30 minutes to 1 hour.

   c. hour.

   d. 2 to 5 minutes.

10. The nurse must be aware that when administering disopyramide (Norpace), the patient may experience the adverse reaction of:

    a. diarrhea and anorexia.

    b. edema of the hands.

    c. postural hypertension.

    d. hypertensive crisis.

11. Quinidine is prescribed for a patient with myasthenia gravis. The nurse must be aware that:

    a. quinidine is contraindicated in patients with myasthenia gravis.

    b. quinidine will help to improve the symptoms of myasthenia gravis.

    c. quinidine must be given with caution in patients with myasthenia gravis.

    d. the risk of cinchonism is increased in this patient.

12. After discontinuing quinidine, the primary care provider prescribes disopyramide. The nurse must administer:

    a. the initial dose of disopyramide before the last dose of quinidine.

    b. the first dose of disopyramide 6 to 12 hours after the last dose of quinidine.

    c. the first dose of disopyramide 24 hours after the last dose of quinidine.

    d. the first dose of disopyramide 3 to 4 hours after the last dose of quinidine.

IV. Crossword Puzzle

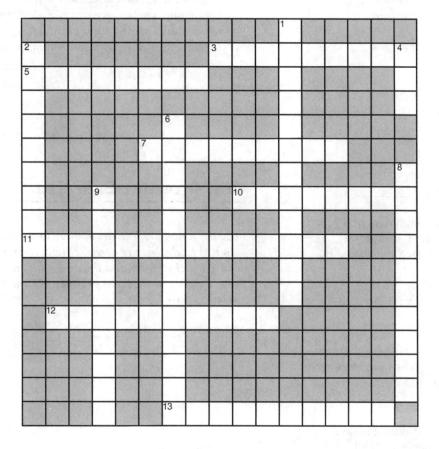

ACROSS CLUES

3. Example of a class 1-B antiarrhythmic drug.
5. Time required for the blood level of a drug to decrease by 50% (two words).
7. Most widely used class III antiarrhythmic drug.
10. The relaxation phase that occurs after systole.
11. Condition when a stimulus passes along a nerve and causes positive ions to move from outside the cell into the cell and the negative ions to move from inside the cell to outside the cell.
12. Disturbance or irregularity in the heart rate, rhythm, or both.
13. Quinidine toxicity.

DOWN CLUES

1. Condition when the nerve cells have positive ions on the outside and negative ions on the inside of the membrane.
2. Term used to describe any stimulus of the lowest intensity that will give rise to a response in a nerve fiber.
4. Provides a record of the electrical activity of the heart (abbreviation).

6. An effect of the antiarrhythmic drugs causing arrhythmias even though they are administered to resolve an existing arrhythmia.
8. Period between the transmission of a nerve impulses along a nerve fiber.
9. Cardiac muscle.

V. Dosage Problems

Solve the following dosage calculations.

1. A patient is receiving lidocaine at a rate of 20 mL/hour. The solution available is 1 gram lidocaine in 500 mL D_5W. Calculate the following:

   a) milligrams/hour _____

   b) milligrams/minute _____

2. A lidocaine drip is infusing at 22 mL/hour. The solution available is 2 grams lidocaine in 250 mL D_5W. Calculate the following:

   a) milligrams/hour _____

   b) milligrams/minute _____

3. A patient is receiving bretylium at 30 micro gtt/minute. The solution available is 2 grams bretylium in 500 mL D_5W. Calculate the following:

   a) milligrams/hour _____

   b) milligrams/minute _____

4. A patient is receiving bretylium at 45 micro gtt/minute. The solution available is 2 grams bretylium in 500 mL D_5W. Calculate the following:

   a) milligrams/hour _____

   b) milligrams/minute _____

5. The physician's order reads: Disopyramide, 600 mg/day, PO, divided doses q6h. How many milligrams would be administered for each dose?

   _____

6. A patient with life-threatening arrhythmias is being treated with sotalol hydrochloride. Appropriate response is occurring with a 320 mg/day dose. Dosing schedule is q12h. Sotalol is available in 160-mg tablets. How many tablets will be administered at each dose? _____

VI. Critical Thinking

1. Charles Green, an 82-year-old retired farmer, was recently diagnosed with atrial fibrillation. His heart rate is irregular, ranging between 120 and 160 beats per minute. At times, Mr. Green is very symptomatic, experiencing weakness, dizziness, and syncope. His physician has prescribed verapamil, a calcium channel blocker. Discuss how atrial fibrillation affects cardiac function and the ability to oxygenate effectively. Explain how verapamil will work to improve cardiac function.

2. Your 58-year-old patient, Mary Clark, is being treated for supraventricular arrhythmias with verapamil. The dosage of verapamil is still being titrated and Ms. Clark requires close monitoring. Discuss your nursing responsibilities for this patient.

VII. Internet Exercise

Use the following Internet address to identify any clinical trials that are currently underway to study cardiac arrhythmias and the drugs used to treat them. Select a clinical trial and print the information to bring to class for discussion.

http://clinicaltrials.gov

CHAPTER 41

Antianginal and Peripheral Vasodilating Drugs

I. Matching

Match each term in Column A with the correct definition or statement in Column B.

COLUMN A

_____ 1. vasodilation

_____ 2. buccal

_____ 3. lumen

_____ 4. transdermal system

_____ 5. prophylaxis

_____ 6. topical

_____ 7. intermittent

_____ 8. atherosclerosis

_____ 9. sublingual

_____ 10. angina

COLUMN B

A. A disease characterized by deposits of fatty plaques on the inner wall of arteries.

B. Inside diameter of artery.

C. An increase in the size of blood vessels.

D. Chest pain or pressure caused by a decreased oxygen supply to the heart muscle.

E. Prevention.

F. Under the tongue.

G. Between the cheek and gum.

H. The route of administration for a medication in ointment form.

I. Adhesive medicated pads containing the drug to be administered.

J. Increased pain in the legs when walking that is relieved with rest.

II. Fill in the Blanks

1. The antianginal and peripheral vasodilating drugs' primary purpose is to _____ _____ _____ to an area by _____ _____ _____.

2. Antianginal drugs relieve _____ _____ or _____ by _____ _____ _____, increasing the _____ supply to the _____.

3. List the two types of antianginal drugs discussed in this chapter.
   a) _____
   b) _____

4. The nitrates have a direct _____ effect on the _____ _____ layer of _____ _____.

5. The calcium channel blockers _____ _____ _____ and _____, which, in turn, deliver more _____ to _____ _____.

6. The nitrates are used to treat _____ _____.

7. _____ _____ _____ are primarily used to prevent _____ _____ associated with certain forms of angina.

8. List the different administration routes for the nitrates.

   a) _____

   b) _____

   c) _____

   d) _____

   e) _____

   f) _____

   g) _____

9. Cilostazol (Pletal) inhibits _____ _____ and _____ vascular beds, particularly in the _____ area.

10. Peripheral vasodilating drugs are chiefly used in the treatment of _____ _____ _____, such as, _____ _____, _____ _____, and _____ _____ _____ _____.

III. Multiple Choice

Circle the letter of the most appropriate answer.

1. During a discussion at a team conference, a nurse correctly states that calcium channel blockers:
   a. promote the movement of calcium ions across the cell membrane.
   b. keep all the calcium within the cell membranes.
   c. inhibit the movement of calcium ions across the cell membranes.
   d. eliminate calcium from around cell membranes.

2. Your patient is being discharged from the hospital with a prescription for sublingual nitroglycerin to be used for treatment of episodes of angina. Patient teaching for this medication should include the instruction to:
   a. place the tablet between the cheek and gum.
   b. keep the medication in a light-proof container.

   c. use tweezers to remove the medication from the container.
   d. always keep the drug in a clear container.

3. A student nurse asks why it is necessary to wear gloves when preparing and administering topical nitroglycerin ointment. You would be correct in stating that the nurse must:
   a. prevent staining of the skin.
   b. prevent the loss of drug effectiveness.
   c. prevent absorption of the drug through the skin.
   d. keep bacterial contamination of the drug at a minimum.

4. When applying topical nitroglycerin ointment, the nurse:
   a. leaves the applied area open to air.
   b. spreads the ointment over a 2 1/4-inch by 3 1/2-inch area.
   c. squeezes the ointment directly onto the skin.
   d. rubs the ointment into the skin until it is absorbed.

5. During a presentation at a team conference, a nurse is asked to explain what the calcium channel blockers are specifically used for. The nurse making the presentation states that these drugs are used:
   a. to prevent anginal attacks.
   b. to abort acute attacks.
   c. to decrease coronary artery blood flow.
   d. along with beta-adrenergic blocking agents.

6. A nurse completing patient teaching for administering sublingual nitroglycerin tells the patient he or she should take no more than:
   a. three doses within a 10-minute period.
   b. three doses within a 30-minute period.
   c. two doses within a 30-minute period.
   d. three doses within a 15-minute period.

7. Patients experiencing severe light-headedness after the use of sublingual nitroglycerin should be instructed to:
   a. lie down, elevate the lower extremities, and breathe deeply.
   b. sit down and place the head between the knees.
   c. lie down, breathe rapidly, and place the hands behind the head.
   d. remain standing and do not try to move for 3 to 5 minutes.

8. When a nitroglycerin transdermal system is prescribed, the nurse applies it:
   a. once a day and leaves it on for 24 hours.
   b. every 4 to 6 hours.
   c. once a day in the morning and leaves it on for 10 to 12 hours.
   d. to slightly damp skin to enhance absorption.

9. When transmucosal nitroglycerin is prescribed, the nurse instructs the patient to:
   a. direct the spray from the canister onto the chest area.
   b. wait 15 minutes between doses.
   c. not use the spray more than three times a day.
   d. direct the spray from the canister under the tongue.

10. Which of the following patient complaints would the nurse recognize as a possible adverse reaction to the nitrates during initial therapy with these drugs?
    a. Abdominal pain   c. Drowsiness
    b. Headache   d. Blurred vision

11. Peripheral vasodilating agents may cause dizziness and light-headedness. Patients are instructed to:
    a. drink extra fluid to eliminate this adverse effect.
    b. remain flat in bed for 1 hour after the drug is given.
    c. ask for assistance when ambulating.
    d. sip ice water until symptoms subside.

IV. Crossword Puzzle

ACROSS CLUES

3. Chest pain or pressure caused by a decreased oxygen supply to the heart muscle.
4. Example of a calcium channel blocker.
5. An increase in the size of blood vessels.
9. Under the tongue.
10. A disease characterized by deposits of fatty plaques on the inner wall of arteries.
12. Between the cheek and gum.
13. The route used for administering medication that is in ointment form.
14. Inside diameter of an artery.

DOWN CLUES

1. Trade name for verapamil.
2. Generic name for Pletal.
6. Drug used for prophylaxis for angina.
7. Example of a peripheral vasodilating drug.
8. Generic name for Cardizem.
11. Mineral necessary for the transmission of nerve impulses.

V. Dosage Problems

Solve the following dosage calculations.

1. A patient with angina pectoris is being treated with an antianginal medication. The patient has demonstrated a good response to diltiazem (Cardizem), 360 mg/day in four divided oral doses. Cardizem is available in 90-mg tablets.

   a) How many milligrams will be administered at each of the four doses? _____

   b) How many tablets will be administered at each dose? _____

2. Mark Allen has been diagnosed with effort-associated angina, and over the last 14 days his medication, nifedipine, has been titrated to obtain the most effective dose. His initial dosage of nifedipine was 10 mg, TID. The dose was gradually increased to 30 mg, QID, which resulted in the desired response.

   a) What will the total daily dose of nifedipine be? _____

   b) Using a drug reference guide, verify if this is a safe dose. _____

3. A patient's dose of verapamil (Calan) is 360 mg/day, PO, in three divided doses. Calan is available in 120 -mg tablets.

   a) How many tablets will be administered at each dose? _____

   b) How many milligrams are given at each dose? _____

VI. Critical Thinking

1. Mrs. Glenn, a patient with newly diagnosed coronary artery disease (CAD), has been started on a nitroglycerin patch that she is to apply in the morning and remove before going to bed at night. Sublingual nitroglycerin, PRN, is ordered for episodes of acute chest pain. Discuss appropriate patient teaching for Mrs. Glenn.

2. Mrs. Morris has nitropaste (nitroglycerin ointment), 1 inch, topically, ordered q6h to decrease blood pressure and control angina. The nurse carefully measures out 1 inch of ointment on the measuring paper and spreads the ointment with her finger. Before she is able to administer the medication, she feels dizzy and unwell. She hands the medication to another nurse and asks her to give it. Identify the medication error(s) and discuss how it could have been prevented.

CHAPTER 42

Antihypertensive Drugs

I. Matching

Match each term in Column A with the correct definition or statement in Column B.

COLUMN A

_____ 1. malignant hypertension

_____ 2. endogenous

_____ 3. isolated systolic hypertension

_____ 4. essential hypertension

_____ 5. vasodilation

_____ 6. hypokalemia

_____ 7. postural hypotension

_____ 8. blood pressure

_____ 9. aldosterone

_____ 10. lumen

_____ 11. secondary hypertension

_____ 12. orthostatic hypotension

_____ 13. hypertension

_____ 14. angiotensin-converting enzyme

_____ 15. hyponatremia

COLUMN B

A. The force of blood against the walls of the arteries.

B. A systolic pressure above 140 mm Hg and a diastolic pressure above 90 mm Hg.

C. Hypertension without a known cause.

D. Hypertension with an identified cause.

E. Hypertension that progresses rapidly and causes organ damage.

F. Increasing the size of the arterial blood vessels.

G. Space or opening within an artery.

H. Substance that converts angiotensin I to angiotensin II.

I. Substances manufactured normally by the body.

J. Endogenous hormone secreted by the adrenal cortex that promotes the retention of sodium and water within the vascular system.

K. Episodes of dizziness and light-headedness that occur when an individual rises suddenly from a sitting or lying position.

L. Hypotension that occurs when an individual has been standing in one place for a long time.

M. Low levels of sodium in the blood.

N. Lower-than-normal levels of potassium in the blood.

O. A condition that develops in older individuals in which the systolic pressure is elevated.

II. Fill in the Blanks

1. List the types of drugs used for the treatment of hypertension.

   a) _____

   b) _____

   c) _____

   d) _____

   e) _____

   f) _____

   g) _____

   h) _____

   i) _____

2. Antihypertensive drugs that have vasodilating activity include:

   a) _____

   b) _____

   c) _____

   d) _____

3. Antihypertensive drugs are used cautiously in patients with _____ or _____ impairment, or _____ imbalances, during _____ and _____, and in _____ patients.

4. The hypotensive effects of most antihypertensive drugs are _____ when administered with _____ and other _____.

5. Administration of _____-_____ diuretics or _____ supplements concurrently with the ACE inhibitors may cause _____.

6. Before therapy with an antihypertensive drug is started, the nurse obtains the _____ _____ and _____ _____ in both arms with the patient in _____, _____, and _____ positions.

7. The nurse also obtains the patient's _____, especially if a _____ is part of therapy or if the physician prescribes a _____ _____ regimen.

8. Each time the _____ _____ is obtained, the nurse uses the _____ arm and the patient is placed in the _____ position.

9. Sublingual nifedipine may be administered by _____ the capsule with a _____ _____ and then squeezing the _____ into the _____ _____.

10. The ACE inhibitors may cause a significant _____ in blood pressure after the _____ dose.

III. Multiple Choice

Circle the letter of the most appropriate answer.

Ms. Jackson, a patient with diabetes, is seen regularly every 4 months in the medical clinic. Today she is exhibiting symptoms of hypertension and the physician has prescribed an antihypertensive drug. Questions 1–3 pertain to Ms. Jackson's case.

1. When developing a teaching plan for Ms. Jackson, the nurse includes warnings to avoid:
   a. foods high in protein.
   b. alcoholic beverages.
   c. exercising.
   d. foods high in carbohydrates.

2. The nurse also teaches Ms. Jackson that some adverse reactions experienced with these drugs will make it necessary for her to:
   a. take the drug in the middle of the day to avoid stomach upset.
   b. eat a diet high in protein.
   c. avoid driving a car if light-headedness or dizziness occurs.
   d. limit her fluid intake if muscle cramps occur.

3. Ms. Jackson is told that she may experience dizziness when rising from a lying position. To eliminate this problem, the nurse tells Ms. Jackson to:
   a. sleep in a sitting position.
   b. use three or four pillows in bed.
   c. sit on the edge of the bed for 1 or 2 minutes before standing up.
   d. rise quickly and stand by the edge of the bed for 1 minute.

4. During the first few days of drug therapy, an elderly patient receiving a diuretic for hypertension will be observed for signs and symptoms of:
   a. fluid overload.   c. hyperkalemia.
   b. hypernatremia.   d. dehydration.

5. When asked at a team conference how diuretics reduce blood pressure, the nurse replies that these drugs:

    a. dilate blood vessels.

    b. decrease potassium excretion.

    c. increase sodium excretion from the body.

    d. promote fluid retention.

6. A transdermal clonidine patch is removed and a new one applied every:

    a. 7 days.   c. 24 hours.

    b. 12 hours.   d. 3 days.

7. An adverse reaction that is usually observed early in therapy for patients being treated with antihypertensives is:

    a. constipation and difficulty urinating.

    b. postural or orthostatic hypotension.

    c. shortness of breath.

    d. diaphoresis.

8. An ongoing assessment of the patient receiving antihypertensives includes checking the patient's _____ _____ immediately before administering the antihypertensive drug.

    a. weight and height   c. blood pressure

    b. pulse rate   d. respiratory rate

9. Ms. Smith is to receive her first dose of an antihypertensive medication. The nurse must include in the assessment:

    a. blood pressure measures in both arms.

    b. the laboratory values for the blood and urine samples.

    c. history of the patient's childhood illnesses.

    d. a list of food Ms. Smith has eaten that day.

10. A nurse is monitoring a patient who is being treated with nitroprusside intravenously. Which of the following would be of the greatest concern to the nurse?

    a. The foil wrapped around the infusion bottle

    b. Very light brownish tint to the solution

    c. Administration tubing not protected from light

    d. The infusion bottle uncovered and exposed to light

11. The nurse must monitor laboratory results for the patient receiving an antihypertensive to identify if the patient is experiencing a(n):

    a. elevated CBC.

    b. electrolyte imbalance.

    c. prolonged PT, PTT.

    d. elevated WBC.

12. When the nurse is completing patient teaching for a patient diagnosed with essential hypertension, it is important to include the following information:

    a. Take your medication until you feel better.

    b. Take your medication only when you are symptomatic.

    c. Essential hypertension cannot be cured, but can be controlled.

    d. Taking your medication correctly will cure your hypertension.

IV. Crossword Puzzle

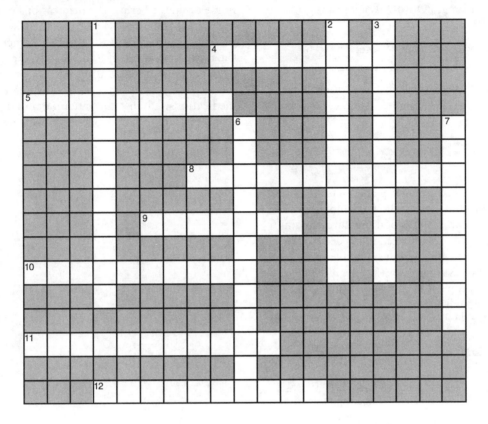

ACROSS CLUES

4. Hypotension characterized by dizziness and light-headedness when rising suddenly from a lying or sitting position.
5. Generic name for Loniten.
8. Low blood sodium.
9. Example of a combination antihypertensive.
10. Generic name for Lasix.
11. Low blood potassium.
12. Word referring to within the body.

DOWN CLUES

1. Increasing the size of the arterial blood vessel.
2. Hypotension that occurs when standing in one place for a long time.
3. Endogenous hormone secreted by the adrenal cortex.
6. High blood pressure.
7. Generic name for Vasotec.

V. Dosage Problems

Solve the following dosage calculations.

1. The physician's order reads: furosemide (Lasix), 80 mg, PO, single dose. The drug is available as an oral solution with a dose strength of 40 mg of Lasix per 5 mL of solution. How many milliliters will be administered for the one-time dose?

   _____

2. The physician's order reads, minoxidil (Loniten), 5 mg, PO, each day. Minoxidil is available as a 2.5-mg tablet. How many tablets would be administered to achieve the prescribed dose of minoxidil? _____

3. The effective dose of enalapril (Vasotec) for a patient diagnosed with hypertension has been established at 15 mg, PO, BID. Enalapril is available in 10-mg and 5-mg tablets.

   a) How many milligrams of Vasotec are to be administered at each dose? _____

   b) How many tablets will be needed for each prescribed dose? _____

VI. Critical Thinking

1. Martin Hall, a 42-year-old carpenter, has returned to the clinic for a follow-up blood pressure check. Mr. Hall's blood pressure remains elevated at 182/94. The physician has decided to begin therapy with an angiotensin-converting enzyme inhibitor. Mr. Hall states, "I can't believe I have high blood pressure. I feel just fine, and I've heard this medicine has some bad side effects." As Mr. Hall's nurse, discuss the information you should give him about hypertension and its effects on the body. Also develop a teaching plan to include nonpharmacological strategies to decrease blood pressure. In addition, discuss what information you could give Mr. Hall about his prescribed medication's side effects.

2. A nursing home resident is having difficulty swallowing his medications in pill form. The nurse decides to crush the medications (Cardizem SR, Lasix, and Slow-K) and mix them with the patient's pudding desert. Consider the actions of the nurse and decide if a medication error has been committed. Use a drug reference text to identify the appropriateness of crushing these medications. Discuss this situation and decide what you would have done in this nurse's place.

CHAPTER 43

Antihyperlipidemic Drugs

I. Matching

Match each term in Column A with the correct definition or statement in Column B.

COLUMN A

_____ 1. cholesterol

_____ 2. bile acid sequestrants

_____ 3. rhabdomyolysis

_____ 4. lipids

_____ 5. garlic

_____ 6. low-density lipoproteins

_____ 7. catalyst

_____ 8. lipoprotein profile

_____ 9. atherosclerosis

_____ 10. high-density lipoproteins

_____ 11. hyperlipidemia

_____ 12. nicotinic acid

_____ 13. triglycerides

_____ 14. lovastatin (Mevacor)

_____ 15. lipoprotein

COLUMN B

A. Increase in the lipids in the blood.

B. Group of fats or fat-like substances found in the blood.

C. Lipid deposits accumulate on the linings of the blood vessels, eventually producing degenerative changes and obstruction of blood flow.

D. Type of lipid found in the blood.

E. Levels of 240 mg/dL of this lipid are associated with atherosclerosis.

F. Lipid-containing protein that transports the triglycerides and cholesterol throughout the body.

G. Type of lipoprotein that transports cholesterol to the peripheral cells.

H. Type of lipoprotein that carries cholesterol from the peripheral cells to the liver, where it is metabolized and excreted.

I. Drugs that bind to bile acids to form an insoluble substance that cannot be absorbed by the intestine and is excreted in the feces.

J. A substance that accelerates a chemical reaction without itself undergoing a change.

K. HMG-CoA reductase inhibitor.

L. Disorder in which muscle tissue is damaged and the contents of the muscle cell are released into the bloodstream.

M. This drug may cause mild to severe facial flushing.

N. Laboratory examination of the levels of total cholesterol, LDL, HDL, and triglycerides.

O. Herbal supplement that lowers serum cholesterol and triglyceride levels.

II. Fill in the Blanks

1. List the two lipids found in the blood.

   a) _____

   b) _____

2. List the types of drugs used to treat hyperlipidemia.

   a) _____

   b) _____

   c) _____

   d) _____

3. Serum cholesterol levels above _____ mg/dL and triglyceride above _____ mg/dL are associated with _____.

4. Elevation of the ____-density lipoproteins _____ the risk of heart disease.

5. HDL is known as the _____ lipoprotein.

III. Multiple Choice

Circle the letter of the most appropriate answer.

1. The nurse knows that colestipol, a bile acid sequestrant, should be:
   a. mixed with some type of food or liquid before administration.
   b. administered 30 minutes before ingesting any type of food.
   c. given at least 1 hour before or 4 hours after meals.
   d. mixed with food or liquids until dissolved before administering.

2. Fluvastatin has been prescribed as adjunct therapy in combination with colestipol granules. The nurse would know to administer the fluvastatin:
   a. together with the colestipol.
   b. immediately before the colestipol.
   c. 2 hours after the colestipol.
   d. immediately after administering the colestipol.

3. Patients taking the bile acid sequestrant, cholestyramine, should be instructed by the nurse to monitor for the common adverse reaction of:
   a. headache.   c. blurred vision.
   b. constipation.   d. hypotension.

4. Which of the following patient complaints would the nurse consider an adverse reaction to long-term treatment with a bile acid sequestrant?
   a. Anxiety   c. Bruising easily
   b. Anorexia   d. Double vision

5. During patient teaching, the nurse explains the difference between "good" cholesterol and "bad" cholesterol and states that it is desirable to see an increase in the:
   a. HDL   c. triglycerides
   b. VLDL   d. LDL

6. When administering nicotinic acid, the nurse will observe the patient for the common adverse reaction to this drug, which is:
   a. hypertensive episodes.
   b. generalized flushing of the skin.
   c. severe nausea and vomiting.
   d. uncontrollable diarrhea.

7. When asked during a team conference how an HMG-CoA inhibitor lowers cholesterol, the nurse correctly answers that it works by inhibiting the manufacture of cholesterol or by:
   a. increasing the secretion of bile acids.
   b. decreasing triglyceride production.
   c. removing cholesterol from the small intestine.
   d. promoting the breakdown of cholesterol.

8. Rhabdomyolysis, a rare condition in which muscle damage results in the release of muscle cell contents into the bloodstream, has been particularly associated with the administration of:
   a. bile acid sequestrants.
   b. nicotinic acid.
   c. HMG-CoA reductase inhibitors.
   d. fibric acid derivatives.

IV. Crossword Puzzle

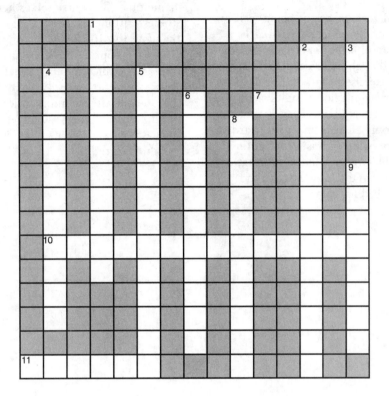

ACROSS CLUES

1. A substance that accelerates a chemical reaction without itself undergoing a change.
7. Trade name for gemfibrozil.
10. Generic name for Questran.
11. Group of fats or fat-like substances.

DOWN CLUES

1. Example of a lipid found in the blood.
2. Increase in the lipids in the blood.
3. Very low density lipoprotein (abbreviation).
4. Small particles of fat in the blood.
5. Type of lipid found in the blood.
6. Generic name for Lescol.
8. Lipid-containing protein that transports the triglycerides and cholesterol throughout the body.
9. Brand name for colestipol.

V. Dosage Problems

Solve the following dosage calculations.

1. The physician has ordered fluvastatin (Lescol), 80 mg/day, PO, in two divided doses. Fluvastatin is available in 40-mg capsules.

   a) How many milligrams of fluvastatin will be administered at each dose? _____

   b) How many capsules will be needed for each dose of medication? _____

2. A patient with triglyceride levels of 750 mg/dL has been prescribed gemfibrozil (Lopid). The dose ordered is 1200 mg daily, PO, in two divided doses, 30 minutes before morning and evening meals. Gemfibrozil is available in 600-mg tablets. How many tablets will be needed for each of the prescribed doses? _____

VI. Critical Thinking

1. Dalton Edwards, 48 years of age, is being seen by his primary health care provider for his yearly physical. His cholesterol has been elevated for the last two visits even though he has changed his diet and started an exercise program. The physician has prescribed niacin (nicotinic acid) to try to reduce his cholesterol level. Discuss what information you should elicit from Mr. Edwards. Discuss also how you will use this information to develop a teaching plan that includes information about high cholesterol and the medication the physician has prescribed for him.

2. Mrs. Kolwell, an 89-year-old nursing home resident, likes to take all of her medications at the same time. The nurse mixes her cholestyramine (Questran) in a large glass of orange juice and hands it to Mrs. Kolwell along with her digoxin, Lasix, captopril, and Slow-K. Mrs. Kolwell uses the orange juice to take all her medications. The nurse monitors the pulse and blood pressure before and after administration, and they are within normal limits. What, if any, additional precautions should the nurse use when Questran is administered?

CHAPTER 44

Anticoagulant and Thrombolytic Drugs

I. Matching

Match each term in Column A with the correct definition or statement in Column B.

COLUMN A

_____ 1. fibrinolytic drugs

_____ 2. hemostasis

_____ 3. Homans' sign

_____ 4. protamine sulfate

_____ 5. prothrombin

_____ 6. thrombolytic drugs

_____ 7. thrombosis

_____ 8. thrombus

_____ 9. anticoagulants

_____ 10. fibrin

COLUMN B

A. Blood clot.

B. Another term used to identify the thrombolytic drugs.

C. Drugs used to prevent the formation and extension of a blood clot.

D. Drugs that dissolve blood clots that have already formed within the wall of a blood vessel.

E. Process that stops bleeding of a blood vessel.

F. The insoluble protein that is essential for clot formation.

G. The formation of a blood clot.

H. Clotting factor II, a substance essential for the clotting of blood.

I. Pain in the calf when the foot is dorsiflexed.

J. A heparin antagonist that counteracts the effects of heparin.

II. Fill in the Blanks

1. List the uses of warfarin.

   a) _____

   b) _____

   c) _____

   d) _____

   e) _____

2. A positive Homans' sign is suggestive of _____
   _____ _____.

3. Symptoms of warfarin overdose could include:

   a) _____

   b) _____

   c) _____

   d) _____

   e) _____

4. Heparin cannot be taken _____ because it is
   _____ by _____ _____ in the
   _____.

5. _____ is the chief complication of
   heparin administration.

6. The most commonly used test to monitor heparin
   therapy is _____ _____
   _____ _____.

7. A patient receiving a thrombolytic will be monitored by the nurse for bleeding every _____ minutes during the first _____ minutes of therapy, every _____ to _____ minutes for the next ____ hours, and at least every _____ hours until therapy is completed.

III. Multiple Choice

Circle the letter of the most appropriate answer.

1. A nurse caring for a patient receiving warfarin (Coumadin) would suspect complications are developing if the patient states:
   a. "My gums bleed when I brush my teeth."
   b. "I can't seem to fall asleep as easily as before."
   c. "I'm having headaches and my vision is blurred."
   d. "My feet swell at the end of the day."

2. A patient assigned to your care is receiving warfarin therapy. As the nurse, you would know that the daily dose of warfarin will be based on the laboratory results of the:
   a. hemoglobin and hematocrit (H&H).
   b. prothrombin time (PT).
   c. activated partial thromboplastin time (APTT).
   d. partial prothromboplastin time (PTT).

3. A nurse educator is presenting information on administering oral anticoagulants. Information concerning adverse reactions would emphasize the following:
   a. Adverse reactions from anticoagulant therapy are not expected for 2 weeks or more.
   b. Careful monitoring of blood coagulation tests will control the possible adverse reactions.
   c. With anticoagulation therapy, bleeding can occur at any time, even when coagulation test results are within normal limits.
   d. Bleeding is usually minimal and no serious problems are expected for the patient.

4. For the patient receiving heparin therapy, the nurse would expect the principal adverse reaction to be:
   a. muscle cramps.   c. nausea.
   b. hemorrhage.   d. edema.

5. At a team conference, a nurse asks what exactly is the action of heparin. You would be correct in stating that heparin:
   a. enhances the absorption of vitamin K.
   b. inhibits the formation of clotting factor I.
   c. inhibits the conversion of fibrinogen to fibrin.
   d. decreases plasma levels of calcium.

6. The nurse would expect the therapeutic dose of heparin would be attained when the APTT is:
   a. 1.5 to 2.5 times normal.
   b. 2.6 to 3 times the normal.
   c. less than 5 seconds.
   d. between 6 and 10 minutes.

7. When following the physician's order to administer heparin subcutaneously, the nurse correctly administers the heparin subcutaneously:
   a. 1/2 inch from the navel.
   b. at an angle of 5 degrees.
   c. using a 2-inch needle.
   d. at a 45- to 90-degree angle.

8. In case of an overdose of heparin, the nurse would be sure that _____ is readily available.
   a. a suction machine   c. vitamin K
   b. protamine sulfate   d. a cardiac monitor

9. At a workshop on the proper techniques for administering heparin, the nurse educator would include which of the following points?
   a. Heparin can be safely administered by any of the follow routes: PO, IV, SC.
   b. Other drugs given by the IV route may be safely given through the needle and tubing used for the heparin administration.
   c. Each time heparin is given, inspect the other needle sites for inflammation, pain, tenderness, and hematoma formation.
   d. Coagulation tests are usually performed 30 minutes after the dose of heparin is given.

10. Which of the following adverse reactions would alert the nurse to possible complications in a patient receiving a thrombolytic drug? The patient:

    a. has bright red blood in his stool.

    b. has complaints of stomach cramps and constipation.

    c. has complaints of headache and a dry cough.

    d. has one episode of nausea and vomiting.

11. The thrombolytic drugs demonstrate their optimal therapeutic effect when administered:

    a. when prothrombin time is within normal limits.

    b. within 4 to 6 hours after thrombus formation.

    c. by the intramuscular route.

    d. when PTT is at 2 to 2.5 times the normal value.

12. When monitoring the INR for a patient receiving warfarin therapy, the nurse would withhold the drug and notify the primary health care provider if the INR exceeds:

    a. 3.   c. 2.5.

    b. 2.   d. 1.5.

13. The nurse explains the effect of acetaminophen and the NSAIDs when taken while undergoing therapy with warfarin by telling the patient that acetaminophen and NSAID-type drugs:

    a. decrease the effect of warfarin.

    b. increase the effect of warfarin.

    c. alter the PT/INR rate.

    d. increase the risk of hypoglycemia.

14. When administering enoxaparin to a surgical patient to prevent embolism after abdominal surgery, the nurse would expect the patient to have:

    a. the first dose 2 hours before surgery.

    b. the medication regimen continued for 14 days after surgery.

    c. the first dose within 36 hours after surgery.

    d. the medication continued postoperatively for 30 days.

15. Which of the following vital signs, if observed by the nurse, would most likely indicate internal bleeding?

    a. Pulse rate of 68 beats/minute

    b. Blood pressure of 180/70 mm Hg

    c. Respiratory rate of 16 breaths/minute

    d. Blood pressure of 90/50 mm Hg

IV. Crossword Puzzle

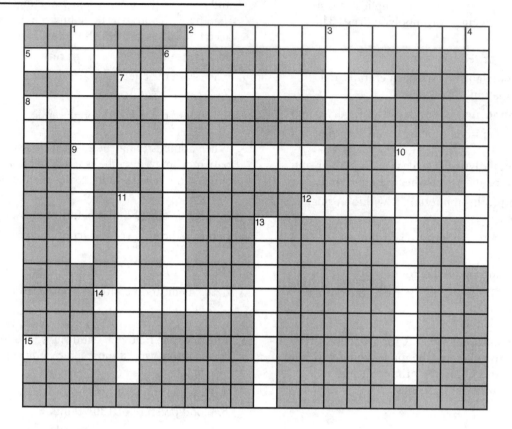

ACROSS CLUES

2. Drugs used to prevent the formation and extension of a blood clot.
5. Heparin is not given by this route.
7. Drugs that dissolve blood clots.
8. Partial prothromboplastin time (abbreviation).
9. Another term for prevention.
12. Blood clot.
14. Yellowish discoloration of the skin.
15. The insoluble protein that is essential for clot formation.

DOWN CLUES

1. Example of a low-molecular-weight heparin.
3. Activated partial thromboplastin time (abbreviation).
4. The formation of a clot.
6. Substance that accounts for most of the action of warfarin.
8. Prothrombin time (abbreviation).
10. Process that stops bleeding of a blood vessel.
11. An oral anticoagulant.
13. The principal adverse reaction seen with the anticoagulants.

V. Dosage Problems

Solve the following dosage calculations.

1. The physician's order reads: Heparin, 750 U, SC, OD. The drug available is heparin, 1000 U per mL. Calculate the dose to be administered.

   _____

2. The physician's order reads: Lovenox, 40 mg, SC, qd. The drug available is Lovenox injection, 30 mg, 0.3 mL. How many milliliters will be administered? _____

3. The physician's order reads: Heparin, 5000 U, SC, BID. The drug available is heparin injection, 20,000 U/mL. How many milliliters will be administered for each dose? _____

VI. Critical Thinking

1. You are caring for a patient who is in traction. She is receiving 5000 U of heparin, SC, twice daily. Discuss why you think this patient is receiving heparin and how you would safely administer this medication.

2. Marty Allen is admitted to your unit with bacterial pneumonia. He is on oral antibiotics and his condition is improving. Mr. Allen also is on Coumadin therapy. You administer his antibiotic and his daily dose of Coumadin and return to the nurse's station to complete your documentation. While checking Mr. Allen's laboratory results for the day, you find his INR was last reported as six (6). What is the medication error that has just occurred, and how will you address this situation?

CHAPTER 45

Agents Used in the Treatment of Anemia

I. Matching

Match each term in Column A with the correct definition or statement in Column B.

COLUMN A

_____ 1. iron deficiency anemia

_____ 2. erythropoietin

_____ 3. vitamin B_{12}

_____ 4. pernicious anemia

_____ 5. anemia

_____ 6. intrinsic factor

_____ 7. folic acid

_____ 8. folinic acid rescue or leucovorin rescue

_____ 9. epoetin alfa

_____ 10. megaloblastic anemia

COLUMN B

A. A hormone that stimulates the formation of red blood cell production.

B. Required for the manufacture of red blood cells in the bone marrow.

C. An anemia caused by a deficiency of folic acid, characterized by the presence of large, abnormal, immature erythrocytes circulating in the blood.

D. When leucovorin is used to diminish the hematological effects of massive doses of methotrexate, allowing normal cells to survive.

E. Essential to growth, cell reproduction, the manufacture of myelin, and blood cell manufacture.

F. A substance produced by cells in the stomach necessary for the absorption of vitamin B_{12} in the intestines.

G. A type of anemia caused by a deficiency of intrinsic factor, resulting in the body being unable to absorb vitamin B_{12}.

H. Condition resulting from the body not having enough iron to supply its needs.

I. Condition in which there is an insufficient amount of hemoglobin to deliver oxygen to the body tissues.

J. Drug used to treat anemia associated with renal failure.

II. Fill in the Blanks

1. The absorption of iron is decreased when administered with these types of drugs:

   a) _____

   b) _____

   c) _____

   d) _____

2. Folic acid is found in what food products?

   a) _____

   b) _____

   c) _____

   d) _____

   e) _____

3. Vitamin B_{12} is essential for:

   a) _____

   b) _____

   c) _____

   d) _____

4. General symptoms of anemia may include:

   a) _____

   b) _____

   c) _____

   d) _____

   e) _____

5. Parenteral iron has resulted in fatal anaphylactic reactions. The nurse should report the adverse reactions of:

   a) _____

   b) _____

   c) _____

   d) _____

   e) _____

6. Iron compounds are _____ in patients with any anemia except _____ _____ anemia.

7. List the two drugs used in the treatment of anemia associated with chronic renal failure (*include generic and trade names*):

   a) _____ _____

   b) _____ _____

8. Patients with pernicious anemia are treated with _____ by the _____ route _____ until stabilized, and then are maintained with _____ injections for the rest of their life.

III. Multiple Choice

Circle the letter of the most appropriate answer.

1. Your patient is suspected of having a deficiency of vitamin B$_{12}$. You would expect that the patient has also developed:

   a. thrombocytopenia.

   b. pernicious anemia.

   c. iron deficiency anemia.

   d. microblastic anemia.

2. A patient tells the nurse that the doctor is prescribing folic acid to treat the megaloblastic anemia that he has been diagnosed with. He asks you to explain what the body needs folic acid for. Your explanation should include the information that folic acid is needed for:

   a. storing iron in the hemoglobin.

   b. manufacturing platelets.

   c. storing iron in the liver.

   d. manufacturing RBCs in the bone marrow.

3. Your patient asks you, "What exactly is iron deficiency anemia?" You would explain that this condition is the result of:

   a. the loss of iron from its storage place, the liver.

   b. a lack of intrinsic factor in the liver that prevents the use of vitamin B$_{12}$.

   c. a loss of iron that is greater than the available iron stored in the body.

   d. loss of iron from red blood cells, but the iron stored remains the same

4. A patient is prescribed ferrous fumarate drops for his iron deficiency anemia. During your patient teaching for the iron supplement, you would be sure to instruct the patient:

   a. to dilute the medication in water or juice and sip through a straw.

   b. to take this medication with an antacid to minimize gastrointestinal upset.

   c. that under no circumstances should the medication be taken with food.

   d. to place the drops on the tongue and swish thoroughly before swallowing.

5. A patient with rheumatoid arthritis has been prescribed iron dextran for his anemia. The nurse explains that some patients with rheumatoid arthritis who receive iron dextran may:

   a. experience moderate relief from the rheumatoid symptoms during treatment.

   b. take a much longer time to respond to the anemia treatment.

   c. experience an acute exacerbation of joint pain and swelling.

   d. notice the symptoms of the arthritis completely resolve during treatment with iron dextran.

6. Maintaining adequate nutrition for the anemic patient may be accomplished by encouraging a diet of:

   a. carbohydrate-rich food.

   b. foods high in iron or folic acid.

   c. foods high in protein and low in carbohydrate.

   d. foods high in fat and low in carbohydrate.

7. The nurse must be aware that the absorption of oral iron medications is decreased when administered concurrently with:

   a. ascorbic acid. c. levodopa.

   b. levothyroxine. d. tetracyclines.

8. Epoetin alfa and darbepoetin alfa are used with caution in patients with:

   a. postural hypotension.

   b. episodic vertigo.

   c. hypertension.

   d. peripheral edema.

9. Intrinsic factor, which is necessary for the absorption of vitamin B_{12} in the intestines, is produced by:

   a. cells in the stomach.

   b. cells in the liver.

   c. pancreatic cells.

   d. the gallbladder.

10. The nurse is admitting a patient with anemia to the unit. While completing the patient history, the nurse discovers the patient is a strict vegetarian, which the nurse knows puts the patient at risk for:

    a. decreased intrinsic factor.

    b. vitamin B_{12} deficiencies.

    c. folic acid deficiency anemia.

    d. erythropoietin deficiency.

IV. Crossword Puzzle

ACROSS CLUES

1. Type of anemia caused by deficiency of intrinsic factor, resulting in the body being unable to absorb vitamin B_{12}.
4. Trade name for epoetin alfa.
5. Trade name for darbepoetin alfa.
7. Inflammation of the tongue.
9. Substance produced by the cells in the stomach that is necessary for the absorption of vitamin B_{12} in the intestines (two words).
10. Required for the manufacture of red blood cells in the bone marrow (two words).

DOWN CLUES

2. Hormone that stimulates the formation of red blood cell production.
3. Type of anemia caused by a deficiency of folic acid and characterized by the presence of large, abnormal, immature erythrocytes circulating in the blood.
6. Insufficient amount of hemoglobin to deliver oxygen to the body tissues.
8. Component of hemoglobin.

V. Dosage Problems

Solve the following dosage calculations.

1. The physician has ordered Epogen, 3000 U, SC, OD, every Monday, Wednesday, and Friday. The Epogen delivered by the pharmacy reads: Epogen 2000 U per mL. How many milliliters of Epogen will be needed for each injection? _____

2. The physician has ordered vitamin K, 10 mg, IM, qd, for 3 days. The vial of vitamin K Reads: 5 mg per mL of solution for injection. How many milliliters of the solution is needed? _____

VI. Critical Thinking

1. Mrs. Morton, a 72-year-old patient who has had chronic renal failure for the past 5 years, has developed severe anemia. Her physician has prescribed epoetin alfa (Epogen) to stimulate red blood cell production. As Mrs. Morton's nurse, you are responsible for teaching her about the medication, including subcutaneous self-administration. Discuss the teaching plan you would develop and include a review of why renal failure causes anemia, along with how Epogen works to increase red blood cell counts. Also, what assessment data should you collect before teaching Mrs. Morton self-injection techniques? Discuss the evaluation process you will use to determine if the Epogen is working. Consider decreased symptoms of the anemia and expected changes in the laboratory values.

2. After a surgical procedure, your patient will be taking ferrous sulfate, 300 mg, TID, with meals. The pharmacy has sent him a month's supply of 300-mg tablets. What information do you need to include in your teaching plan for this drug before the patient is discharged?

CHAPTER 46

Diuretics

I. Matching

Match each term in Column A with the correct definition or statement in Column B.

COLUMN A

_____ 1. postural hypotension

_____ 2. hypokalemia

_____ 3. loop diuretics

_____ 4. edema

_____ 5. diuretic

_____ 6. glaucoma

_____ 7. orthostatic hypotension

_____ 8. osmotic diuretics

_____ 9. hyperkalemia

_____ 10. dehydration

_____ 11. carbonic anhydrase inhibitors

_____ 12. filtrate

_____ 13. potassium-sparing diuretics

_____ 14. hyponatremia

_____ 15. glycosuria

COLUMN B

A. A drug that increases the excretion of urine by the kidneys.

B. Retention of excess fluid in the body tissues.

C. Fluid removed from the blood during the filtering process of the kidneys.

D. Decrease the production of aqueous humor in the eye, which in turn decreases intraocular pressure.

E. Inhibit the reabsorption of sodium and chloride in the distal and proximal tubules of the kidneys and in the loop of Henle.

F. Diuretics that increase the density of the filtrate in the glomerulus.

G. Diuretics that depress the excretion of potassium by the kidneys.

H. A condition that creates an increase in the intraocular pressure of the eye that, if left untreated, can result in blindness.

I. Dizziness and light-headedness when rising suddenly from a sitting or lying position.

J. Glucose in the urine.

K. Hypotension that occurs after standing in one place for a long time.

L. Increase in potassium levels in the blood.

M. Low levels of potassium in the blood.

N. When too much water is lost from the body.

O. Lower than normal levels of sodium in the blood.

II. Fill in the Blanks

1. List the five general types of diuretics.

   a) _____

   b) _____

   c) _____

   d) _____

   e) _____

2. List the two carbonic anhydrase inhibitors discussed in this chapter (*include generic and trade names*).

   a) _____ _____

   b) _____ _____

3. List the loop diuretics discussed in this chapter (*include generic and trade names*).

   a) _____ _____

   b) _____ _____

c) _____ _____

d) _____ _____

4. List the potassium-sparing diuretics discussed in this chapter (*include generic and trade names*).

a) _____ _____

b) _____ _____

c) _____ _____

5. Before administering a diuretic, the nurse assesses the _____ _____ and _____ the patient.

6. If a patient has peripheral edema, the nurse inspects the involved _____ and records the _____ and _____ of edema in the patient's _____.

7. The type of ongoing assessment the nurse will perform for the patient being treated with diuretics depends on:

a) _____

b) _____

c) _____

d) _____

8. Before the first dose of the diuretic is administered, the nurse will explain:

a) _____

b) _____

c) _____

III. Multiple Choice

Circle the letter of the most appropriate answer.

1. A nurse is presenting an in-service program on caring for the patient with glaucoma. Some of the information presented includes the effects of osmotic diuretics when used for glaucoma, which include:

a. dilation of the pupil.

b. lowering of intraocular pressure.

c. dehydration of the patient.

d. an increase in intraocular pressure.

2. Ms. Martin is receiving acetazolamide (Diamox) for acute glaucoma. Which of the following assessments will be made by the nurse while Ms. Martin is receiving the Diamox?

a. Monitoring blood pressure every 2 hours

b. Determining her intake and output ratio

c. Asking her if the pain is relieved or lessened

d. Measuring her intraocular pressure

3. Your patient is being discharged home with a prescription for a diuretic that is to be taken one time daily. When completing the patient teaching for this type of drug, the nurse will instruct the patient to take the diuretic:

a. before going to bed.

b. with the noon meal.

c. with the evening meal.

d. early in the morning.

4. Instructions for the patient receiving a potassium-sparing diuretic include the signs of hyperkalemia that should be monitored for. These include:

a. diarrhea.   c. hypotension.

b. cold, clammy skin.   d. leg and foot cramps.

5. When monitoring a patient for possible dehydration due to excessive diuresis after administration of a diuretic, the nurse will observe for:

a. poor skin turgor, dry mucous membranes.

b. hypertension, increased urine output.

c. hyperthermia, productive cough.

d. bradycardia, edema of the extremities.

6. Mr. Moss has several health problems for which he is taking medication. Currently, he is being treated with a digitalis glycoside and a diuretic. Which of the following would indicate that Mr. Moss has developed hypokalemia?

a. Weight gain of more than 5 pounds

b. Development of a cardiac arrhythmia

c. Complaints of excessive thirst

d. Edema of the lower extremities

7. Daily assessments of the patient beginning diuretic therapy would include:

    a. obtaining a daily weight.

    b. monitoring vital signs hourly.

    c. advising the patient to limit fluids.

    d. monitoring blood glucose levels.

8. A nursing intervention that can help prevent a fluid volume deficit in the elderly or confused patient who is taking a diuretic is to:

    a. offer liquid nourishment at bedtime.

    b. have fluids in the patient's room.

    c. have fluids on the meal tray.

    d. frequently offer fluids during waking hours.

9. When teaching the patient who has been prescribed a diuretic, the nurse can help to prevent an electrolyte imbalance by advising the patient to:

    a. exercise each day.

    b. avoid eating fresh fruits.

    c. eat a well-balanced diet.

    d. eat a low-protein diet.

10. The nurse advises the patient who is being treated with a diuretic to avoid:

    a. resting during the day.

    b. eating fresh vegetables.

    c. exercise or cardiac stimulation.

    d. drinking alcohol.

11. A patient with diabetes has been prescribed a loop diuretic. The nurse will need to advise this patient:

    a. that less insulin will most likely be required.

    b. that blood glucose levels may be elevated.

    c. not to use a glucometer to check the blood glucose.

    d. to increase the evening meal carbohydrate intake.

12. Mr. Barnes is receiving a thiazide diuretic and digoxin, a cardiac glycoside. The nurse will monitor Mr. Barnes closely for:

    a. signs and symptoms of hypernatremia.

    b. a decrease in respiratory rate.

    c. signs and symptoms of hyperkalemia.

    d. development of cardiac arrhythmias.

13. The nurse is aware that short-term use of the carbonic anhydrase inhibitors:

    a. can cause crystalluria and fever.

    b. can result in paresthesias and anorexia.

    c. rarely causes adverse reactions.

    d. usually causes a photosensitivity reaction.

14. Mannitol is a diuretic that the nurse will administer:

    a. intravenously.   c. IM.

    b. orally.   d. SC.

IV. Crossword Puzzle

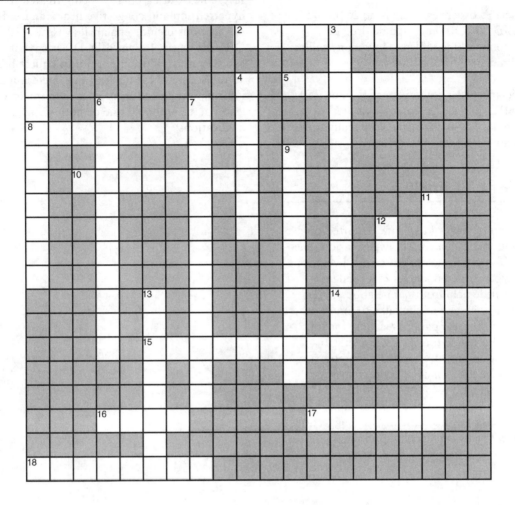

ACROSS CLUES

1. Trade name for torsemide.
2. A commonly prescribed loop diuretic.
5. Diuretic that acts by inhibiting the reabsorption of sodium and chloride ions in the ascending portion of the loop of Henle and the distal tubules.
8. Drug that increases the secretion of urine.
10. Example of an osmotic diuretic.
14. Type of diuretic that increases the density of the filtrate in the glomerulus.
15. Example of a potassium-sparing diuretic
16. Lasix is what type of diuretic?
17. Another name for open-angle glaucoma.
18. Fluid removed from the blood during the filtering process of the kidneys.

DOWN CLUES

1. When too much water is lost from the body.
3. Generic name for Aldactone.
4. Most diuretics act on the kidney nephron
   _____.
6. An example of a potassium-sparing diuretic.
7. An example of a carbonic anhydrase inhibitor.
9. Glucose in the urine.
11. Generic name for Bumex.
12. Retention of excess fluid in the body tissues.
13. Condition that creates an increase in the intraocular pressure of the eye that, if left untreated, can result in blindness.

V. Dosage Problems

Solve the following dosage calculations.

1. The physician's order reads: Lasix 80 mg, slow IV, now. The available drug is furosemide, 40 mg/5 mL. How many milliliters of Lasix will the

nurse administer? _____

2. The physician's order reads: Spironolactone 75 mg, PO, BID, QOD. The available drug is spironolactone, 50-mg tablets. How many tablets will be administered at each dose? _____

3. The physician's order reads: Acetazolamide 250 mg, PO, BID, QOD. The available drug is acetazolamide, 125-mg tablets. How many tablets will be administered at each dose? _____

VI. Critical Thinking

1. Sally Hall, an 82-year-old widow, is started on a thiazide diuretic to control her hypertension. She also has a history of osteoarthritis. She lives alone with her two cats and manages independently with only a little help from her neighbors. Her son lives out-of-state, but she talks to him on the phone weekly. Discuss patient teaching for this drug and include how the drug will work to reduce the blood pressure. Also discuss how a diuretic and its effects may affect activities and normal daily functions for Ms. Hall. Identify factors, including the diuretic therapy, that may pose safety risks for this patient. Give suggestions for how these risks might be minimized.

2. One of your assigned patients has a diagnosis of severe heart disease. He is being treated for hypertension and congestive heart failure. His medications include enalapril (Vasotec) 10 mg, QID and Lasix 40 mg, BID. Discuss what assessment data are important to collect before administering these medications. Determine what information gained from your assessment would lead you to withhold one or both of his medications.

CHAPTER 47

Urinary Anti-infectives and Miscellaneous Urinary Drugs

I. Matching

Match each term in Column A with the correct definition or statement in Column B.

COLUMN A

_____ 1. cystitis

_____ 2. dysuria

_____ 3. neurogenic bladder

_____ 4. overactive bladder

_____ 5. prostatitis

_____ 6. pyelonephritis

_____ 7. urge incontinence

_____ 8. UTI

_____ 9. urinary urgency

_____ 10. anti-infectives

COLUMN B

A. Involuntary contractions of the detrusor or bladder muscle.

B. Term describing drugs used to fight infection.

C. Inflammation of the bladder.

D. Inflammation of the prostate gland.

E. Infection caused by pathogenic microorganisms of one or more structures of the urinary tract.

F. Painful or difficult urination.

G. Accidental loss of urine caused by a sudden, unstoppable urge to void.

H. A strong and sudden urge to urinate.

I. Altered bladder function due to a nervous system abnormality.

J. Inflammation of the kidneys and renal pelvis.

II. Fill in the Blanks

1. List and define common disorders associated with the urinary system.

   a) _____

   b) _____

   c) _____

   d) _____

2. Anti-infectives used in the treatment of urinary tract infections are drugs that have an effect on _____ in the _____ _____.

3. List the urinary anti-infectives (*include the generic and trade names*).

   a) _____ _____

   b) _____ _____

   c) _____ _____

   d) _____ _____

   e) _____ _____

   f) _____ _____

4. Nitrofurantoin may be _____ or _____, depending on the _____ of the drug in the urine.

5. When trimethoprim is combined with _____ (_____), the _____ effects associated with a _____ may also occur.

6. Oxybutynin (Ditropan) acts by _____ the _____ muscle and reducing _____.

7. When nitrofurantoin is administered with _____ there is a delay in gastric emptying, _____ the _____ of nitrofurantoin.

8. Phenazopyridine treats the _____ of _____ but does not treat the _____ of the _____.

9. When a patient is diagnosed with a UTI, the nurse assesses for and documents _____, urinary _____, bladder _____, or other symptoms associated with the _____ system.

10. Signs and symptoms of acute pulmonary reaction include:

    a) _____

    b) _____

    c) _____

    d) _____

    e) _____

III. Multiple Choice

Circle the letter of the most appropriate answer.

1. Patients prescribed nitrofurantoin for a UTI must be advised by the nurse that it is very important to take the drug:
   a. with limited amounts of fluid.
   b. with food or milk.
   c. early in the morning.
   d. with a diet that is low in sodium.

2. A nurse assistant (NA) asks how she can determine if an elderly patient is drinking extra fluid. You can advise the NA to:
   a. ask a family member to write down what the patient drinks.
   b. have the patient keep a record of her fluid intake.
   c. check the urine during the day to see if it appears concentrated or dilute.
   d. have the patient save an early morning specimen.

3. Signs and symptoms that may indicate the patient has developed an acute pulmonary reaction associated with the administration of nitrofurantoin would include:
   a. dyspnea, cough, chest pain.
   b. bradycardia, malaise, increased urine output.
   c. abdominal distention, bloody sputum, hypertension.
   d. edema, fever, increased respiratory rate.

4. A patient prescribed nalidixic acid (NegGram) for a urinary tract infection asks what he should do to prevent a photosensitivity reaction. The nurse would be correct in stating:
   a. take vitamin C with this drug.
   b. avoid prolonged exposure to sunlight or ultraviolet light.
   c. drink extra fluids to prevent this reaction.
   d. do not go outside during daylight hours.

5. To ensure compliance to the prescribed treatment regimen for a urinary tract infection, the nurse stresses the importance of:
   a. taking the drug until the patient feels better.
   b. eating a diet high in citrus fruit and milk.
   c. taking one's temperature daily.
   d. taking the drug for the prescribed length of time.

6. At a team meeting, a nurse asks the question, "Why is phenazopyridine (Pyridium) given for UTIs?" The most correct answer would be that:
   a. this drug is an antiseptic used to treat the UTI.
   b. Pyridium is an analgesic used to treat the discomfort of a UTI.
   c. it is a drug used to acidify the urine.
   d. this is one of the urinary anti-infectives.

7. A patient with a UTI asks the nurse why drinking extra fluids is so important in the treatment of the UTI. The best answer the nurse could give would be:

   a. extra fluid helps keep the urine alkaline.

   b. bacteria are more easily flushed from the genitourinary tract.

   c. fluids help to stop the bacteria from multiplying.

   d. the extra fluid makes the urine more acidic.

8. Patient teaching for the medication fosfomycin would include the instructions:

   a. take this drug on an empty stomach.

   b. chew the tablet thoroughly before swallowing.

   c. dissolve in 90 to 120 mL of water and drink immediately.

   d. mix the powder with hot milk and drink.

9. The nurse caring for the patient with a UTI would notify the primary health care provider if the:

   a. urine output increases.

   b. urine appears clear and dilute.

   c. Pyridium has caused the urine to appear red.

   d. urine output decreases and urine is concentrated during daytime hours.

10. A patient has been admitted for treatment of a severe UTI. The nurse knows to collect a sample of urine for a _____ test before the medication is started.

    a. CBC.   c. H&H

    b. PT.   d. C&S.

11. A nurse caring for an elderly patient who is being treated with flavoxate (Urispas) for urge incontinence will be aware of the possible adverse reaction of:

    a. mental confusion.

    b. hypertension.

    c. vaginitis.

    d. decreased production of tears.

12. Individuals with frequent UTIs are encouraged to include in their daily diet:

    a. orange juice.   c. cranberry juice.

    b. tea and coffee.   d. carbonated sodas.

IV. Crossword Puzzle

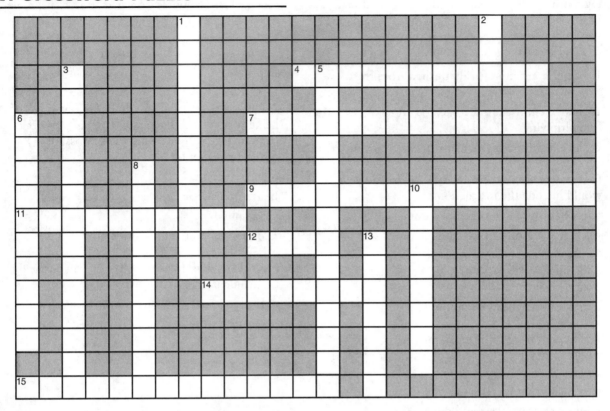

ACROSS CLUES

4. Trade name for methamine mandelate.
7. Slows or retards the multiplication of bacteria.
9. A urinary tract analgesic.
11. Inflammation of the urethra.
12. Type of incontinence characterized by accidental loss of urine due to a sudden, unstoppable urge to void.
14. Inflammation of the bladder.
15. Inflammation of the kidneys and the renal pelvis.

DOWN CLUES

1. Inflammation of the prostate gland.
2. Urinary tract infection (abbreviation).
3. Pregnancy Category D urinary anti-infective.
5. Drugs that fight infection.
6. Generic name for Ditropan.
8. Brand name for nitrofurantoin.
10. Trade name for phenazopyridine.
13. Painful or difficult urination.

V. Dosage Problems

Solve the following dosage calculations.

1. The physician's order reads: Phenazopyridine 200 mg, PO, TID, after meals. The available drug is Pyridium, 100-mg tablets. How many tablets will be administered at each dose? _____

2. The physician's order reads: Oxybutynin 5 mg, PO, TID. The available drug is Ditropan Syrup, 5 mg/5 mL.

   a) How many milliliters are administered at each dose? _____

   b) How many doses of medication will be given in each 24-hour period? _____

3. The physician's order reads: Nitrofurantoin 75 mg, PO, QID. The available drug is Nitrofurantoin Oral Suspension, 25 mg/5 mL.

   a) How many milliliters will be administered for each dose? _____

   b) What is the total milligram dosage for the 24-hour period? _____

VI. Critical Thinking

1. Connie Mann, 15 years of age, visits the walk-in clinic with the symptoms of urgency, frequency, and dysuria. A routine urinalysis indicates the presence of a bacterial infection. The physician prescribes nitrofurantoin for 10 days and phenazopyridine for 2 days. Discuss the patient teaching that will be necessary for these two medications and the data needed to determine if Connie's UTI is responding to treatment.

2. A patient recovering from urologic surgery is to be started on the combination drug, trimethoprim-sulfamethoxazole (Bactrim DS), twice daily. He takes no other medications and reports an allergy to eggs, nuts, sulfa, and morphine. The unit dose of Bactrim, provided by the pharmacy, is a tablet containing 160 mg of trimethoprim and 800 mg of sulfamethoxazole. The nurse administers one tablet at 9:00 AM. for his morning dose. What medication error has just occurred, and how could it have been prevented? How would you respond to this error, and what actions will you take?

CHAPTER 48

Drugs That Affect the Gastrointestinal System

I. Matching

Match each term in Column A with the correct definition or statement in Column B.

COLUMN A

_____ 1. antacids

_____ 2. antiflatulents

_____ 3. emetic

_____ 4. gallstone-solubilizing

_____ 5. gastric stasis

_____ 6. gastroesophageal reflux disease

_____ 7. hypersecretory

_____ 8. proton pump inhibitor

_____ 9. docusate

_____ 10. hydrochloric acid

_____ 11. photophobia

_____ 12. antidiarrheals

_____ 13. ipecac

_____ 14. paralylic ileus

_____ 15. *Helicobacter pylori*

COLUMN B

A. Used to treat diarrhea.

B. Against flatus or gas in the intestinal tract.

C. Drug that induces vomiting.

D. Gallstone-dissolving drugs.

E. Used to prevent dry, hard stools.

F. Drugs that block the last step in acid production.

G. Implicated as a causative organism of chronic gastritis and peptic and duodenal ulcers.

H. Aversion to bright light, an adverse reaction to the anticholinergics.

I. Intestinal atony; diminished or absent bowel signs; lack of peristalsis or movement in the intestine.

J. An over-the-counter emetic for use at home.

K. A substance secreted by some cells in the stomach that aids in the initial digestive process.

L. A drug that works against acids.

M. Failure to move food normally out of the stomach.

N. A reflux or backup of gastric contents into the esophagus.

O. Excessive gastric secretion of hydrochloric acid in the stomach.

II. Fill in the Blanks

1. The antacids containing _____ and _____ have a _____ effect and produce diarrhea.

2. List the four different elements that antacids may contain.

   a) _____

   b) _____

   c) _____

   d) _____

3. Antacids containing _____ and _____ tend to produce constipation.

4. List the three ways antacids may interfere with other drugs.

   a) _____

   b) _____

   c) _____

5. _____ and _____
   increase the motility of the upper
   gastrointestinal tract.

6. Dexpanthenol administration may cause:

   a) _____

   b) _____

   c) _____

7. List the histamine H_2 antagonists (*include the generic and trade names*).

   a)_____ _____

   b)_____ _____

   c)_____ _____

   d)_____ _____

8. Charcoal is an _____ that reduces
   the amount of _____ gas.

9. The emetic, ipecac, causes _____
   because of its local _____ effect on the
   _____ and by stimulation of the
   _____ center in the _____.

10. Relief from the heartburn associated with
    gastroesophageal reflux disease may be obtained
    from (*include the generic and trade names*):

    a) _____ _____

    b) _____ _____

III. Multiple Choice

Circle the letter of the most appropriate answer.

1. The physician has prescribed an antacid to the medication regimen of an elderly patient. The nurse will give the antacid:
   a. with the other drugs.
   b. in the early morning and at bedtime.
   c. 2 hours before or 2 hours after administration of other medications.
   d. 30 minutes before or 30 minutes after giving other drugs.

2. Your patient has been prescribed docusate sodium, a stool softener, for her constipation. She asks you how a stool softener works to relieve constipation. You would be correct in stating that these drugs work by:
   a. promoting water retention in the fecal mass.
   b. lubricating the intestinal walls.
   c. promoting sodium retention in the fecal mass.
   d. stimulating the walls of the intestines.

3. A nursing student is discussing her patient's medication regimen with the charge nurse. The student asks why patients are prescribed digestive enzymes. The correct answer would be that these drugs are used:
   a. for patients with a fat intolerance and diarrhea.
   b. for those who have chronic indigestion or constipation.
   c. to aid in the digestion of saturated fats and carbohydrates.
   d. as a replacement therapy for those with pancreatic enzyme deficiency.

4. Diphenoxylate (Lomotil), a narcotic-related antidiarrheal, is combined with atropine, an anticholinergic, in an effort to:
   a. increase gastric motility.
   b. discourage abuse of the drug.
   c. prevent fluid loss.
   d. decrease gastric secretions.

5. When an anticholinergic drug is prescribed for treatment of a peptic ulcer, the nurse observes the patient for adverse effects, which may include:
   a. dry mouth, urinary retention.
   b. edema, tachycardia.
   c. weight gain, increased respiratory rate.
   d. diarrhea, anorexia.

6. When caring for the patient receiving a magnesium-containing antacid, the nurse must be alert to the possible development of:
   a. diarrhea.   c. fever.
   b. respiratory acidosis.   d. blurred vision.

7. The nurse is caring for a patient just admitted with severe diarrhea. The physician has ordered an antidiarrheal, which the nurse will administer:

a. hourly until diarrhea resolves.

b. with food.

c. twice a day, morning and night.

d. after each diarrhea episode.

8. A physician has ordered an emetic to be administered to a patient being treated in the emergency department. The nurse must be alert to the possibility that the patient may:

a. retain fluid.   c. aspirate vomitus.

b. become violent.   d. develop diarrhea.

9. Before or immediately after administration of an emetic, the nurse will place the patient:

a. face down.

b. in a supine position.

c. upright.

d. in a side-lying position.

10. The physician has ordered mineral oil, PRN, for a patient. The nurse will administer this medication:

a. on an empty stomach in the evening.

b. in the morning with breakfast.

c. with any kind of food or milk.

d. with or immediately after the evening meal.

11. Patient teaching for the antacids should include the instructions to:

a. chew the tablet completely before swallowing.

b. drink a full glass of water after swallowing the tablet.

c. make sure not to chew or bite the tablet.

d. allow the tablet to dissolve in the mouth.

12. Patients taking a bulk-producing laxative should be instructed by the nurse to:

a. refrain from drinking fluids for 1 hour.

b. take a second dose in 30 minutes.

c. immediately drink a full glass of water.

d. allow the tablet to dissolve in the mouth.

13. While completing your patient's medication history, you discover that he uses mineral oil frequently as a laxative. As this patient's nurse, you should explain that frequent ingestion of mineral oil can:

a. increase serum potassium levels.

b. interfere with absorption of vitamins A, D, E, and K.

c. increase the absorption of fats.

d. produce severe fluid retention.

14. The nurse administers a magnesium-containing antacid cautiously in patients with:

a. decreased renal function.

b. claudication.

c. hepatic impairment.

d. cardiac disease.

15. The nurse should advise the patient not to use high doses of laxatives and not to use them for an extended period of time in order to avoid:

a. hypertension.   c. headache.

b. flu-like symptoms.   d. diarrhea.

IV. Crossword Puzzle

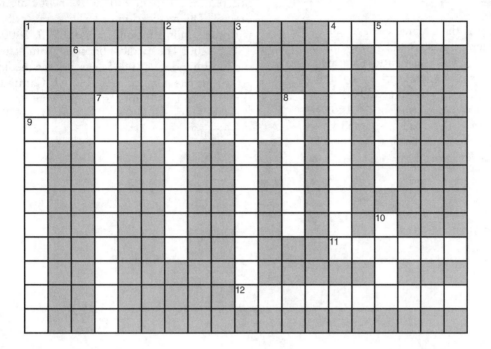

ACROSS CLUES

4. Antacid consisting of aluminum and magnesium hydroxide.
6. Trade name for ranitidine.
9. Generic name for Nexium.
11. Drug used to induce vomiting.
12. Generic name for Tagamet.

DOWN CLUES

1. A narcotic-related antidiarrheal.
2. Pancreatic enzyme.
3. Acid secreted in the stomach that aids in the initial digestive process.
4. Example of an antacid.
5. Drug used to reduce or neutralize the acidity of the stomach.
7. Generic name for Prilosec.
8. Trade name for famotidine.
10. Gastroesophageal reflux disease (abbreviation).

V. Dosage Problems

Solve the following dosage calculations.

1. The physician's order reads: Ranitidine 75 mg, PO, as needed for heartburn. The available drug is Zantac Syrup, 15 mg/mL. How many milliliters will be administered at each dose? _____

2. The physician's order reads: Dexpanthenol 500 mg, IM, now, repeat in 2 hours, then give every 6 hours. The available drug is dexpanthenol injection, 250 mg/mL. How many milliliters will be administered with each injection? _____

3. The physician's order reads: Omeprazole 60 mg, PO, qd. The available drug is Prilosec DR capsules, 20 mg. How many capsules will the patient take at each dose? _____

VI. Critical Thinking

1. You are working as the telephone triage nurse in the emergency department. A caller, 69 years of age, complains of severe constipation, stating, "My stomach hurts so much I can hardly stand it. Do you think I should try some milk of magnesia?" Discuss other data that need to be obtained from this patient. Why wouldn't you recommend milk of magnesia for this patient? What is your suggestion to him?

2. Sucralfate (Carafate) 1 gram, PO, AC and HS, is ordered for a patient with active peptic ulcer disease. The medication order was transcribed with the administration times of 0900, 1300, 1800, 2200. The medication nurse administered the morning dose at 0845. Discuss the medication error that has just occurred. How is Carafate supposed to be administered, and what are its actions? How can an error like this be avoided in the future?

CHAPTER 49

Antidiabetic Drugs

I. Matching

Match each term in Column A with the correct definition or statement in Column B.

COLUMN A

_____ 1. lipodystrophy

_____ 2. secondary failure

_____ 3. hypoglycemia

_____ 4. glucagon

_____ 5. diabetes mellitus

_____ 6. glucometer

_____ 7. hyperglycemia

_____ 8. insulin

_____ 9. glycosylated hemoglobin

_____ 10. diabetic ketoacidosis

_____ 11. *Escherichia coli*

_____ 12. type 1 diabetes

COLUMN B

A. A hormone produced by the pancreas; acts to maintain blood glucose levels within normal levels.

B. A chronic disorder in which there is insufficient insulin produced by beta cells of the pancreas or cellular resistance to insulin.

C. Insulin dependent.

D. Human insulin is derived from a biosynthetic process using strains of _____.

E. Low blood glucose or sugar.

F. _____ (HbA$_{1c}$) is a blood test used to monitor the patient's average blood glucose level over a 3- to 4-month period.

G. Device used to monitor blood glucose levels.

H. Hormone produced by the pancreas that acts to stimulate the conversion of glycogen to glucose in the liver.

I. A potentially life-threatening deficiency of insulin resulting in severe hyperglycemia that requires prompt diagnosis and treatment.

J. Occurs when sulfonylurea loses its effectiveness.

K. Higher than normal blood glucose or sugar.

L. Atrophy of the subcutaneous fat at overused insulin injection sites.

II. Fill in the Blanks

1. A patient taking metformin will be monitored by the nurse for signs and symptoms of lactic acidosis, which include:

   a) _____

   b) _____

   c) _____

   d) _____

   e) _____

2. List the three properties of insulin that are clinically important.

   a) _____

   b) _____

   c) _____

3. Insulin preparations are classified as:

   a) _____

   b) _____

   c) _____

4. Hypoglycemia may occur:

a) _____

b) _____

c) _____

5. Hyperglycemia can occur:

a) _____

b) _____

c) _____

6. Before withdrawing insulin from the vial, the nurse must check the label for:

a) _____

b) _____

c) _____

d) _____

7. Methods of terminating a hypoglycemic reaction include the administration of one or more of these items:

a) _____

b) _____

c) _____

d) _____

e) _____

8. List the symptoms of a possible hyperglycemic episode that the nurse should report immediately.

a) _____

b) _____

c) _____

d) _____

e) _____

f) _____

g) _____

h) _____

i) _____

III. Multiple Choice

Circle the letter of the most appropriate answer.

1. Regular insulin and lente insulin are to be administered to your patient in a single injection. You will be correct if you:

   a. withdraw the regular insulin into the syringe first.

   b. shake the vial vigorously before withdrawing the insulin.

   c. withdraw the lente insulin into the syringe first.

   d. refrigerate the regular insulin for 30 minutes before administration.

2. If the nurse observes an episode of hypoglycemia:

   a. the physician is contacted for the method to be used to terminate the episode.

   b. it must be corrected as soon as the symptoms are recognized.

   c. the patient is placed on bed rest until the physician arrives.

   d. the temperature is taken before notifying the physician.

3. Which of the following would be an appropriate nursing action used to terminate a hypoglycemic episode?

   a. Give the patient a banana to eat.

   b. Administer 1 or 2 glasses of carbonated beverage.

   c. Have the patient drink orange juice diluted with 1 glass of water.

   d. Give the patient hard candy or honey.

4. During an in-service on administering insulin, a nurse asks about the storage of insulin. The correct answer for this nurse would be to store insulin:

   a. in the freezer.

   b. at room temperature, away from heat and light.

   c. in a warm, dark area.

   d. in the coldest section of the refrigerator.

5. Patient teaching for the patient with diabetes should include:

   a. check your urine daily for the presence of glucose or use a glucose monitoring device once a month.

   b. eat two meals a day, with your largest meal being at noon.

   c. wear identification, such as Medic-Alert, to inform medical personnel of your insulin use or hypoglycemic drug.

   d. to lose weight, use a commercial weight loss product.

6. As a nurse, you would know all insulins can be administered:

   a. SC.   c. orally.

   b. IV.   d. orally and IM.

7. Which of the following symptoms exhibited by a patient would alert the nurse to a possible hyperglycemic episode?

   a. Rapid, shallow respirations; headache

   b. Fatigue, weakness, confusion

   c. Thirst, abdominal pain, nausea

   d. Pale, moist skin; elevated temperature

8. The nurse will correctly collect a sample of capillary blood for glucometer testing by:

   a. obtaining the blood sample from the palm of the hand.

   b. collecting several drops of blood for a good sample.

   c. retrieving the blood sample from the vein in the hand.

   d. collecting a hanging drop of blood and distributing it over the entire pad.

9. When teaching the patient how to prevent lipodystrophy when self-administering insulin, the nurse would stress the importance of:

   a. immediately reporting any itching at the injection site.

   b. rotating injection sites and areas.

   c. massaging the injection site to enhance absorption.

   d. administering insulin only by the intravenous route.

10. The physician would be notified if your patient's blood glucose level is:

    a. 70 mg/dL.   c. 120 mg/dL.

    b. 100 mg/dL.   d. 280 mg/dL.

11. Which of the following would be included in a teaching plan for a diabetic patient taking human insulin?

    a. There is less chance of developing lipodystrophy when using human insulin.

    b. Human insulin appears to cause fewer allergic reactions than insulin obtained from animal sources.

    c. Human insulin must be administered by the oral route.

    d. Larger doses of human insulin are required because it is less potent than insulin from animal sources.

12. For patients being treated with oral hypoglycemics, the nurse must be aware that hypoglycemic episodes:

    a. may be less intense than reactions seen with insulin administration.

    b. will most likely occur 1 to 2 hours after a meal.

    c. may be more intense than reactions seen with insulin administration.

    d. occur more frequently in patients being treated with oral hypoglycemics.

13. During a team conference, the nurse explains that the oral hypoglycemic agents:

    a. work in the same manner as insulin.

    b. have fewer adverse reactions than insulin.

    c. cannot be substituted for insulin.

    d. can be used to treat type 1 diabetes.

14. In managing hyperglycemia, the nurse would report blood glucose levels that are consistently over:

    a. 200 mg/dL.   c. 180 mg/dL.

    b. 70 mg/dL.   d. 120 mg/dL.

15. During initial therapy with a hypoglycemic agent, the nurse will monitor the patient for a hypoglycemic reaction:

    a. daily.

    b. every 2 to 4 hours.

    c. after meals.

    d. every 10 to 15 minutes.

IV. Crossword Puzzle

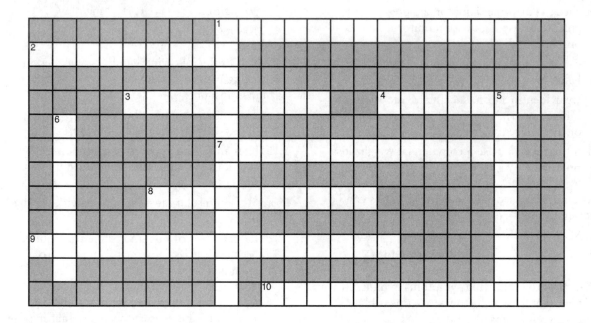

ACROSS CLUES

1. Higher than normal blood glucose or sugar.
2. _____ failure occurs when the sulfonylureas lose their effectiveness.
3. Example of a biguanide antidiabetic drug.
4. Hormone produced by the pancreas that acts to stimulate the conversion of glycogen to glucose in the liver.
7. Atrophy of the subcutaneous fat at overused insulin injection sites.
8. Device used to monitor blood glucose levels.
9. Chronic disorder where there is insufficient insulin produced by beta cells of the pancreas or cellular resistance to insulin.
10. Oral antidiabetic drug.

DOWN CLUES

1. Low blood glucose or sugar.
5. Generic name for Micronase.
6. Hormone produced by the pancreas which acts to maintain blood glucose levels within normal limits.

V. Dosage Problems

Solve the following dosage calculations.

Calculate the dose of insulin where necessary, and shade in the correct dose on the picture of the syringe provided. Insulin labeled 100 U/mL is available for all problems regardless of type of insulin stated.

1. The physician's order reads: Humulin Regular, 10 U, SC, AC, 0730.

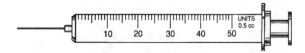

2. The physician's order reads: Humulin Regular, 8 U, SC and 12 U, SC. Humulin NPH AC 0730.

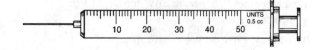

3. The physician's order reads: Glyburide 5 mg each day, PO, with breakfast. The available drug is Micronase, 2.5-mg tablets. How many tablets will be administered with each dose? _____

4. A patient is on a sliding scale for insulin doses. The physician ordered Humulin Regular insulin q6h as follows:

Finger stick blood
glucose

	0–180	No coverage
	180–240	2 U SC.
	241–300	4 U SC.
	301–400	6 U SC.
	>400	8 U SC and repeat finger stick in 2 hours

At 1130, the patient's finger stick is 364. Shade in the area on the syringe that will indicate the dosage the patient is to receive.

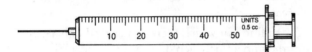

VI. Critical Thinking

1. Angela Clark, an 11-year-old, has been diagnosed with diabetes and prescribed daily insulin injections. She lives in a single-parent home and attends public school. Her mother feels very unsure of her ability to understand and learn about her daughter's insulin. How would you approach this situation? Discuss the patient and family teaching that needs to be completed in relation to insulin and its role in managing diabetes.

2. A patient on oral hypoglycemic medication asks you to explain how his Micronase works to keep his blood glucose at a safe level. Discuss how you would teach this patient about his medication, and how you would determine if the information was understood by the patient. Include information about diabetes and nonpharmacological management of the disease.

CHAPTER 50

Pituitary and Adrenocortical Hormones

I. Matching

Match each term in Column A with the correct definition or statement in Column B.

COLUMN A

_____ 1. adrenal insufficiency

_____ 2. corticosteroids

_____ 3. cryptorchism

_____ 4. Cushing's syndrome

_____ 5. diabetes insipidus

_____ 6. feedback mechanism

_____ 7. glucocorticoids

_____ 8. gonadotropins

_____ 9. gonads

_____ 10. buffalo hump

_____ 11. mineralocorticoids

_____ 12. rhynile

_____ 13. somatotropic hormones

_____ 14. anovulatory

_____ 15. hyperstimulation syndrome

COLUMN B

A. Hormones secreted by the anterior pituitary that influence the organs of reproduction.

B. Failure to produce an ovum or failure to ovulate.

C. Failure of the testes to descend into the scrotum.

D. Sudden ovarian enlargement accompanied by ascites.

E. Growth hormone secreted by the anterior pituitary.

F. Disease resulting from the failure of the pituitary to secrete vasopressin, or from surgical removal of the pituitary.

G. A flexible calibrated plastic tube used to administer desmopressin nasally.

H. Hormones secreted by the adrenal glands that regulate the functions of the immune system; regulate glucose, fat, and protein metabolism; and control the anti-inflammatory response.

I. Disease due to the overproduction of endogenous glucocorticoids.

J. Hormones that are important in controlling sodium and water balance.

K. Method by which the body maintains most hormones at a relatively constant level in the bloodstream.

L. A condition in which there is a critical deficiency of the mineralocorticoids and the glucocorticoids, requiring immediate treatment.

M. The organs of reproduction.

N. Term referring to the hormones that are produced by the adrenal glands.

O. A hump that forms on the back of the neck and is a sign of Cushing's syndrome.

II. Fill in the Blanks

1. A patient taking clomiphene will need to monitor for symptoms of ovarian stimulation, which may include:

   a) _____

   b) _____

   c) _____

2. The nurse must teach parents whose child is taking growth hormone to monitor for signs and symptoms of diabetes, which include:

   a) _____

   b _____

   c) _____

3. Excessive _____ and excessive

   _____ characterize diabetes insipidus.

4. Before administering the first dose of vasopressin for diabetes insipidus, the nurse will assess and document the patient's:

   a) _____

   b) _____

   c) _____

   d) _____

5. Before administering vasopressin to relieve abdominal distention, the nurse will assess and document the patient's:

   a) _____

   b) _____

   c) _____

   d) _____

   e) _____

6. Patients taking lypressin for treatment of

   diabetes insipidus learn to adjust their

   medication dosage based on the _____

   of urination and _____ of thirst.

7. When the patient has diabetes insipidus, the nurse measures fluid intake and output and observes patient for signs of dehydration, which include:

   a) _____

   b) _____

   c) _____

   d) _____

   e) _____

8. Examples of the glucocorticoids include:

   a) _____

   b) _____

   c) _____

   d) _____

   e) _____

9. Adverse reactions that may occur with long-term treatment with the glucocorticoids include the signs and symptoms of a Cushing-like state, which include:

   a) _____

   b) _____

   c) _____

   d) _____

   e) _____

   f) _____

   g) _____

   h) _____

   i) _____

10. Examples of the gonadotropin drugs include:

    a) _____

    b) _____

    c) _____

    d) _____

III. Multiple Choice

Circle the letter of the most appropriate answer.

Ms. Chapman has severe rheumatoid arthritis, which has not responded well to therapy with anti-inflammatory agents. Her physician has prescribed a glucocorticoid in an attempt to prevent further joint destruction, as well as to relieve the symptoms of the disorder. Questions 1–7 pertain to Ms. Chapman's case.

1. When administering a glucocorticoid, the nurse must be aware that administration over a period of as little as 5 to 10 days will result in:

   a. shutting off the pituitary release of ACTH.

   b. drug tolerance.

   c. increasing the amount of endogenous glucocorticoids secreted by the adrenal glands.

   d. drug sensitivity.

2. There is a possibility that Ms. Chapman will experience adverse effects with the administration of the glucocorticoids. The nurse must be aware that these can include:

   a. hypotension, hyperkalemia.

   b. paresthesias, occipital headaches.

   c. osteoporosis, hypertension.

   d. sodium and fluid loss.

3. Ms. Chapman may experience electrolyte imbalance. The nurse will monitor laboratory results for:

   a. hypercalcemia, hyperkalemia.

   b. hypernatremia, hypokalemia.

   c. hypocalcemia, hyperkalemia.

   d. hyponatremia, hypocalcemia.

4. Nursing personnel and visitors with any type of infection should avoid contact with Ms. Chapman because:

   a. of her possible decreased resistance to infection.

   b. she may harbor infectious bacteria that may be transmissible.

   c. she has an infectious form of arthritis.

   d. her WBC count will be elevated, rendering her susceptible to disease.

5. Ms. Chapman also has insulin-dependent diabetes. While on the glucocorticoid therapy, the nurse may have to:

   a. make frequent adjustments in her insulin dosage, per physician's orders.

   b. provide a diet high in carbohydrates and low in protein.

   c. monitor her urine for increased protein.

   d. perform blood glucose testing every 2 hours.

6. Patients who are not diabetic and are on glucocorticoid therapy have their urine and blood checked weekly for glucose because of the possibility of:

   a. developing ketoacidosis.

   b. false-positive urine tests for glucose.

   c. aggravating latent diabetes.

   d. increasing excretions of ketones.

7. The physician has decided to discontinue the glucocorticoids after 3 weeks of treatment. The nurse will expect the drug to be discontinued by:

   a. stopping the dose immediately, which will shock the pituitary into secreting ACTH quickly.

   b. gradually switching to a milder drug before discontinuing the glucocorticoid.

   c. giving one last large dose and then discontinuing the drug.

   d. tapering the drug dosage over a period of several days.

8. A patient is to begin receiving clomiphene and the nurse is explaining the adverse reactions that may occur with this drug, which include:

   a. sedation.   c. hypertension.

   b. vasomotor flushes.   d. edema.

9. Which of the following assessments would be most important for the nurse to make when a child receiving growth hormone comes to the physician's office or the clinic for an evaluation?

   a. Diet history

   b. Blood pressure, pulse, respirations

   c. Abdominal girth

   d. Height and weight

10. The patient receiving ACTH will need to be monitored for the development of the cushingnoid appearance, which is indicated by:

    a. pallor of the skin.

    b. moon face, hirsutism.

    c. kyphosis, periorbital edema.

    d. exophthalmos, weight loss.

11. Mr. Lyons has developed severe abdominal distention. The nurse expects the physician to prescribe:

    a. lypressin (Diapid).

    b. desmopressin (DDAVP).

    c. vasopressin (Pitressin Synthetic).

    d. fludrocortisone (Florinef).

12. At a staff meeting, a nurse states that vaso-pressin is prescribed for the treatment of:
    a. diabetes mellitus.
    b. diabetes insipidus.
    c. electrolyte imbalances.
    d. dehydration.

13. After administration of vasopressin, the nurse would observe the patient every 10 to 15 minutes for signs of overdosage, which may include:
    a. excessive urinary output.
    b. nausea, diarrhea, excessive perspiration.
    c. dry skin, flushing hypothermia.
    d. blanching of the skin, nausea, abdominal cramps.

14. At a team conference, a discussion begins about the mineralocorticoids and a nurse states that these corticosteroids perform an important role in:
    a. glucose metabolism.
    b. promoting the release of ACTH from the pituitary.
    c. conserving sodium and increasing the secretion of potassium.
    d. promoting the excretion of aldosterone.

15. Parents of a child starting treatment with soma-trem are told by the nurse that during the first year of treatment, they can expect growth of about:
    a. 5 cm/year.   c. 7 cm/year.
    b. 6 cm/year.   d. 8 cm/year.

IV. Crossword Puzzle

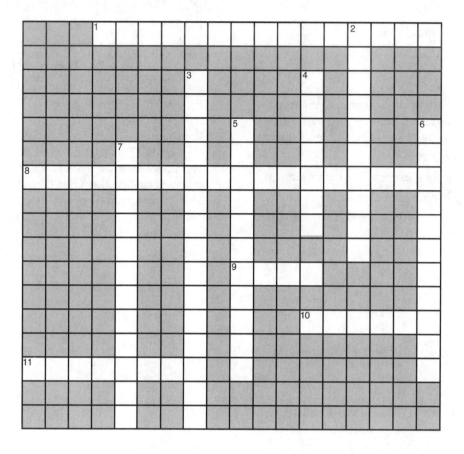

ACROSS CLUES

1. Drug that has both glucocorticoid and mineralocorticoid activity.
8. Hormones that are important in controlling salt and water balance.
9. Anterior pituitary hormone that stimulates the adrenal cortex to produce and secrete adrenocortical hormone.
10. Organs of reproduction.
11. Disease due to the overproduction of endogenous glucocorticoids.

DOWN CLUES

2. Generic name of a synthetic growth hormone product.
3. Posterior pituitary.
4. A flexible calibrated plastic tube used to administer desmopressin nasally.
5. Failure to produce an ovum or failure to ovulate.
6. Hormone produced by the posterior pituitary gland.
7. Failure of the testes to descend into the scrotum.

V. Dosage Problems

Solve the following dosage calculations.

1. A child weighing 66 pounds is placed on treatment with somatrem. The prescribed dosage is 0.1 mg/kg, IM, three times a week. The vial contains 5 mg of somatrem that is to be diluted with 1 milliliter of bacteriostatic water for injection. Resultant solution yields a strength of 5 mg/mL.

   a) How many kilograms does the child weigh?
   _____

   b) What is the milligram dose for the child?
   _____

   c) How many milliliters of solution will be needed for the prescribed dose? _____

2. The physician's order reads: Vasopressin 5 U, IM, at 3-hour intervals. The available drug is Vasopressin, 20 U/mL. How many milliliters will be administered each dose? _____

3. The physician's order reads: Prednisone 30 mg, PO, daily before 0900. The available drug is Prednisone Syrup, 5 mg/mL. How many milliliters are needed for the prescribed dose?

_____

VI. Critical Thinking

1. Harry Graham has been receiving high-dose corticosteroid therapy (hydrocortisone 80 mg BID) for the last month. You receive an order to taper Mr. Graham's dose as follows: Decrease hydrocortisone dose by 20 mg each day for 3 days. Day 4, decrease by 10 mg per day and give every other day. You are caring for Mr. Graham on the third day and administer 40 mg for his morning dose. Discuss what medication error just occurred and suggest what could have been done to prevent this type of error.

2. Beth Ross, a 62-year-old teacher, was admitted for elective abdominal surgery. Her medication history reveals daily use of prednisone. Individualize a postoperative plan of care for Beth considering her chronic steroid use.

CHAPTER 51

Thyroid and Antithyroid Drugs

I. Matching

Match each term in Column A with the correct definition or statement in Column B.

COLUMN A

_____ 1. euthyroid

_____ 2. goiter

_____ 3. hyperthyroidism

_____ 4. hypothyroidism

_____ 5. iodine

_____ 6. iodism

_____ 7. myxedema

_____ 8. thyroid gland

_____ 9. thyroid storm

_____ 10. thyrotoxicosis

_____ 11. agranulocytosis

_____ 12. iodine allergy

_____ 13. antithyroid drugs

_____ 14. thyroxine

_____ 15. triiodothyronine

COLUMN B

A. Symptoms include swelling of parts of the face and body, fever, joint pain, and difficulty breathing, which requires immediate medical attention.

B. Excessive amounts of iodine in the body.

C. Decrease in the number of neutrophils, basophils, and eosinophils.

D. Inhibits the body's ability to manufacture thyroid hormones.

E. Located in the neck, anterior to the trachea, and secretes thyroid hormones.

F. Characterized by high fever, extreme tachycardia, and an altered mental state.

G. A decrease in the amount of thyroid hormone manufactured and secreted.

H. Essential element for the manufacture of the two thyroid hormones.

I. T_4, a hormone secreted by the thyroid gland.

J. An increase in the amount of thyroid hormone manufactured and secreted by the thyroid gland.

K. Term used to describe the normal thyroid.

L. Severe form of hypothyroidism.

M. Enlargement of the thyroid gland

N. Another name for thyrotoxicosis.

O. T_3, a hormone secreted by the thyroid gland.

II. Fill in the Blanks

1. Thyroid hormones are used as _____ therapy when the patient is _____.

2. The _____ effects of _____ _____ _____ therapy may not be apparent for _____ weeks or _____, but _____ effects may be apparent in as little as _____ hours.

3. Thyroid hormones are administered _____ a day, _____ in the _____ and preferably before _____.

4. Symptoms of iodism may include:

   a) _____

   b) _____

   c) _____

   d) _____

   e) _____

   f) _____

5. Iodine solutions should be _____ through a _____ because they may cause _____ discoloration.

III. Multiple Choice

Circle the letter of the most appropriate answer.

Ms. Jackson has been diagnosed with hypothyroidism and her physician has prescribed a thyroid hormone. Questions 1–5 pertain to Ms. Jackson's case.

1. Ms. Jackson asks the nurse why the doctor has prescribed a thyroid hormone. The nurse explains that the use of a thyroid hormone is an attempt to:
   a. increase the manufacture of endogenous thyroid hormones.
   b. block the secretion of thyroxine from the thyroid gland.
   c. change the iodine uptake of the thyroid gland.
   d. create normal thyroid function (euthyroid).

2. During initial therapy, the most common adverse reactions the nurse would expect Ms. Jackson to experience are signs of:
   a. Stevens-Johnson syndrome.
   b. hypothyroidism.
   c. congestive heart failure.
   d. hyperthyroidism.

3. The nurse is aware of the importance of informing Ms. Jackson that the full effects of the thyroid therapy may not be evident for:
   a. several weeks or more.
   b. 24 to 48 hours.
   c. 8 to 10 months.
   d. 1 to 3 days.

4. During Ms. Jackson's thyroid therapy, she will be monitored for the signs that will indicate how well she is responding to therapy. Which of the following would be a positive indication to the nurse that Ms. Jackson is responding well to treatment?
   a. Weight loss, mild diuresis, sense of well-being
   b. Decrease in pulse rate and metabolism; absence of tremors
   c. Decrease in anxiety; increase in blood pressure; irregular menses
   d. Weight gain, improved appetite, decrease in blood pressure

5. The nurse is planning her discharge teaching for Ms. Jackson. It will be important for Ms. Jackson to know:
   a. she should take the medication at bedtime.
   b. the brand of drug can be changed without checking with the physician.
   c. the dosage of the drug may require periodic adjustment.
   d. a weight gain of 8 to 10 pounds is normal.

6. A patient is to receive strong iodine solution (Lugol's solution). The nurse would administer the drug correctly when it is measured in:
   a. drops and mixed with fruit juice or water.
   b. milliliters and given twice daily.
   c. grams and given at bedtime.
   d. drops and placed directly on the tongue.

7. The nurse would suspect complications are developing in a patient receiving methimazol (Tapozole) if which of the following symptoms are exhibited?
   a. Cough, periorbital edema, constipation
   b. Fever, sore throat, bleeding from injection site
   c. Unsteady gait, blurred vision, insomnia
   d. Constipation, anorexia, blurred vision

8. When monitoring the patient receiving radioactive iodine, it is very important for the nurse to understand which of the following?
   a. Why the patient will be NPO
   b. Unusual bowel habits of the patient
   c. Directions of the Nuclear Medicine department with regard to precautions to take
   d. Laboratory results of the thyroid function tests

9. When a patient is experiencing hyperthyroidism, he will exhibit certain symptoms that the nurse would recognize, which may include:

   a. intolerance to cold, weight loss, tachycardia.

   b. increased appetite, weight loss, bradycardia.

   c. lethargy, puffy face, flushed skin.

   d. nervousness, tachycardia, moderate hypotension.

10. When caring for the patient receiving radioactive iodine, the nurse would suspect the patient is experiencing an adverse reaction if he makes this statement:

    a. "My body hurts all over."

    b. "My throat hurts when I swallow."

    c. "I'm sleepy most of the day."

    d. "I'm unable to sleep at night."

IV. Crossword Puzzle

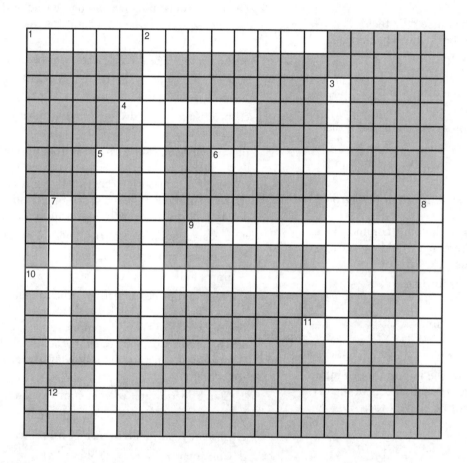

ACROSS CLUES

1. Drug of choice for hypothyroidism.
4. Excessive amounts of iodine in the body.
6. Enlargement of the thyroid gland.
9. Normal thyroid.
10. T_3, a hormone secreted by the thyroid gland.
11. Essential element for the manufacture of the two thyroid hormones.
12. Potentially the most serious adverse reaction to propylthiouracil.

DOWN CLUES

2. A decrease in the amount of thyroid hormones produced.
3. A severe form of hyperthyroidism.
5. Another name for thyrotoxicosis.
7. Located in the neck anterior to the trachea and secretes thyroid hormones.
8. Severe form of hypothyroidism.

V. Dosage Problems

Solve the following dosage calculations.

1. The physician's order reads: Levothyroxine 50 mcg, PO, daily. The available drug is Synthroid, 0.05-mg scored tablets. How many tablets will the nurse administer? _____

2. The physician's order reads: Synthroid 25 mcg, PO, QOD. The available drug is levothyroxine, 0.05-mg scored tablets. How many tablets will the nurse administer? _____

3. The physician's order reads: Propylthiouracil 300 mg/day, PO, in three divided doses. The available drug is PTU, 50-mg tablets.

   a) How many milligrams will be given at each dose? _____

   b) How many tablets will be needed for the prescribed dose? _____

VI. Critical Thinking

1. Mr. Adams has been taking Synthroid for approximately 2 years. During the last year, he has retired and is now living on a fixed income and has no insurance to help pay for his medication. Two months ago, he asked his pharmacist to refill his Synthroid with a less expensive generic medication. When he returned to the clinic today for his regular visit, he was complaining of fatigue, weight gain, dry skin, and cold intolerance. Discuss what you suspect is occurring with Mr. Adams and give suggestions as to how it could have been avoided.

2. Gail Lawrence is a 55-year-old woman who has just been diagnosed with chronic (Hasimoto's) thyroiditis and is to begin treatment with levothyroxine (Synthroid) 0.1 mg daily. You are the patient educator in your clinic and it is your responsibility to educate Ms. Lawrence about her hypothyroidism and thyroid replacement therapy. Discuss the information you need to share with the patient with regard to the signs and symptoms of hypothyroidism and its impact on functional abilities. You have only approximately 10 minutes to spend with Ms. Lawrence. What would be your priority to include in your teaching? Also discuss the importance of compliance with the treatment protocol and follow-up for hypothyroidism and drug management.

CHAPTER 52

Male and Female Hormones

I. Matching

Match each term in Column A with the correct definition or statement in Column B.

COLUMN A

_____ 1. anabolism

_____ 2. androgens

_____ 3. catabolism

_____ 4. endogenous

_____ 5. estradiol

_____ 6. chloasma

_____ 7. estrogen

_____ 8. Testoderm

_____ 9. menarche

_____ 10. progesterone

_____ 11. progestins

_____ 12. testosterone

_____ 13. virilization

_____ 14. saw palmetto

_____ 15. gynecomastia

COLUMN B

A. Herb used to relieve the symptoms of benign prostatic hypertrophy.

B. Male hormone that stimulates the development of the accessory sex organs.

C. Tissue-building process.

D. Male hormones, testosterone and its derivatives.

E. Tissue-depleting process.

F. Acquisition of the male sexual characteristics by a female.

G. Breast enlargement.

H. Produced by the body.

I. The most potent of the endogenous estrogens.

J. Female hormone necessary for the development of the placenta.

K. Hormone that promotes the development of the female accessory sex organs.

L. Female hormone secreted by the corpus luteum, placenta, and adrenal cortex.

M. Age of onset of first menstruation.

N. Pigmentation of the skin.

O. Testosterone transdermal system.

II. Fill in the Blanks

1. List the two endogenous female hormones.

   a) _____

   b) _____

2. List the three endogenous estrogen hormones.

   a) _____

   b) _____

   c) _____

3. The synthetic _____ are usually preferred for medical use because of the _____ effectiveness of _____ when administered _____.

4. The benefits of contraceptive hormones, not related to contraception, include:

   a) _____

   b) _____

   c) _____

   d) _____

5. Estrogens may be administered by any of these routes:

    a) _____

    b) _____

    c) _____

    d) _____

    e) _____

6. The anabolic steroids are _____ drugs chemically related to the _____.

7. The transdermal _____ system is used as _____ therapy when endogenous _____ is _____ or _____.

III. Multiple Choice

Circle the letter of the most appropriate answer.

1. A new nurse asks about the use of androgen therapy to treat women with inoperable metastatic breast cancer. You would be correct in stating that this therapy may be used with women who:

    a. have not had an oophorectomy.

    b. are 1 to 5 years past menopause.

    c. have not had chemotherapy.

    d. do not wish to have radiation therapy.

2. A teaching plan for a patient who is to begin treatment with estrogen should include information about the uses of estrogen. These uses include:

    a. relief of moderate to severe vasomotor symptoms of menopause.

    b. aid in weight loss for the severely obese.

    c. treatment of bladder infections.

    d. treatment of osteoporosis in women before menopause.

3. During a discussion with another nurse about the uses of androgens, you would be correct in stating that the androgens may be used to treat:

    a. female infertility.

    b. prostatic cancer.

    c. problems associated with pregnancy.

    d. selected cases of delayed puberty in the male patients.

4. Mr. Thomas is being seen in the clinic today with symptoms of benign prostatic hypertrophy (BPH). The nurse is aware that the type of drug usually prescribed to treat the symptoms of BPH is:

    a. progestins.

    b. androgens.

    c. androgen hormone inhibitors.

    d. estrogens.

5. While reviewing information on the uses of anabolic steroids, a nurse reads that these drugs may be used to:

    a. promote weight gain when a severe illness causes weight loss.

    b. supplement the endogenous androgens.

    c. encourage weight loss in severe obesity.

    d. reduce the size of the prostate.

6. A nursing student asks the charge nurse about the estrogens and their potency. The nurse would correctly reply that the most potent estrogen is:

    a. estrone.   c. estriol

    b. progesterone.   d. estradiol.

7. During a staff meeting, a question is asked about specific actions of the estrogens. A nurse correctly replies that the estrogens:

    a. promote ovulation.

    b. thicken cervical mucus.

    c. promote fluid retention.

    d. induce protein catabolism.

8. Female patients receiving androgens for inoperable breast carcinoma are closely observed for common adverse reactions associated with androgen therapy, which include:

    a. virilization, menstrual irregularities.

    b. abdominal distention, peripheral edema.

    c. excessive weight gain, signs of anemia.

    d. hypotension, decreased sodium levels.

9. Which of the following adverse reactions might the patient taking estrogen report?

a. Increased appetite, hair loss

b. Virilization, constipation

c. Nausea, breakthrough bleeding

d. Deepening of the voice, light-headedness

10. Patients prescribed oral contraceptives are advised not to smoke. Smoking will increase the risk of:

a. pregnancy.

b. ovarian carcinoma.

c. extreme weight gain.

d. cardiovascular effects such as thromboembolism.

11. Patient teaching for oral contraceptives should include information about the best time to take the drug, which is:

a. between noon and the evening meal.

b. with the evening meal or at bedtime.

c. with the noon meal.

d. in the morning before breakfast.

12. Diabetic patients taking estrogen or progestin are observed for a(n):

a. increased incidence of hypoglycemic reactions.

b. rise in blood glucose levels.

c. marked increase in appetite.

d. sharp decrease in blood glucose levels.

13. The nurse is teaching a patient about the estradiol transdermal system and where the patch is to be applied. The nurse tells the patient to apply the patch on:

a. the dry skin of the forearm.

b. the outer thigh.

c. either breast.

d. the abdomen below the waistline.

14. A patient is asking questions about the Norplant System of birth control. The nurse explains the capsules are placed under the skin of the upper arm and are effective for:

a. 5 years.   c. 12 months.

b. 6 months.   d. 3 years.

15. A patient is to receive medroxyprogesterone acetate as a contraceptive. She asks how the drug is given and how long it lasts. The nurse states that the drug is administered:

a. orally every 25 days.

b. intramuscularly every 5 years.

c. intramuscularly every 6 months.

d. intramuscularly every 3 months.

IV. Crossword Puzzle

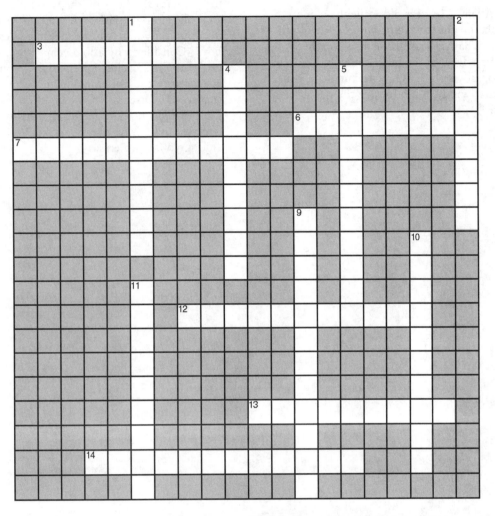

ACROSS CLUES

3. Pigmentation of the skin.
6. Age of onset of first menstruation.
7. Breast enlargement in the male.
12. Herb used to relieve the symptoms of benign prostatic hypertrophy. (Two words)
13. The most potent of the endogenous estrogens.
14. Male hormone.

DOWN CLUES

1. Tissue-depleting process.
2. Female hormone secreted by the corpus luteum and placenta.
4. Testosterone transdermal system.
5. An androgen hormone inhibitor.
9. Acquisition of male sexual characteristics by the female.
10. Produced by the body.
11. Tissue-building process.

V. Dosage Problems

Solve the following dosage calculations.

1. The physician's order reads: Depo-Provera, 0.6 g, IM, once a week. The available drug is Depo-Provera, 400 mg/mL. How many milliliters will be needed for the dose ordered? _____

2. The physician's order reads: Fluoxymesterone, 2.5 mg, PO, qd. The available drug is fluoxymesterone, 5-mg tablets. How many tablets will be administered for each dose? _____

VI. Critical Thinking

1. Bethany Allen, a 16-year-old, calls the clinic because she forgot to take her birth control pill yesterday. What effect will this have on the therapeutic effects of the birth control pills? How should you advise her? What teaching can you provide that will help her to take the medication regularly?

2. You are working as the school nurse for the local junior high school. The wrestling coach asks you to talk with the boys on the wrestling team about anabolic steroids. How will you prioritize the information you need to give the adolescent boys? Consider why adolescents might want to use anabolic steroids. Discuss what you will say in regard to the potential dangers of anabolic steroid use. Discuss what suggestions you could offer the coach on strategies that might be effective in limiting the use of anabolic steroids among young athletes.

CHAPTER 53

Drugs Acting on the Uterus

I. Matching

Match each term in Column A with the correct definition or statement in Column B.

COLUMN A

_____ 1. preeclampsia

_____ 2. ergotism

_____ 3. uterine atony

_____ 4. uterine relaxants

_____ 5. water intoxication

_____ 6. oxytocic drugs

_____ 7. eclampsia

_____ 8. antepartum

COLUMN B

A. Marked relaxation of the uterine muscles.

B. Drugs used to induce uterine contractions similar to normal labor.

C. Before birth of the baby.

D. A condition of pregnancy characterized by hypertension, headaches, albuminuria, and edema of the lower extremities.

E. A condition characterized by convulsive seizures and coma.

F. Overdosage of ergonovine.

G. Fluid overload, fluid volume excess.

H. Useful in management of preterm labor.

II. Fill in the Blanks

1. Oxytocic drugs are given _____ the delivery of the placenta and are used to prevent _____ and _____ hemorrhage due to _____ _____.

2. Immediately before starting an infusion of oxytocin, the nurse assesses the _____ _____ _____ and the mother's _____ _____, _____, and _____ _____.

3. The nurse assesses and records the activity of the uterus, which includes the _____, _____, and _____ of any contractions.

4. Signs and symptoms of water intoxication may include:

   a) _____

   b) _____

   c) _____

   d) _____

   e) _____

   f) _____

   g) _____

5. List the two drugs currently used as uterine relaxants (*include generic and trade names*).

   a) _____ (_____)

   a) _____ (_____)

6. Yutopar and Brethine are used as uterine

_____ in the management of _____

_____.

7. List the tasks that the nurse performs at 15- to 30-minute intervals for the patient receiving uterine relaxants.

a) _____

b) _____

c) _____

d) _____

e) _____

8. List the three drugs used as uterine stimulants (*include generic and trade names*).

a) _____ (_____)

b) _____ (_____)

c) _____ (_____)

III. Multiple Choice

Circle the letter of the most appropriate answer.

1. At a team conference, the staff is discussing the medications ergonovine and methylergonovine. A nurse correctly states that these drugs are given:

a. to induce an abortion.

b. before contractions are 2 to 3 minutes apart.

c. after delivery of the placenta.

d. to induce labor.

2. When a patient is receiving ergonovine, the nurse monitors the patient for which of the following adverse reactions?

a. Nausea, vomiting, elevated blood pressure

b. Constipation, hypotension, jaundice

c. Edema, confusion, agitation

d. Tachycardia, hypotension, diarrhea

3. The physician has ordered administration of oxytocin for your patient. As a nurse, you would know that this drug will be administered:

a. by means of an IV infusion pump.

b. by IV push.

c. as an intermittent IV push.

d. undiluted.

4. The nurse monitoring a patient receiving oxytocin would know to contact the physician if:

a. uterine contractions last longer than 5 to 10 seconds.

b. urinary output is 50 mL/hour.

c. there is a marked change in the rhythm of uterine contractions.

d. uterine contractions are 4 to 5 minutes apart.

5. Patients receiving oxytocin require close observation by the nurse, who will be monitoring for:

a. fetal bradycardia, uterine rupture, cardiac arrhythmias.

b. uterine relaxation, hemorrhage, maternal bradycardia.

c. maternal jaundice, uterine rupture, hemorrhage.

d. fetal jaundice, insomnia, hypertension.

6. The nurse is aware that oxytocin may be administered as a nasal spray in situations in which there is a need to:

a. slow the delivery of the placenta.

b. encourage uterine atony.

c. stimulate the milk ejection reflex.

d. control postpartum hemorrhage.

7. When your patient is receiving oxytocin, you must be alert for the signs and symptoms of water intoxication, which may include:

a. anxiety, nervousness.

b. decreased respirations, nausea.

c. uterine atony, abdominal cramping.

d. wheezing, coughing.

8. A patient is prescribed terbutaline for preterm labor. The nurse would instruct the patient to notify the health care provider if contractions occur:

a. 1 or 2 times per hour.

b. 4 to 6 times per hour.

c. 2 to 3 times per hour.

d. once every hour.

9. When administering terbutaline (Brethine), the nurse would be alert for which of the following adverse reactions?

   a. Hypotension and diarrhea

   b. Transient fever and nausea

   c. Hypertension and hypokalemia

   d. Nausea and drowsiness

10. The nurse administering terbutaline to a patient for preterm labor is aware that the drug will be continued for at least _____ hours after uterine contractions have ceased.

   a. 2   c. 8

   b. 6   d. 2

IV. Crossword Puzzle

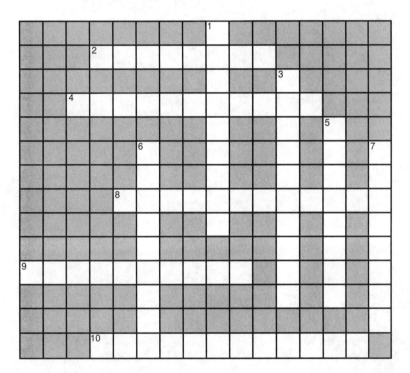

ACROSS CLUES

2. Drug used to induce uterine contractions.
4. Beta adrenergic agonist used for the treatment of preterm labor.
8. Marked relaxation of the uterine muscles (two words).
9. Drug used after the delivery of the placenta to prevent postpartum hemorrhage.
10. A condition of pregnancy characterized by hypertension, headaches, albuminuria, and edema of the lower extremities.

DOWN CLUES

1. A condition characterized by convulsive seizures and coma.
3. Before the birth of the baby.
5. Ergot poisoning.
6. Example of a uterine relaxant.
7. An endogenous hormone produced by the posterior pituitary gland.

V. Dosage Problems

Solve the following dosage calculations.

1. The physician's order reads: Terbutaline, 0.25 mg, SC, lateral deltoid area; if no significant improvement in 15 minutes, give another 0.25 mg SC; if no improvement in 15 minutes following second dose, call physician. The available drug is terbutaline, 1 mg/mL. How many milliliters will be administered for the first injection? _____

VI. Critical Thinking

1. Kathy Jones has just been admitted to the labor and delivery unit for induction of labor. She is 1 week past her due date and the baby is mature enough for safe delivery. The physician has ordered oxytocin. Discuss your assessment of Kathy before you begin the Pitocin therapy and your ongoing assessment during the induction process.

CHAPTER 54

Immunologic Agents

I. Matching

Match each term in Column A with the correct definition or statement in Column B.

COLUMN A

_____ 1. helper T4 cells

_____ 2. antibody

_____ 3. globulins

_____ 4. immunity

_____ 5. passive immunity

_____ 6. antigen

_____ 7. active immunity

_____ 8. artificially acquired active immunity

_____ 9. immune globulins

_____ 10. humoral immunity

_____ 11. antigen–antibody response

_____ 12. naturally acquired active immunity

_____ 13. attenuated

_____ 14. vaccine

_____ 15. toxin

_____ 16. antitoxin

_____ 17. booster

_____ 18. antivenins

COLUMN B

A. Proteins found in the blood that contain antibodies.

B. When the body forms antibodies after exposure to specific antigens.

C. When the body is exposed to a disease, contracts the disease, and manufactures antibodies that provide future immunity to the disease.

D. Weakened.

E. Additional dose of vaccine that will maintain the desired immunity.

F. Provides immediate immunity to an antigen but lasts only a short time.

G. When killed or weakened antigens are injected, which stimulates the formation of antibodies against the disease.

H. Used to produce artificial active immunity.

I. Substance that works in the same manner as antibodies.

J. Solutions obtained from human blood containing antibodies that have been formed by the body to specific antigens.

K. Used for passive, transient protection from the toxic effects of bites from spiders and snakes.

L. The resistance an individual has against disease.

M. When an antigen enters the body and specific antibodies neutralize the specific invading antigen.

N. A substance, usually a protein, that stimulates the body to produce antibodies.

O. A globulin produced as a defense against an antigen.

P. Cells in the bloodstream that identify and destroy antigens.

Q. Special lymphocytes that produce circulating antibodies to act against a foreign substance.

R. A poisonous substance produced by some bacteria.

II. Fill in the Blanks

1. List the T lymphocytes involved in cell-mediated immunity and briefly describe their function.

   a) _____

   b) _____

   c) _____

   d) _____

2. Immunity refers to the ability of the _____ to _____ and resist _____ that are potentially _____.

3. List the two types of active immunity.

   a) _____

   b) _____

4. Before administration of any _____, the nurse obtains an _____ history.

5. List the information the nurse documents after administering a vaccine.

   a) _____

   b) _____

   c) _____

   d) _____

6. VAERS _____ and _____ information from reports of _____ reactions following _____.

III. Multiple Choice

Circle the letter of the most appropriate answer.

1. At a team conference, the nurse explains that naturally acquired active immunity is attained when the individual:
   a. receives a vaccine containing attenuated antibodies.
   b. receives a vaccine containing killed antigens.
   c. contracts the disease and forms antibodies against the disease.
   d. forms antibodies after receiving live antigens.

2. Which of the following statements would alert the nurse to the possibility of an allergy to the diphtheria antitoxin vaccine? "My daughter is allergic to _____."
   a. eggs
   b. several animals
   c. pollen and ragweed
   d. milk

3. In discussing the meaning of vaccines, the nurse correctly states that vaccines contain:
   a. only live antigens.
   b. attenuated or killed antigens.
   c. only killed antigens.
   d. immune globulins.

4. The nurse informs the patient that he will receive hepatitis B immune globulin to provide _____ immunity.
   a. active
   b. naturally acquired
   c. passive
   d. artificially acquired

5. A parent asks what type of immunity is obtained from the tetanus toxoid. The nurse explains that a tetanus toxoid provides a type of immunity called:
   a. passive immunity.
   b. naturally acquired active immunity.
   c. artificially acquired active immunity.
   d. cell-mediated immunity.

6. Because of certain serious, possibly fatal, adverse reactions associated with human immune globulin IV products, individuals who are _____ should not be given IGIV human.
   a. under the age of 15 years.
   b. between the ages of 30 and 45 years.
   c. over 65 years of age.
   d. under the age of 20 years.

7. At what age should children receive their first diphtheria, tetanus, and pertussis vaccine?
   a. 1 month
   b. 2 months
   c. 3 months
   d. 6 months

---

8. Immunity against diphtheria is produced by use of a(n):

    a. toxin.
    b. antitoxin.
    c. attenuated vaccine.
    d. immunoglobulin.

9. An example of a killed virus used for immunization is the cholera vaccine. This vaccine protects patients who receive it from acquiring cholera for about:

    a. 3 to 6 months.
    b. 1 year.
    c. 1 month.
    d. 6 to 8 weeks.

10. When discussing the possibility of adverse reactions after receiving a vaccine, the nurse tells the parents of a young child that:

    a. adverse reactions may be severe and that the child should be monitored closely for 24 hours.

    b. adverse reactions are usually mild.

    c. the child will develop a hypersensitivity reaction.

    d. adverse reactions include nausea, vomiting, and headache.

IV. Crossword Puzzle

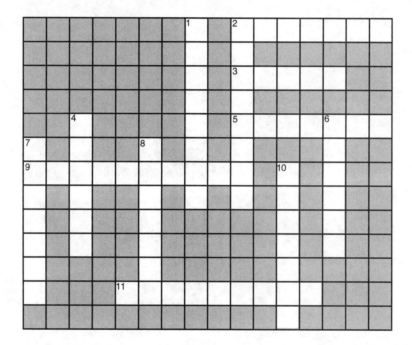

ACROSS CLUES

2. A substance that stimulates the body to produce antibodies.
3. Poisonous substance produced by some bacteria.
5. Additional dose of vaccine that will maintain the desired immunity.
9. Weakened.
11. Proteins found in the blood that contain antibodies.

DOWN CLUES

1. The resistance an individual has against disease.
2. A globulin produced as a defense against an antigen.
4. Type of immunity in which the body forms antibodies.
6. A weakened or killed toxin that is capable of stimulating the formation of antitoxins.
7. Type of immunity obtained from the administration of immune globulins.
8. Antibody-mediated immunity.
10. Used to produce artificial active immunity.

V. Critical Thinking

1. You are working in an urgent care clinic when a 33-year-old construction worker comes in with a puncture wound in his left foot, which he received when he stepped on a nail. Prioritize and explain why prioritizing is important.

2. A young mother brings her 6-week-old infant into the clinic for a well-baby checkup and her first vaccination. After examining the infant, you spend some time discussing how the young woman is adjusting to motherhood. During the discussion, the young woman asks why vaccinations are started so early with infants and if they are really necessary before the child is old enough for school. Discuss how you would answer the mother.

CHAPTER 55

Antineoplastic Drugs

I. Matching

Match each term in Column A with the correct definition or statement in Column B.

COLUMN A

_____ 1. alopecia

_____ 2. anorexia

_____ 3. anemia

_____ 4. chemotherapy

_____ 5. leukopenia

_____ 6. mucositis

_____ 7. stomatitis

_____ 8. vesicant

_____ 9. thrombocytopenia

_____ 10. aberrant

_____ 11. alkylating drugs

_____ 12. antimetabolites

_____ 13. antimitotics

_____ 14. hyperuricemia

_____ 15. metastasis

COLUMN B

A. Treatment with antineoplastic drugs for malignant diseases.
B. Abnormal.
C. Drugs that interfere with the process of cell division of malignant and normal cells.
D. Elevated blood uric acid levels.
E. Loss of hair.
F. Decrease in white blood cells.
G. Decrease in thrombocytes.
H. Loss of appetite resulting in inability to eat.

I. Drugs that interfere with the various metabolic functions of cells.
J. Decrease in red blood cells.
K. Inflammation of the mouth.
L. Drugs that interfere with or stop cell division.
M. Inflammation of the oral mucous membranes.
N. Drug that can cause tissue necrosis if it infiltrates or extravasates out of the blood vessel and into the soft tissue.
O. Spreading of cancer to other sites.

II. Fill in the Blanks

1. List the types of antineoplastic drugs covered in this chapter.

   a) _____

   b) _____

   c) _____

   d) _____

   e) _____

   f) _____

2. Cancer cells have no biological _____ controls that _____ their aberrant _____ or _____.

3. Chemotherapy is administered at the time the cell is _____ as part of a _____ to optimize _____ _____.

4. Normal cells that are also rapidly dividing cells, which may be affected by the chemotherapy agent, include:

a) _____

b) _____

c) _____

d) _____

e) _____

f) _____

5. List two examples of alkylating drugs (*include generic and trade names*).

a) _____ _____

b) _____ _____

6. List examples of the antibiotic antineoplastics (*include generic and trade names*).

a) _____ _____

b) _____ _____

c) _____ _____

7. List examples of the antimetabolite drugs (*include generic and trade names*).

a) _____ _____

b) _____ _____

8. Examples of hormones used as neoplastic drugs include (*list generic and trade names if indicated*):

a) _____ _____

b) _____ _____

c) _____ _____

9. Examples of the mitotic inhibitors include (*list generic and trade names*):

a) _____ _____

b) _____ _____

10. Examples of miscellaneous antineoplastics include (*list generic and trade names*):

a) _____ _____

b) _____ _____

11. List the signs and symptoms of an extravasation.

a) _____

b) _____

c) _____

d) _____

III. Multiple Choice

Circle the letter for the most appropriate answer.

Ms. Martin, age 48 years, is admitted to the oncology unit of the hospital for chemotherapy. The following questions pertain to Ms. Martin's case.

1. Before the administration of the antineoplastic drug, the nurse explains to Ms. Martin that antineoplastic drugs generally affect:

a. only the malignant cells.

b. all cells that rapidly proliferate.

c. only superficial cancer cells.

d. cells that slowly proliferate.

2. The nurse tells Ms. Martin that antineoplastic drugs:

a. are given as single drugs only.

b. may be given in combination with other antineoplastic drugs.

c. work best when two drugs are given a week apart.

d. will be given with meals to slow absorption.

3. While Ms. Martin is receiving chemotherapy, the nurse should remember that:

a. the occurrence of serious adverse reactions is rare.

b. these drugs are not toxic when given in recommended doses.

c. the development of adverse reactions almost always depends on the type of malignancy being treated.

d. these drugs are potentially toxic.

4. Ms. Martin is to be given cisplatin (Platinol). Before administration, the nurse will expect the physician to prescribe that Ms. Martin:

   a. be placed in isolation.

   b. receive enemas until clear.

   c. be hydrated with 1 to 2 liters of IV fluid.

   d. receive a sedative.

5. When preparing a parenteral form of antineoplastic drug, the nurse must:

   a. wear plastic disposable gloves.

   b. avoid touching the outside of the bottle once the diluent is added.

   c. prepare the drug 24 hours before use.

   d. wrap the solution in heavy wrap or foil to prevent exposure to light.

6. Which of the following would indicate to the nurse that Ms. Martin is developing thrombocytopenia?

   a. A platelet count greater than 1,000,000/mm^3

   b. A platelet count less than 100,000/mm^3

   c. A white blood cell count greater than 2000/mm^3

   d. A white blood cell count less than 2000/mm^3

7. Ms. Martin is allowed to ambulate and meets another patient, Ms. Allen, in the hallway. Ms. Martin notes that the patient has lost most of her hair. Nurses should consider alopecia to be a:

   a. minor problem that is no cause for concern because the hair will grow back.

   b. personal problem that is best not to mention.

   c. serious problem because the hair will not grow back.

   d. personal problem that may cause great emotional concerns on the part of the patient.

8. Ms. Martin has a significant drop in her platelet count. The nurse would modify her care plan to include:

   a. observing her daily for signs of increased urine output.

   b. watching for signs of electrolyte imbalance.

   c. the prevention of bleeding and bruising episodes.

   d. placing her in isolation.

9. Ms. Martin has frequent blood counts, which are necessary to allow the nurse to:

   a. monitor her response to a diet high in iron.

   b. determine the bone marrow–depressing effects of the antineoplastic drug.

   c. determine if she has an infection.

   d. monitor the effectiveness of the drug.

10. The patient in the room next to Ms. Martin is receiving melphalan (Alkeran). One adverse reaction associated with the administration of this drug is hyperuricemia. When this reaction is known to occur, the nurse will:

    a. place the patient in reverse isolation.

    b. watch for signs of pulmonary edema.

    c. assess for changes in the heart rate and rhythm.

    d. encourage the patient to drink at least 2000 mL of water per day.

IV. Matching: Antineoplastic Drugs

Match the antineoplastic drug with the correct classification (some letters will be used more than once).

COLUMN A

_____ 1. Plicamycin (Mithracin)

_____ 2. Testolactone (Teslac)

_____ 3. Mechlorethamine (Mustargen)

_____ 4. Bleomycin (Blenoxane)

_____ 5. Fluorouracil (5-FU) (Adrucil)

_____ 6. Medroxyprogesterone (Depo-Provera)

_____ 7. Vincristine (Oncovin)

_____ 8. Chlorambucil (Leukeran)

_____ 9. Estramustine phosphate sodium (Emcyt)

_____ 10. Methotrexate (Rheumatrex)

COLUMN B

A. Alkylating agent

B. Antibiotic

C. Antimetabolite

D. Androgen

E. Estrogen

F. Progestin

G. Mitotic inhibitor

V. Crossword Puzzle

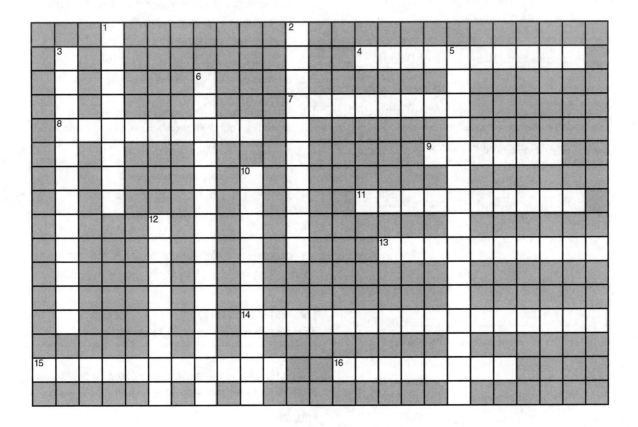

ACROSS CLUES

4. Inflammation of the mouth.
7. Abnormal.
8. Inflammation of the oral mucous membranes.
9. Condition caused by decrease in red blood cells.
11. A decrease in white blood cells.
13. Treatment aimed at relieving symptoms.
14. Decrease in thrombocytes.
15. Example of a mitotic inhibitor.
16. Loss of hair.

DOWN CLUES

1. Drug that can cause tissue necrosis if it infiltrates or extravasates out of the blood vessel and into the soft tissue.
2. Spreading of cancer to other sites.
3. Therapy with antineoplastic drugs.
5. Drugs used to treat malignancy.
6. Classification of methotrexate.
10. Classification of chlorambucil.
12. Loss of appetite resulting in inability to eat.

VI. Critical Thinking

1. Your patient, Sarah Hall, is to begin her chemotherapy today, the combination treatment of bleomycin and a myelosuppressive drug. Severe allergic reactions can occur with these drug combinations, which include hypotension and pulmonary toxicity (eg, interstitial pneumonitis and pulmonary fibrosis). Discuss how you plan to explain these reactions to Ms. Hall and reassure her that the adverse reactions will be identified and managed. Decide how much information to give Ms. Hall and explain your reasoning.

CHAPTER 56

Topical Drugs Used in the Treatment of Skin Disorders

I. Matching

Match each term in Column A with the correct definition or statement in Column B.

COLUMN A

_____ 1. antipsoriatics

_____ 2. antiseptics

_____ 3. dermis

_____ 4. epidermis

_____ 5. germicide

_____ 6. immunocompromised

_____ 7. keratolytic

_____ 8. necrotic

_____ 9. proteolysis

_____ 10. proteolytic

_____ 11. purulent exudates

_____ 12. superinfection

_____ 13. psoriasis

COLUMN B

A. Outermost layer of the skin.

B. Patients with an immune system incapable of fighting bacteria.

C. Layer of the skin immediately below the epidermis.

D. An overgrowth of bacterial or fungal microorganisms not affected by the antibiotic being administered.

E. Drug that kills bacteria.

F. Drug that stops, slows, or prevents the growth of microorganisms.

G. Dead (tissue).

H. Drugs used to treat psoriasis.

I. A chronic skin disease manifested by bright red patches covered with silvery scales or plaques.

J. Pus-containing fluid

K. Removal of dead soft tissues.

L. Enzyme that aids in the reduction of proteins into simpler substances and hastens the removal of soft dead tissue.

M. Drug that removes excess growth of the epidermis.

II. Fill in the Blanks

1. List the types of drugs included in the topical anti-infectives.

   a) _____

   b) _____

   c) _____

2. List examples of the topical antibiotics (*include generic and trade names*).

   a) _____ _____

   b) _____ _____

   c) _____ _____

   d) _____ _____

3. List the two topical antiviral drugs currently available for use (*include generic and trade names*).

   a) _____ _____

   b) _____ _____

4. Benzalkonium solutions are _____

   or _____ depending on their

   _____.

5. Topical _____ and

   _____ are primarily used to

   _____ the number of _____ on

   skin _____.

6. Examples of corticosteroids include (*list generic and trade names*):

   a)_____ _____

   b)_____ _____

   c)_____ _____

   d)_____ _____

   e)_____ _____

7. An example of a topical enzyme is (*include generic and trade name*) _____

   _____.

8. Examples of conditions that may respond to the application of a topical enzyme include:

   a) _____

   b) _____

   c) _____

9. Examples of the keratolylics include (*list generic and trade names*):

   a)_____ _____

   b)_____ _____

10. Topical anesthetics temporarily

    _____ the conduction of

    _____ from _____ nerve

    fibers.

III. Multiple Choice

Circle the letter of the most appropriate answer.

1. Unless ordered otherwise, previous applications of a topical anti-infective are _____ before a new application is made.
   a. removed with gauze or cotton ball
   b. treated with an antiseptic
   c. removed with soap and warm water
   d. irrigated with normal saline

2. To prevent accidents, an antiseptic or germicide container is:
   a. clearly labeled as to contents.
   b. kept in the closet of the patient's room.
   c. kept in the bathroom adjoining the patient's room.
   d. labeled with the name of the product, the strength and, when applicable, the date of the preparation of the solution.

3. Nursing management of the patient prescribed any topical drug for a skin disorder includes:
   a. covering the area with an occlusive dressing after each application.
   b. informing the patient that topical drugs cannot be absorbed through the skin.
   c. inspecting the area immediately before the next application of the drug.
   d. applying the drug on and 1 inch around the area to be treated.

4. When asked at a team conference to explain how topical anesthetics relieve pain, the nurse correctly answers that these drugs temporarily:
   a. inhibit the conduction of impulses in motor nerve fibers.
   b. reduce swelling around the affected area.
   c. stimulate sensory nerve fibers.
   d. inhibit the conduction of impulses from sensory nerve fibers.

5. Patients using a topical gel such as lidocaine viscous for oral anesthesia are instructed to:
   a. not eat food for 1 hour after application.
   b. drink extra fluids.
   c. hold the gel in the mouth for 1 hour.
   d. apply the gel with a finger.

6. When applying a topical drug, which of the following requires contacting the physician as soon as possible?

   a. Decreased redness of the affected area

   b. Momentary stinging or burning when the drug is applied

   c. Prolonged, intense itching after the drug is applied

   d. Staining of the skin of the affected area

IV. Crossword Puzzle

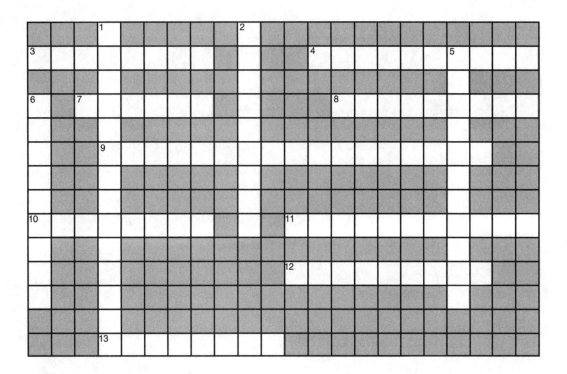

ACROSS CLUES

3. Exudate containing pus.
4. Drug that stops, slows, or prevents the growth of microorganisms.
7. Layer of the skin immediately below the epidermis.
8. Generic name for Zovirax.
9. Patients with an immune system incapable of fighting bacteria.
10. Another word for hypersensitivity.
11. Drug that removes excess growth of the epidermis.
12. Outermost layer of skin.
13. Dead tissue.

DOWN CLUES

1. Overgrowth of bacteria or fungal microorganisms not affected by the antibiotic being used.
2. Drug that kills bacteria.
5. Removal of dead soft tissue.
6. A chronic skin disease manifested by bright red patches covered with silvery scales or plaques.

V. Critical Thinking

1. You are working in the operating room. A surgeon asks for acetic acid for irrigation of a wound. You go to the stock supply and locate where acetic acid is usually stored. The bottle has been previously used and the label is difficult to read. What should you do?

2. A patient who has been prescribed a topical ointment is beginning to demonstrate signs of increased skin sensitivity to the medication. She is complaining of increasing redness, discomfort, and itching. Discuss nursing intervention that may help to make the patient more comfortable and relieve some or all of her symptoms. Also, discuss symptoms that need to be reported to the physician immediately.

CHAPTER 57

Otic and Ophthalmic Preparations

I. Matching

Match each term in Column A with the correct definition or statement in Column B.

COLUMN A

_____ 1. cycloplegia

_____ 2. intraocular pressure

_____ 3. miosis

_____ 4. mydriasis

_____ 5. mydriatic

_____ 6. myopia

_____ 7. ophthalmic

_____ 8. otic

_____ 9. ptosis

_____ 10. uveitis

COLUMN B

A. Ear.

B. Pressure within the eye.

C. Dilation of the pupil.

D. Eye

E. Paralysis of the cilliary muscles, resulting in an inability to focus the eye.

F. Drooping of the upper eyelid.

G. An inner eye inflammation.

H. Drugs that dilate the eye.

I. Nearsightedness.

J. Contraction of the pupil of the eye.

II. Fill in the Blanks

1. List the three categories that otic preparations are divided into.

   a) _____

   b) _____

   c) _____

2. Otic preparations are instilled in the external _____ canal and may be used to _____ pain, treat _____ and _____ and aid in the removal of _____ _____.

3. After examining the patient's ear, the nurse will document a description of any _____ or the presence of _____ _____.

4. List the two types of glaucoma.

   a) _____

   b) _____

5. The alpha$_2$-adrenergic drugs act to _____ aqueous humor production and _____ the outflow of aqueous humor.

6. The sympathomimetic drugs lower the _____ _____ by _____ the outflow of aqueous humor in the eye and are used to treat _____.

III. Multiple Choice

Circle the letter of the most appropriate answer.

1. Mary Jackson has been prescribed an otic solution that must be kept refrigerated. The nurse will warm the solution before administering it by:
   a. holding the container in the palms of the hands for a few minutes.
   b. heating it in a microwave oven.
   c. placing the container in running hot water.
   d. letting it stand in a warm room for 3 minutes.

2. Before instilling ear drops, the patient is told that:
   a. the solution is kept in the ear for 30 minutes.
   b. there may be a temporary decrease in hearing in the treated ear.
   c. the solution should be allowed to run out in 30 seconds.
   d. there will be a loss of hearing for 30 minutes.

3. When instilling an otic drug into the ear of an adult, the earlobe is pulled:
   a. down and back.   c. forward.
   b. forward and up.   d. up and back.

4. You are helping a new nurse to instill an otic solution in the ear of a patient who is sitting. You would be correct to instruct the nurse to tell the patient to:
   a. keep his head upright.
   b. tilt his head forward.
   c. tilt his head toward the untreated side.
   d. tilt his head backward.

5. After instilling an otic solution, the drug is allowed to remain in the ear canal for:
   a. 30 seconds.   c. 15 minutes.
   b. 2 to 3 minutes. d. 30 minutes.

6. When the label of an otic solution lists benzocaine as one of the contents, the nurse recognizes this drug as being a(n):
   a. local anesthetic.   c. analgesic.
   b. emollient.   d. anti-infective.

7. Which of the following instructions would be included in a teaching plan for the patient prescribed an otic solution?
   a. Contact the physician if a temporary change in hearing occurs after the drug is instilled.
   b. Keep the drug in a warm, but not hot, place.
   c. Do not insert anything into the ear unless advised to do so by the physician.
   d. If symptoms are not relieved in 12 hours, contact the physician.

8. The nurse has just brought a patient's ophthalmic solution to his room to administer it. Before instilling the solution, the nurse tells the patient:
   a. that a temporary stinging or burning may be felt.
   b. that eyes are squeezed tightly shut as soon as the solution is instilled.
   c. immediately to wipe his eye using pressure to squeeze out excess medication.
   d. to sit upright and bend his head slightly forward.

9. The nurse will correctly administer an ophthalmic solution by instilling it into the:
   a. inner canthus.
   b. upper conjunctival sac.
   c. lower conjunctival sac.
   d. outer canthus.

10. Depending on the physician's order, an ophthalmic ointment is dropped into the lower conjunctival sac or applied to the:
    a. inner canthus.
    b. lower lid margin.
    c. area above the eyelashes.
    d. outer canthus.

11. When looking up an ophthalmic drug, the nurse reads that it is a beta-adrenergic blocking agent, which is used in the treatment of:
    a. eye infection.
    b. decreased intraocular pressure.
    c. dry eyes.
    d. glaucoma.

12. Patients admitted for treatment of acute glaucoma are assessed every 2 hours for:

    a. relief of pain.

    b. changes in the intraocular pressure.

    c. changes in the vital signs.

    d. improvement in the color of the sclera.

13. When asked at a team conference to describe the action of beta-adrenergic blocking drugs when a patient has glaucoma, the nurse correctly answers that these drugs:

    a. close the space between the anterior and posterior chambers of the eye.

    b. decrease production of aqueous humor.

    c. dilate the pupil.

    d. increase the production of vitreous humor.

IV. Crossword Puzzle

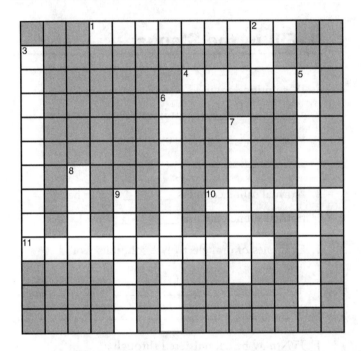

ACROSS CLUES

   1. Dilation of the pupil.
   4. Nearsightedness.
  10. Constriction of the pupil.
  11. Paralysis of the cillary muscle.

DOWN CLUES

   2. Abbreviation for intraocular pressure.
   3. Drugs that dilate the pupil.
   5. Type of drug that may result in a superinfection.
   6. Referring to the eye.
   7. An inner eye inflammation.
   8. Referring to the ear.
   9. Drooping of the upper eyelid.

V. Critical Thinking

1. Susan Jackson, a 42-year-old data entry specialist, has made an appointment to have her eyes examined because she has been having difficulty seeing her computer screen clearly. She has not had her eyes checked for over 10 years. When she arrives at the office, she asks why it was necessary for someone to accompany her for the examination. You explain that the examination will include using medication to dilate her eyes that will impair her ability to drive for several hours. Discuss what you would tell Ms. Jackson about the examination and about the medication that will be used for the dilation. Also discuss what teaching you need to do for this patient in regard to regular check-ups and glaucoma testing.

2. Sylvia Arnold, an 82-year-old widow, is diagnosed in your clinic with open-angle glaucoma. She is given a prescription of timolol maleate (Timoptic) eye drops to decrease her intraocular pressure. Discuss what assessments need to be made and what teaching is important before Mrs. Arnold leaves the clinic.

CHAPTER 58

Fluids and Electrolytes

I. Matching

Match each term in Column A with the correct definition or statement in Column B.

COLUMN A

_____ 1. electrolyte

_____ 2. extravasation

_____ 3. fluid overload

_____ 4. half-normal saline

_____ 5. hypocalcemia

_____ 6. hypokalemia

_____ 7. hyponatremia

_____ 8. infiltration

_____ 9. normal saline

_____ 10. protein substrates

_____ 11. substrate

_____ 12. dextrose

COLUMN B

A. A substance that is the basic component of an organism.

B. More fluid than the body can accommodate in the circulatory system.

C. Escape of fluid from a blood vessel into surrounding tissue.

D. Collection of fluid into tissues.

E. Electrically charged substance essential to the normal functioning of all cells.

F. Low blood levels of calcium.

G. IV solution containing 0.45% NaCl.

H. Low blood levels of sodium.

I. Low blood levels of potassium.

J. IV solution containing 0.9% NaCl.

K. A carbohydrate used to provide a source of calories and fluid.

L. Amino acid preparations that act to promote the production of proteins.

II. Fill in the Blanks

1. IV solutions are used to replace _____ and _____ that have been lost and to provide _____ by their _____ content.

2. Normal saline contains _____ NaCl; half-normal saline contains _____ NaCl.

3. Examples of oral electrolyte solutions would include:

   a) _____

   b) _____

4. TPN may be administered through a _____ vein or through a _____ _____ _____.

5. At no time should any IV solution be _____ at a _____ rate, unless there is a specific _____ order to do so.

6. During the first _____ minutes of infusion of a fat solution, the nurse carefully observes the patient for _____ _____, _____, _____, _____, or signs of a _____ reaction.

7. _____ overloading of calcium in the
_____ circulation results in acute
_____ syndrome. Symptoms of this
syndrome include elevated plasma _____,
_____, _____, severe
_____ and _____, _____, and, if
left untreated, _____.

8. The _____ _____ reflex is tested _____
each dose of magnesium sulfate.

9. The maximum recommended
_____ of potassium is _____
mEq/1000 mL of IV solution.

10. A too rapid infusion of an amino
acids–carbohydrate mixture may result in
_____, _____, _____
_____, and _____ _____
_____.

III. Multiple Choice

Circle the letter of the most appropriate answer.

1. Charlie Martin, 89 years old, 3 weeks post
bowel surgery, is readmitted with a draining fis-
tula of the bowel. A nasogastric tube is con-
nected to low suction. The nurse will monitor
this patient for signs and symptoms of:
a. high serum bicarbonate.
b. increased sodium levels.
c. decreased potassium levels.
d. increased calcium levels.

2. Unless physician orders specify exactly, the nurse
is aware that 1000 mL of IV solution is allowed
to infuse over a period of _____ hours.
a. 1 to 2   c. 1 to 3
b. 2 to 3   d. 4 to 8

3. The nurse monitoring a patient receiving an IV
of 1000 mL of 5% dextrose and water finds the
fluid to have infused at a too rapid rate over the
last hour. The patient will need to be monitored
for:
a. abdominal distention.
b. signs and symptoms of fluid overload.
c. a decreased urine output.
d. signs and symptoms of a fluid deficit.

4. A patient has developed hypokalemia and the
physician has ordered IV potassium for treatment. The nurse knows that when potassium is
administered IV, it is:
a. always diluted in an IV solution before
administering.
b. given undiluted over a 5-minute period.
c. piggybacked into any available IV line.
d. given diluted in normal saline over a 15-
minute period.

A team meeting is being held to discuss questions the
staff has concerning IV solutions and electrolyte
therapy. Questions 5–10 pertain to issues discussed
at the meeting.

5. When asked about the use of plasma protein
fractions, the nurse correctly states that their
uses include treatment of:
a. head injuries.   c. dehydration.
b. calcium imbalances. d. hypoproteinemia.

6. When asked to define protein substrates, a nurse
correctly states that they are:
a. triglycerides.
b. small-molecule proteins.
c. amino acids.
d. high-density lipoproteins.

7. A nurse assistant asks why the physician ordered
a plasma expander when he admitted Ms.
Moore. A nurse states that these IV solutions are
used to:
a. expand plasma volume when shock is due to
burns or other trauma.
b. remove high-density proteins from the blood.
c. treat fluid overload.
d. keep the blood pressure normal when shock
is due to electrolyte imbalance.

8. A new nurse comments that she is having a difficult time understanding the role of bicarbonate.
The team leader explains that this electrolyte:

   a. plays an important role in the function of
   muscles.

   b. is necessary for the transmission of nerve
   impulses.

   c. plays an important role in the acid-base
   balance.

   d. is necessary for the clotting of blood.

9. During a discussion of the uses of magnesium
sulfate, a nurse correctly states that this electrolyte is useful in preventing and controlling:

   a. seizures in obstetrical patients with
   pregnancy-induced hypertension.

   b. dehydration in patients with third-degree
   burns.

   c. cardiac arrest during a myocardial infarction.

   d. urinary shutdown in patients with drug
   overdose.

10. A nurse assistant asks why Mr. Teale received
1000 mL of normal saline. A nurse states that
the saline solution was used because he had
hyponatremia that was caused by:

    a. dehydration.

    b. a diet high in sodium.

    c. chronic constipation.

    d. severe vomiting and diarrhea.

11. The doctor has ordered a patient's IV fluid to be
changed from dextrose 5% to normal saline.
The nurse obtains the solution labeled, sodium
chloride _____%.

    a. 1.5   c. 0.45

    b. 0.9   d. 0.225

12. A nursing intervention that can be used to help
prevent or correct a fluid volume deficit is to:

    a. explain to the patient the physiological need
    for fluid.

    b. allow the patient to ambulate during the day.

    c. offer oral fluids at regular intervals.

    d. encourage small, frequent meals.

13. An essential component in a plan of care for the
patient receiving IV potassium is checking the
IV site for extravasation. A complication of
extravasation of IV fluid containing potassium
is:

    a. paralysis of the upper extremities.

    b. local tissue necrosis.

    c. severe headache.

    d. thrombus formation.

14. The physician has ordered calcium IV for a
patient with severe hypocalcemia. The nurse is
aware that the patient will have to:

    a. have his vital signs monitored every 30
    minutes.

    b. be encouraged to drink large quantities of
    fluid.

    c. be weighed daily.

    d. be placed in a sitting position for the IV
    administration.

15. The nurse will be correct when she administers
the patient's oral potassium:

    a. on an empty stomach.

    b. at bedtime.

    c. with a sip of orange juice.

    d. immediately after meals or with food.

16. When magnesium sulfate is administered IM, it
is injected into the:

    a. deltoid muscle.

    b. triceps muscle.

    c. gluteus muscle.

    d. abdominal muscle.

IV. Crossword Puzzle

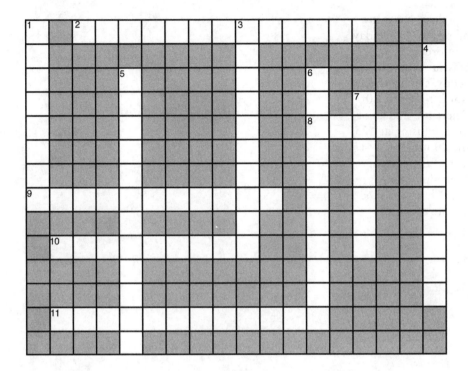

ACROSS CLUES

2. Escape of fluids from a blood vessel into surrounding tissues.
8. Liquid part of the blood.
9. An electrically charged article.
10. Solutions used to expand plasma volume
11. Low blood sodium.

DOWN CLUES

1. Carbohydrate used to provide calories.
3. Amino acids used in certain disease states are called protein _____.
4. Electrolyte that plays a vital role in acid-base balance of the body.
5. Collection of fluid into tissues.
6. Low potassium blood levels.
7. Electrolyte necessary for functioning of nerves and muscles.

V. Dosage Problems

Solve the following dosage calculations.

1. The physician's order reads: Potassium chloride, 10 mEq/1000 mL IV fluid × 2 L. The available drug is potassium chloride, 40 mEq/20 mL (2 mEq/mL). How many milliliters of the potassium chloride will be added to each bag of IV fluid?

   _____

2. 10 mEq of potassium chloride is added to a 500-mL bag of D_5W to be administered at the rate of 2 mEq/hour.

   a) many milliliters of solution are needed to deliver 2 mEq of potassium? _____

   b) Calculate the drops per minute needed to deliver 2 mEq/hour. The administration set delivers 20 gtt/mL. _____

VI. Critical Thinking

1. Martha Hunt, a postoperative patient, has a low serum potassium on her second postoperative day (2.1 mEq/mL), and her physician orders an additional 20 mEq of KCl (potassium chloride) to be added to her IV fluid. Currently, she has 1000 cc 5% dextrose with 0.45% NaCl, to which 20 mEq of KCl has been added. There are 200 cc of the solution remaining in the bag, infusing at 125 cc/hour. The nurse draws up the 20 mEq of additional potassium and adds it to the current infusion without changing the infusion rate. Discuss what has just happened. What would be the correct method to use to initiate the drug order?

Answer Key

1 General Principles of Pharmacology

MATCHING
1. F   2. D   3. J   4. A   5. C   6. H
7. I   8. E   9. G   10. B

MULTIPLE CHOICE
1. c   2. b   3. d   4. c   5. b   6. d   7. a   8. a
9. b   10. b

CROSSWORD SOLUTION
Across

2. Brand name
5. Toxic
6. Pharmaceutic
8. Complementary
10. Tolerance
12. Hypersensitivity
13. Synergist
14. Cumulative
15. Biotransformation

Down

1. Generic
3. Angioedema
4. Polypharmacy
5. Teratogen
7. Half-life
9. Anaphylactic
11. Antagonist

2 The Administration of Drugs

MATCHING
1. F   2. H   3. A   4. I   5. C   6. J   7. D   8. E
9. G   10. B

MULTIPLE CHOICE
1. c   2. d   3. a   4. c   5. b   6. d   7. a   8. a
9. d   10. b   11. d   12. a

FILL IN THE BLANKS
1. a) right drug b) right dose c) right patient d) right
   time e) right route f) right documentation
2. a) standing—Lanoxin 0.25 mg PO QID
   b) single—Valium 10 mg IVP @ 10:00 AM
   c) PRN—Demerol 100 mg IM q4h PRN for pain
   d) STAT—Morphine 10 mg IV STAT
3. a) oral b) parenteral c) topical d) transdermal
   e) inhalation

4. a) recording the administration of the drug
   b) recording any information concerning the
   administration of the drug
   c) evaluating and recording the patient's response to
   the drug
   d) observing the adverse reactions
5. Medication errors occur when the patient receives the
   wrong dose, the wrong drug, an incorrect dosage of
   the drug by the wrong route, or if the drug is given at
   the wrong time.
6. Drugs administered by the transdermal route are
   readily absorbed from the skin and have systemic
   effects. This type of drug system maintains a relatively
   constant blood concentration and reduces the
   possibility of toxicity.
7. Drug droplets, vapors, or gases are administered
   through the mucous membranes of the respiratory
   tract with the use of a nebulizer or a positive pressure
   breathing machine. Examples of drugs administered
   through inhalation include bronchodilators,
   mucolytics, and some anti-inflammatory drugs.

CROSSWORD SOLUTION
Across

4. Transdermal
13. Infiltration
15. Six rights
16. Intradermal
17. Parenteral

Down

1. Z track
2. Single
3. Inhalation
5. Documentation
6. Standing
7. Intravenous
8. Buccal
9. Pyxis
10. Extravasation
11. Intramuscular
12. Drug error
14. Oral

3 Review of Arithmetic and Calculation of Drug Dosages

REVIEW OF ARITHMETIC
A. Fractions

1. Numerator; denominator
2. a. Part of a whole; any number less than a whole
   b. A fraction having a numerator the same as or larger
   than the denominator.

3. c; d; h; I
4. The numerator and denominator are not expressed in like terms.

B. Mixed Numbers and Improper Fractions

1. A whole number and a proper fraction

2. a. $\frac{13}{8}$ b. $\frac{8}{3}$ c. $\frac{9}{2}$ d. $\frac{73}{6}$

   e. $\frac{16}{3}$ f. $\frac{15}{2}$ g. $\frac{73}{8}$ h. $\frac{41}{2}$

   i. $\frac{25}{3}$

3. a. $2\frac{2}{7}$ b. $1\frac{5}{9}$ c. $10\frac{1}{3}$ d. $4\frac{1}{4}$

   e. $2\frac{2}{5}$ f. $2\frac{4}{13}$ g. $2\frac{2}{3}$ h. $4\frac{2}{3}$

   i. $1\frac{4}{5}$

C. Adding Fractions With Like Denominators

1. a. $\frac{1}{2}$ b. $\frac{4}{5}$ c. $\frac{5}{7}$ d. $\frac{1}{2}$

   e. 1   f. $\frac{4}{5}$ g. $\frac{2}{3}$ h. $1\frac{1}{3}$

   i. $\frac{1}{2}$

D. Adding Fractions With Unlike Denominators

1. a. $\frac{22}{15}$ or $1\frac{7}{15}$ b. $\frac{3}{14}$ c. $\frac{24}{35}$

   d. $\frac{25}{24}$ or $1\frac{1}{24}$ e. $\frac{7}{10}$ f. $\frac{1}{2}$

   g. $\frac{3}{64}$ h. $\frac{1}{2}$

2. a. $1\frac{1}{2}$ b. $1\frac{2}{9}$ c. $1\frac{7}{45}$ d. $1\frac{5}{8}$

   e. $1\frac{9}{22}$ f. $1\frac{7}{15}$

E. Adding Mixed Numbers or Fractions With Mixed Numbers

1. a. $3\frac{9}{20}$ b. $2\frac{1}{6}$ c. $6\frac{3}{4}$ d. $3\frac{2}{3}$

   e. $2\frac{3}{8}$ f. $4\frac{5}{8}$

F. Comparing Fractions

1. a. $\frac{4}{5}$ b. $\frac{5}{8}$ c. $\frac{2}{3}$ d. $\frac{3}{8}$

   e. $\frac{1}{2}$ f. $\frac{1}{2}$

2. grain $\frac{1}{4}$

G. Multiplying Fractions

1. a. $\frac{1}{8}$ b. $\frac{1}{3}$ c. $\frac{8}{15}$ d. $\frac{35}{48}$

   e. $\frac{2}{25}$ f. $\frac{1}{9}$

H. Multiplying Whole Numbers and Fractions

1. a. $2\frac{2}{3}$ b. $\frac{3}{5}$ c. $2\frac{1}{2}$ d. 6

   e. $3\frac{1}{3}$ f. 6

I. Multiplying Mixed Numbers

1. a. $5\frac{5}{8}$ b. $8\frac{1}{8}$ c. $24\frac{3}{4}$ d. $9\frac{1}{3}$

   e. $28\frac{1}{2}$ f. $12\frac{1}{2}$

J. Multiplying a Whole Number and a Mixed Number

1. a. $13\frac{7}{8}$ b. 6   c. $8\frac{1}{2}$ d. $3\frac{1}{3}$

   e. $7\frac{1}{2}$ f. $4\frac{3}{4}$

2. 20 ounces
3. 10½ ounces
4. 750 milliliters

K. Dividing Fractions

1. a. 2   b. $\frac{1}{2}$ c. $2\frac{7}{10}$ d. 4

   e. $\frac{3}{10}$ f. $1\frac{1}{4}$ g. 10   h. $\frac{1}{125}$

L. Dividing Fractions and Mixed Numbers

1. a. 5   b. $9\frac{1}{3}$ c. 22   d. $6\frac{1}{24}$

   e. $\frac{3}{40}$ f. $\frac{8}{25}$

2. a. $\frac{3}{5}$ b. $1\frac{9}{13}$ c. $1\frac{8}{9}$ d. 4

   e. 2   f. $\frac{11}{20}$

3. a. 4   b. $\frac{1}{32}$ c. $\frac{1}{24}$ d. $\frac{1}{3}$

   e. $\frac{1}{12}$ f. 24

4. a. $\frac{8}{11}$ b. $\frac{3}{4}$ c. $1\frac{1}{19}$ d. $1\frac{19}{21}$

   e. $1\frac{2}{3}$ f. $2\frac{2}{5}$

M. Ratios

1. A way of explaining a part of a whole or the relationship of one number to another.

2. a. 1:4, $\frac{1}{4}$ b. 1:100, $\frac{1}{100}$ c. 1:10, $\frac{1}{10}$

   d. 2:5, $\frac{2}{5}$ 20

3. a. $\frac{1}{200}$ b. $\frac{1}{1000}$ c. $\frac{1}{5}$ d. $\frac{1}{20}$

4. a. 1:10
   b. 1:250
   c. 3:400

d. 1:2000
5. ½ strength
6. weaker
7. a. $\frac{1}{32}$

N. Percentage

1. Parts per hundred
2. a. 54 parts per hundred
   b. 35 parts per hundred
   c. 80 parts per hundred
   d. 25 parts per hundred
3. 87
4. 87 parts per hundred; $\frac{87}{100}$

5. a. $\frac{11}{50}$ b. $\frac{1}{2}$ c. $\frac{37}{1000}$ d. $\frac{9}{10}$

   e. $\frac{1}{10}$ f. $\frac{41}{100}$

6. a. 80% c. $66\frac{2}{3}$% c. 10% d. $37\frac{1}{2}$%

   e. 25% f. $16\frac{2}{3}$%

7. a. 0.2% b. 2% c. 0.4% d. $12\frac{1}{2}$%

   e. 0.1% f. 0.5%
8. a. 1:20 b. 1:4 c. 3:10 d. 1:100
   e. 3:1000 f. 1:125
9. 0.4%
10. 0.025%
11. 1:10

O. Proportion

1. a. 20 b. 16 c. 4 d. 80
   e. 10 f. 28
2. a. Proportion: 30 minutes : 20 miles :: 60 minutes :
   X miles
   Solution: X = 40 miles
   b. Proportion: 15 minutes : 1 miles :: 30 minutes :
   X mile(s)
   Solution: X = 2 miles
   c. Proportion: 15 grains : 1 gram :: 30 grains :
   X gram(s)
   Solution: X = 2 grams
   d. Proportion: 2. 2 pounds : 1 kilogram :: X pounds :
   45 kilograms
   Solution: X = 99 pounds
   e. Proportion: 30 milligrams : 1/2 grain ::
   90 milligrams : X grain(s)
   Solution: X = 1 1/2 grains
   f. Proportion: 1 milligram : 1/60 grain :: 5 milligrams :
   X grain(s)
   Solution: X = 1/12 grain

P. Decimals

1. A fraction in which the denominator is 10 or some
   power of 10.
2. a. A decimal with numbers only to the right of the
   decimal.
   b. A decimal with numbers to the left and right of the
   decimal.

3. a. 0.9 b. 0.005 c. 3. 4 d. 0.1
4. a. Three tenths
   b. One and seven tenths
   c. Seven hundredths
   d. Six and nine tenths
5. a. 3 b. 151 c. 2.6 d. 34.7
6. a. 8.6 b. 12 c. 1.3 d. 9.2
7. a. 1 b. 3.2 c. 6.5 d. 28.8
8. a. 4.32 b. 7.2 c. 7 d. 1.98
   e. 28.6 f. 0.124
9. a. 0.52 b. 2.08 c. 3 d. 0.76
   e. 0.706 (0. 71) f. 0.066 (0.07)

10. a. $\frac{3}{10}$ b. $\frac{7}{20}$ c. $\frac{3}{500}$ d. $\frac{1}{2}$

CALCULATION OF DRUG DOSAGES

A. Systems of Measurement

1. Metric system; apothecaries' system; household
   measurements
2. Metric system
3. Gram
4. Liter
5. Meter

B. Conversion Between Systems

1. a. 2 g
   b. gr 1/30
   c. 60 mL
   d. 1 pt
   e. 2 mL
   f. 4 g
   g. 1000 mL

C. Converting Within a System

1. a. 2 L
   b. 0.03 g
   c. 0.65
   d. 0.5 mg
   e. 200 mcg
   f. 0.1 g
   g. 100 mg
   h. 0.5 g

D. Oral Dosages of Drugs

1. a. 2 tablets
   b. 1 tablet
   c. 1 tablet
   d. 2 capsules
   e. 2 tablets
   f. 2 tablets
   g. 2 capsules (500 mg) each dose
2. a. 300 mg
   b. 4
   c. 2000 mg; 2 g
   d. 0.5 g
   e. 150 mg
3. a. 2½ mL
   b. 20 mL
   c. 2½ mL
   d. 10 mL

E. Parenteral Dosages of Drugs

1. a. 0.75 mL or 12 minims
   b. 0.5 mL or 8 minims
   c. 1.5 mL
   d. 2 mL
   e. 0.5 ml or 8 minims
   f. 6 mL
   g. 5 mL
   h. 2 mL
2. a. four doses
   b. One 1000 mL and one 500 mL container or three 500 mL containers
   c. 1 g vial 2 mL, 3 g vial 6 mL, 6 g vial 12 mL

F. Calculating IV Flow Rates

1. a. 28 to 29
   b. 83
   c. 20 to 21
   d. 30
   e. 2160 mL
   f. 104 mL
   g. 16.6 or 17 mL/h
   h. 24 or 25

G. Oral or Parenteral Drug Dosages Based on Weight

1. a. 4.5
   b. 83
   c. 55.9
   d. 63.6
   e. 10
   f. 27.27 or 27.3
2. a. 220
   b. 88
   c. 44
   d. 121
3. a. 227 mg; 4.5 mL
   b. 7.6 mg
   c. 368 mg/day; 93 mg
   d. 2.89 (or 2.9) mg; 1.45 (1.5) mL

H Temperatures

1. a. 33.3° C
   b. 38.3° C
   c. 38.88° (or 38.9°) C
   d. 37.3° C
2. a. 99.5° F
   b. 100.4° F
   c. 101.1° F
   d. 102° F

4 The Nursing Process

MATCHING
1. E   2. C   3. F   4. D   5. I   6. A
7. H   8. G   9. J   10. B

MULTIPLE CHOICE
1. d   2. b   3. a   4. d   5. b   6. a   7. c
8. d   9. a   10. c

FILL IN THE BLANKS
1. a) assessment b) nursing diagnosis c) planning d) implementation e) evaluation
2. a) initial b) on-going
3. a) subjective b) objective
4. a) Effective Therapeutic Regimen Management
   b) Risk for Ineffective Therapeutic Regimen Management
   c) Noncompliance with Drug Reginem
   d) Deficient Knowledge
5. a) extended therapy for chronic illness causes patients to become discouraged
   b) troublesome adverse reactions
   c) ack of understanding of the purpose of the drug
   d) forgetfulness
   e) misunderstanding of oral or written instructions on how to take the drug
   f) weak–relationships
   Or these: lack of funds to obtain drug; mobility problems; lack of family support; cognitive deficits; visual or hearing deficits; lack of motivation

CROSSWORD SOLUTION
Across
1. Evaluation
5. Subjective
7. Diagnosis
9. Noncompliant
10. Plan
11. Implementation

Down
2. Assessment
3. Ongoing
4. Anxiety
6. Objective
8. Initial

5 Patient and Family Teaching

MATCHING
1. C   2. F   3. G   4. D   5. A   6. B
7. H   8. J   9. E   10. I

MULTIPLE CHOICE
1. b   2. c   3. d   4. c   5. d   6. a   7. c   8. b
9. c   10. d

FILL IN THE BLANKS
1. a) information the patient or family needs to know about a particular drug
   b) the patient's or family member's ability to learn, accept, and use information
   c) any barriers or obstacles to learning
2. a) dosage regimen b) adverse reactions
   c) family members d) basic drug information
   e) drug containers f) drug storage
3. a) cognitive—thought, recall, decision making, drawing conclusion
   b) affective-attitudes, feelings, beliefs, opinions
   c) psychomotor—physical skills

CROSSWORD SOLUTION

Across

3. Physical
4. Learning
7. Individualized
8. Label
9. Affective
10. Motivation

Down

1. Water
2. Cognitive
5. Medi-Alert
6. Teaching

6 Anti-infectives

MATCHING

1. I   2. H   3. J   4. F   5. A   6. E   7. G   8. C
9. B   10. D

MULTIPLE CHOICE

1. c   2. a   3. b   4. b   5. d   6. a   7. c   8. b
9. b   10. d

CROSSWORD SOLUTION

Across

2. Allergic
4. Anorexia
6. Crystalluria
7. Leukopenia
8. Thrombocytopenia
9. Aplastic
10. Anti-infective

Down

1. Pruritus
3. Bacteriostatic
5. Stomatitis

FILL IN THE BLANKS

1. a) agranulocytosis b) thrombocytopenia c) aplastic anemia d) leukopenia
2. a) agranulocytosis—decrease in or lack of granulocytes, a type of white blood cells
   b) thrombocytopenia—decrease in number of blood platelets
   c) aplastic anemia—anemia due to deficient red blood cell production in the bone marrow
   d) leukopenia—decrease in number of white blood cells
3. a) antibacterial—active against bacteria
   b) anti-infective—treats infections caused by certain bacteria
   c) bacteriostatic—slow or retard the multiplication process of bacteria.
4. a) mafenide (Sulfamylon) b) silver sulfadiazine (Silvadene)

5. a) with renal impairment b) with hepatic impairment c) with bronchial asthma d) with allergies e) who are diabetic and taking oral hypoglycemic drugs f) who are pregnant

DOSAGE PROBLEMS

1. 4 tablets; 1 tablet every 6 hours
2. 800 milligrams
3. 1 tablet every 4 hours
4. ½ tablet

7 Penicillins

MATCHING

1. E   2. G   3. D   4. L   5. I   6. F
7. A   8. K   9. M   10. O   11. C   12. N
13. H   14. J   15. B

MULTIPLE CHOICE

1. c   2. d   3. a   4. b   5. a   6. d   7. c   8. b
9. d   10. b   11. d   12. b

CROSSWORD SOLUTION

Across

1. Leukopenia
10. Bactericidal
11. Penicillinase
12. Pathogenic

Down

2. Prophylaxis
3. Phlebitis
4. Anaphylactic
5. Nonpathogenic
6. Sensitivity
7. Stomatitis
8. Superinfection
9. Glossitis

FILL IN THE BLANKS

1. a) allergy history b) history of all medical/surgical treatments c) drug history d) symptoms of present infection
2. a) Diarrhea
   b) Risk for Impaired Skin Integrity
   c) Risk for Impaired Oral Mucous Membranes
   d) Risk for Imbalanced Body Temperature
3. a) natural penicillins—penicillin G and penicillin V
   b) penicillinase-resistant penicillins—cloxacillin, dicloxacillin, nafcillin
   c) aminopenicillins—ampicillin, bacampicillin, amoxicillin
   d) extended-spectrum penicillins—mezlocillin, piperacillin, ticarcillin
4. a) Augmentin b) Timentin c) Zosyn d) Unasyn
5. a) diarrhea b) blood or mucus in the stool c) fever d) abdominal cramps

DOSAGE PROBLEMS

1. 20 milliliters
2. 12.5 milliliters
3. 0.8 milliliter (0.83 milliliter rounded)
4. 4 milliliters
5. 0.6 milliliter
6. 2.4 milliliters
7. 2 teaspoons
8. 146 to 292 milligrams per day recommended dosage. Dose ordered is 125 milligrams three times per day = 375 milligrams; this is not a safe dose.

8 Cephalosporins

MATCHING
1. H   2. D   3. G   4. E   5. A   6. J
7. B   8. C   9. I   10. F

FILL IN THE BLANKS

1. Cephalosporins may be differentiated according to the microorganisms that are sensitive to them.
2. Cephalosporins are valuable in treating bacteria that have become resistant to penicillin.
3. Cephalosporins affect the bacterial cell wall, making it defective and unstable, resulting in the bacteria's destruction.
4. The most common adverse reactions seen with cephalosporins are nausea, vomiting, and diarrhea.
5. Because of the close relation of the cephalosporins to penicillin, a patient who is allergic to penicillin may also be allergic to the cephalosporins.

MULTIPLE CHOICE
1. d   2. c   3. b   4. a   5. b   6. c   7. a   8. b
9. b   10. d

DOSAGE PROBLEMS

1. a) 25 to 50 milligrams per kilogram per day b) 400 to 800 milligrams per day c) yes d) 6 milliliters of solution
2. 1 milliliter of solution
3. 0.83 milliliter (round to 0.8 milliliter)
4. 2 capsules
5. 7.5 milliliters
6. 20 milliliters

CROSSWORD SOLUTION
Across

2. Thrombophlebitis
3. Nephrotoxicity
5. Hemoccult
8. Rocephin
9. Intramuscular
10. Diarrhea
11. Lesions
12. Cephalosporins

Down

1. Cefoxitin
4. Streptococci
6. Cephalexin
7. Cefaclor

9 Tetracyclines, Macrolides, and Lincosamides

MATCHING
1. D   2. B   3. E   4. H   5. A   6. F
7. J   8. I   9. G   10. C

MULTIPLE CHOICE
1. b   2. d   3. b   4. c   5. b   6. c
7. a   8. b   9. d   10. b   11. d   12. d

CROSSWORD SOLUTION
Across

1. *Helicobacter pylori*
5. Myasthenia gravis
6. *Chlamydia trachomatis*
7. Macrolides
8. Demeclocycline
9. Lincosamides
10. Rickettsiae

Down

2. Calcium
3. Staphylococci
4. Tetracyclines

FILL IN THE BLANKS

1. a) tetracyclines
   1. doxycycline (Vibramycin)
   2. minocycline (Minocin)
   3. tetracycline (Sumycin)

   b) macrolides
   1. azithromycin (Zithromax)
   2. clarithromycin (Biaxin)
   3. erythromycin (E-mycin)

   c) lincosamides
   1. clindamycin (Cleocin)
   2. lincomycin (Lincocin)

2. a) nausea b) vomiting c) diarrhea d) epigastric distress e) stomatitis f) sore throat g) skin rashes h) photosensitivity reactions
3. Tetracyclines are contraindicated in children because they may cause permanent discoloration of the teeth.
4. Foods high in calcium impair absorption of the tetracyclines.
5. The macrolides are particularly effective against infections of the respiratory and genital tracts.
6. Macrolides are used as prophylaxis treatment before dental and other procedures in patients allergic to penicillin.
7. Macrolides are primarily eliminated from the body by the liver and should be used with caution in patients with liver dysfunction.
8. Use of antacids decreases the absorption of most macrolides.

9. <u>Lincosamides</u> have a high potential for toxicity.
10. The <u>neuromuscular</u> <u>blocking</u> <u>action</u> of <u>lincosamides</u> poses a danger to patients with myasthenia gravis.

DOSAGE PROBLEMS

1. 2 milliliters
2. a) 140 milliliters b) 200 milliliters c) 200 milligrams per 5 milliliters d) 10 days
3. 20 milliliters; 10 milliliters
4. 20 milliliters
5. 1500 milligrams
6. 2 milliliters

10 Fluoroquinolones and Aminoglycosides

MATCHING

1. D   2. B   3. I   4. E   5. G   6. J
7. A   8. H   9. F   10. C

MULTIPLE CHOICE

1. a   2. a   3. c   4. d   5. c   6. b   7. b   8. b
9. c   10. d   11. c   12. d

FILL IN THE BLANKS

1. a) ciprofloxacin (Cipro) b) enoxacin (Penetrex)
   c) gatifloxacin (Tequin) d) lomefloxacin (Maxaquin)
   e) moxifloxacin (Avelox) f) ofloxacin (Floxin)
   g) sparfloxacin (Zagam)
2. a) nausea b) diarrhea c) headache d) abdominal pain or discomfort e) dizziness
3. a) amikacin (Amikin) b) gentamicin (Garamycin)
   c) kanamycin (Kantrex) d) neomycin (Mycifradin)
   e) netilmicin (Netromycin) f) tobramycin (Nebcin)
   g) streptomycin
4. a) theophylline—increase in serum theophylline levels
   b) cimetidine—interferes with elimination of fluoroquinolones
   c) NSAIDs—risk of seizures
   d) antacids, iron salts, zinc—decrease absorption of fluoroquinolones
   e) drugs that increase the QT interval—risk of severe cardiac arrhythmias
   f) oral anticoagulants—increased effects of the oral anticoagulant
5. <u>Kanamycin</u>, <u>neomycin</u>, and <u>paromomycin</u> are used orally in the management of hepatic coma.
6. a) nephrotoxicity b) ototoxicity c) neurotoxicity
7. An aminoglycoside used for long-term treatment of tuberculosis is <u>streptomycin</u>.
8. a) numbness b) skin tingling c) circumoral paresthesia d) peripheral paresthesia e) tremors f) muscle twitching g) convulsions h) muscle weakness i) neuromuscular blockade
9. a) identify and record the signs and symptoms of the infection
   b) obtain a thorough allergy history
   c) take and record vital signs
10. a) level of consciousness b) ability to swallow

CROSSWORD SOLUTION
Across

2. Neurotoxicity
9. Ciprofloxacin
10. Fluoroquinolones
11. Hematuria
12. Proteinuria
13. Aminoglycoside
14. Nephrotoxicity

Down

1. Streptomycin
3. Circumoral
4. Neomycin
5. Bactericidal
6. Hepatic coma
7. Achilles
8. Ototoxicity

DOSAGE PROBLEMS

1. 2 milliliters
2. 3 tablets
3. ½ tablet
4. a) Yes b) 3 milliliters
5. a) 9 milliliters b) 400 milligrams per milliliter c) 1.25 milliliters

11 Miscellaneous Anti-infectives

MATCHING

1. G   2. K   3. C   4. L   5. F   6. N
7. H   8. O   9. B   10. A   11. E   12. I
13. M   14. D   15. J

FILL IN THE BLANKS

1. a) chloramphenicol (Chloromycetin) b) linezolid (Zyvox) c) meropenem (Merrem IV)
   d) metronidazole (Flagyl) e) pentamidine isethionate (Pentam 300, parenteral form/NebuPent, aerosol form) f) spectinomycin (Trobicin) g) vancomycin (Vancocin)
2. Administration of <u>chloramphenicol</u> is recommended to be done in a hospital setting because of the serious and sometimes fatal <u>blood</u> <u>dyscrasias</u> that can occur.
3. <u>Linezolid</u> is an anti-infective that is effective in treating VRE and MRSA.
4. a) pseudomembranous colitis b) thrombocytopenia
5. <u>Meropenem</u> is contraindicated in patients allergic to cephalosporin and penicillin.
6. The most serious adverse reactions associated with metronidazole are associated with the <u>CNS</u>, and include <u>seizures</u> and <u>numbness</u> of the <u>extremities</u>.
7. a) leukopenia b) hypoglycemia c) thrombocytopenia d) hypotension
8. The two, possibly irreversible, adverse reactions that may be seen with vancomycin are <u>nephrotoxicity</u> and <u>ototoxicity</u>.

MULTIPLE CHOICE

1. b   2. d   3. c   4. a   5. d   6. a   7. b   8. d
9. a   10. b

CROSSWORD SOLUTION

Across

1. Chloramphenicol
6. Thrombocytopenia
10. Hypoglycemia
11. NebuPent
12. Penicillin
13. Vancomycin

Down

1. Cimetidine
2. Metronidazole
3. MRSA
4. Pentamidine
5. VRE
7. Anaerobic
8. Hypotension
9. Flagyl

DOSAGE PROBLEMS

1. 2 capsules
2. ½ milliliter
3. 20 milliliters of solution; no; 2 vials
4. a) 60 kilograms b) 900 milligrams c) 9 milliliters d) 450 milligrams e) 4.5 milliliters

12 Antitubercular Drugs

MATCHING

1. C	2. F	3. M	4. J	5. B	6. G
7. O	8. E	9. K	0. I	11. N	12. A
13. L	14. H	15. D			

MULTIPLE CHOICE

| 1. c | 2. a | 3. b | 4. a | 5. c | 6. d | 7. d | 8. b |
| 9. a | 10. c | | | | | | |

FILL IN THE BLANKS

1. a) ethambutol b) isoniazid c) pyrazinamide d) rifampin e) streptomycin
2. a) ciprofloxacin b) ofloxacin c) levofloxacin d) sparfloxacin
3. The drugs used to treat tuberculosis do not <u>cure</u> the disease, but they render the patient <u>noninfectious</u> to <u>others</u>.
4. Second-line tuberculosis drugs are used to treat <u>extrapulmonary</u> <u>tuberculosis</u> and <u>drug-resistant</u> <u>organisms</u>.
5. Some patients treated with ethambutol experience <u>optic</u> <u>neuritis,</u> which appears to be dose related and usually disappears with <u>discontinuation</u> of the drug.
6. Severe and sometimes fatal <u>hepatitis</u> has been associated with isoniazid therapy.
7. Isoniazid toxicity may develop and can be identified by the common symptom of <u>peripheral</u> <u>neuropathy</u>.
8. a) nephrotoxicity b) ototoxicity c) numbness d) tingling e) tinnitus f) nausea g) vomiting h) vertigo i) circumoral paresthesia

DOSAGE PROBLEMS

1. 6 milliliters
2. 2 tablets
3. 4 tablets
4. a) 300 to 600 milligrams b) yes c) 30 kilograms
5. 2½ milliliters
6. 6 tablets

CROSSWORD SOLUTION

Across

3. Primary
5. Vertigo
6. Gout
7. Extrapulmonary
8. Fluoroquinolones
11. Isoniazid
12. Tuberculosis
13. Ethambutol

Down

1. Anaphylactoid
2. Bacteriostatic
4. Hemolysis
9. Rifampin
10. Tinnitus

13 Leprostatic Drugs

MATCHING

| 1. C | 2. F | 3. D | 4. A | 5. E | 6. B |

MULTIPLE CHOICE

| 1. b | 2. d | 3. a | 4. c | 5. b |

CROSSWORD SOLUTION

Across

3. Hemolysis
5. Rifampin
7. *Mycobacterium leprae*
8. Hansen's

Down

1. Clofazimine
2. Compliance
4. Dapsone
6. Leprosy

14 Antiviral Drugs

MATCHING

1. C	2. I	3. K	4. F	5. B	6. E
7. O	8. M	9. H	10. N	11. G	12. A
13. J	14. L	15. D			

FILL IN THE BLANKS

1. Virus can reproduce only within a <u>living</u> <u>cell</u>.
2. a) acyclovir (Zovirax) b) amantadine (Symmetrel)
   c) didanosine (Videx) d) ribavirin (Virazole)
   e) zanamivir (Relenza) f) zidovudine (AZT, Retrovir)
3. Use of a drug for a specific disorder or condition that is not officially approved by the Food and Drug Administration (FDA) is called an <u>unlabeled</u> <u>use</u>.
4. a) initial and recurrent mucosal and cutaneous herpes simplex virus (HSV)-1 and HSV-2 infections in immunocompromised patients, encephalitis, and herpes zoster
   b) human immunodeficiency virus (HIV; combined with other drugs)
   c) cytomegalovirus (CMV) retinitis
   d) genital herpes
   e) influenza A respiratory tract illness
   f) respiratory syncytial virus (RSV)
   g) viral herpes infections
5. Antiviral drugs are given <u>systemically</u> or as <u>topical</u> drugs.
6. a) determining the patient's state of health and resistance to infection.
   b) identifying and recording patient's symptoms and complaints.
   c) taking and recording the patient's vital signs.
   d) inspecting the skin for lesions (e.g., mouth, face, eyes, genitalia) before treatment begins.
7. a) allowing patient the time to talk and ask questions about methods of treatment, especially if an IV drug is used.
   b) explaining all treatment methods to the patient and family members.
   c) preparing the antiviral drugs according to the manufacturers' directions.
   d) following the administration orders of the primary care physician.
   e) preventing trauma if platelet count is low.
   f) administering analgesics as prescribed when needed.
8. a) Risk for Nutritional Imbalance: Less than Body Requirements
   b) Risk for Impaired Skin Integrity
   c) Risk for Injury
   d) Risk for Infection (immunosuppression)

MULTIPLE CHOICE

1. a 2. c 3. d 4. a 5. b 6. c 7. d 8. a
9. c 10. b

CROSSWORD SOLUTION

Across

2. Jaundice
7. HIV
8. Anticholinergic
9. RSV
11. Crystalluria
13. Ribavirin
14. Influenza
15. Granulocytopenia

Down

1. Asthenia
3. Erythema
4. Photosensitivity
5. Exacerbation
6. Retinitis
10. Viruses
12. Remission

DOSAGE PROBLEMS

1. 2 blisters
2. ½ tablet
3. 2 tablets
4. 50 milligrams
5. a) 1200 milligrams b) 4 milliliters c) yes d) 1. 9 or 2. 0 milligrams per milliliter

15 Antifungal Drugs

MATCHING

1. C 2. L 3. E 4. I 5. J 6. B
7. F 8. A 9. M 10. H 11. G 12. K
13. O 14. N 15. D

FILL IN THE BLANKS

1. a) amphotericin B (Fungizone) b) fluconazole (Diflucan) c) flucytosine (Ancobon) d) griseofulvin (Grisactin) e) ketoconazole (Nizoral) f) miconazole (Monistat)
2. Antifungal drugs may be <u>fungicidal</u> or <u>fungistatic</u>.
3. Antifungal drugs are used to treat <u>superficial</u> and <u>deep</u> <u>fungal</u> infections.
4. fever, shaking chills, headache, malaise, anorexia, joint/muscle pain, abnormal renal function, nausea, vomiting, and anemia
5. Fluconazole administration may result in abnormal <u>liver</u> <u>function</u>.
6. Flucytosine administration requires periodic <u>renal</u> <u>function</u> <u>tests</u>.
7. Miconazole, a Pregnancy Category C antifungal, is used during the <u>first</u> <u>trimester</u> only when essential.
8. a) Assess the patient for signs of the infection.
   b) Inspect for superficial fungal infections of the skin or skin structures and describe them in the patient's record.
   c) Document any skin lesions to obtain an accurate database.
   d) Describe any vaginal discharge.
   e) Describe any changes to the mucous membranes.
   f) Take and record vital signs.
   g) Weigh the patient.
9. a) Disturbed Body Image
   b) Risk for Ineffective Tissue Perfusion: Renal
   c) Risk for Infection
   d) Impaired Skin Integrity
10. Amphotericin B is reconstituted with <u>sterile</u> <u>water</u> because any other diluent may cause <u>precipitation</u>.

MULTIPLE CHOICE
1. c   2. c   3. a   4. d   5. a   6. b   7. d   8. b
9. c   10. a

CROSSWORD SOLUTION
Across
1. Superficial
3. Systemic
9. Fungicidal
12. Tinea corporis
13. Miconazole
14. Fungus

Down
2. Fungistatic
4. *Candida albicans*
5. Hypokalemia
6. Tinea cruris
7. Fluconazole
8. Onychomycosis
10. Tinea pedis
11. Fever

DOSAGE PROBLEMS
1. 500 milligrams per dose, 1000 milligrams total for two doses
2. a) 80 kilograms b) 20 milligrams per day to 120 milligrams per day c) no
3. a) solution b) 1 milliliter c) 3 milliliters
4. a) 2800 milligrams b) 28 tablets c) 14 tablets d) hepatic toxicity
5. a) 12,000 milligrams b) 3000 milligrams c) 6 capsules

16 Antiparasitic Drugs

MATCHING
1. E   2. D   3. K   4. H   5. N   6. B
7. I   8. M   9. F   10. O   11. L   12. C
13. J   14. G   15. A

FILL IN THE BLANKS
1. a) albendazole (Albenza) b) mebendazole (Vermox) c) pyrantel (Antiminth) d) thiabendazole (Mintezol)
2. a) chloroquine (Aralen HCL) b) doxycycline (Vibramycin) c) quinine
3. a) chloroquine (Aralen HCL) b) iodoquinol (Yodoxin) c) metronidazole (Flagyl) d) paromomycin (Humatin)
4. Diagnosis of a helminth infection is made by examination of the stool for ova and all or part of the helminth.
5. When pinworm infection is suspected, the nurse takes a specimen from the anal area, preferably early in the morning, using a cellophane tape swab.
6. Parenteral injection of chloroquine is avoided because the drug can cause respiratory distress, shock, and cardiovascular collapse when given intramuscularly or intravenously.

7. Paromomycin may be absorbed in large amounts by patients with bowel disease, causing ototoxicity and renal impairment.
8. Diagnosis of amebiasis is made by examining the stool, as well as by considering the patient's symptoms.
9. The nurse immediately delivers all stool specimens saved for amebiasis examination to the laboratory because the organisms die when the specimen cools.
10. Ingesting of alcohol while taking metronidazole may cause a mild to severe reaction with symptoms of severe vomiting, headache, nausea, abdominal cramps, flushing and sweating.

CROSSWORD SOLUTION
Across
4. Thrombocytopenia
10. Merozoites
12. Ameba
13. Helminth
14. Quinine

Down
1. Vermox
2. Pinworms
3. Parasite
5. Pyrantel
6. Fansidar
7. Sporozoites
8. Anopheles
9. Amebiasis
11. Malaria

MULTIPLE CHOICE
1. b   2. a   3. c   4. d   5. a   6. d   7. b   8. a
9. d   10. d   11. c   12. b

DOSAGE PROBLEMS
1. a) two 500-milligram tablets b) 1500 milligrams c) 9 tablets
2. a) two tablets b) 800 milligrams c) 112 tablets d) 126 days e) approximately 4 months
3. a) 4 tablets b) 28 tablets
4. a) 360 milligrams b) 720 milligrams c) son—two capsules; mother—four capsules

17 Nonnarcotic Analgesics: Salicylates and Nonsalicylates

MATCHING
1. C   2. F   3. L   4. H   5. A   6. O   7. E   8. N
9. J   10. G   11. M   12. I   13. B   14. K   15. D

FILL IN THE BLANKS
1. a) celecoxib (Celebrex) b) rofecoxib (Vioxx)
2. a) gastric upset b) heartburn c) nausea d) vomiting e) anorexia f) gastrointestinal bleeding
3. a) curry powder b) paprika c) licorice d) prunes e) raisins f) tea

4. Aspirin may increase the risk of bleeding during heparin administration.

5. Acetaminophen has analgesic and antipyretic activity but does not possess anti-inflammatory action.

6. a) dizziness b) tinnitus c) impaired hearing d) nausea e) vomiting f) flushing g) sweating h) rapid deep breathing i) tachycardia j) diarrhea; or mental confusion, lassitude, drowsiness, respiratory depression, or coma

7. a) nausea b) vomiting c) anorexia d) malaise e) diaphoresis f) abdominal pain g) confusion h) liver tenderness i) hypotension j) arrhythmias k) jaundice l) acute hepatic and renal failure

8. Pain is subjective and the patient's report of pain should always be taken seriously.

9. The nonnarcotic analgesics are a group of drugs used to relieve pain without the possibility of causing physical dependency.

10. Loss of blood through the gastrointestinal tract occurs with salicylate use.

MULTIPLE CHOICE
1. b   2. a   3. c   4. c   5. a   6. b   7. d   8. c
9. d   10. c

CROSSWORD SOLUTION
Across

1. Tinnitus
3. Aspirin
8. Reye
9. Pain
13. Prostaglandins
14. Acetaminophen

Down

2. Salicylism
4. Salicylates
5. Aggregation
6. Asterixis
7. Pancytopenia
10. Analgesics
11. Mucomyst
12. Jaundice

DOSAGE PROBLEMS
1. a) 30 milliliters b) 4000 milligrams c) no
2. a) two 500-milligram tablets b) one 250-milligram and one 500-milligram tablet or one and one-half 500-milligram tablets c) 2500 milligrams
3. a) 3 milliliters b) 600 milligrams

18 Nonnarcotic Analgesics: Nonsteroidal Anti-inflammatory Drugs (NSAIDs)

MATCHING
1. B   2. D   3. A   4. E   5. C

MULTIPLE CHOICE
1. b   2. b   3. a   4. c   5. b

FILL IN THE BLANKS
1. a) celecoxib (Celebrex) b) ibuprofen (Advil) c) naproxen (Naprosyn) d) rofecoxib (Vioxx)
2. The NSAIDs are so named because they do not belong to the steroid group of drugs.
3. The NSAIDs have anti-inflammatory, antipyretic, and analgesic effects.
4. a) relief of signs and symptoms of osteoarthritis, rheumatoid arthritis, and other musculoskeletal disorders
   b) mild to moderate pain relief
   c) primary dysmenorrhea
   d) fever reduction
5. Adverse reactions to the NSAIDs may affect the special senses. The nurse should know to monitor for visual disturbances, blurred or diminished vision, diplopia, swollen or irritated eyes, photophobia, reversible loss of color vision, tinnitus, taste changes, rhinitis.

DOSAGE PROBLEMS
1. 20 milliliters
2. 187.5 milligrams
3. a) 250 milligrams b) 12.5 milliliters

CROSSWORD SOLUTION
Across

7. Ibuprofen
8. Celebrex
10. Osteoarthritis

Down

1. Cyclooxygenase
2. Rhinitis
3. Tinnitus
4. Naproxen
5. Dysmenorrhea
6. Rofecoxib
9. NSAID

19 Narcotic Analgesics

MATCHING
1. C   2. H   3. E   4. J   5. D   6. A
7. I   8. F   9. G   10. B

FILL IN THE BLANKS
1. Narcotic antagonists compete with the narcotics at the receptor sites and are used to reverse the depressant effects of the narcotic analgesics.
2. a) morphine b) codeine c) hydrochlorides of opium alkaloids d) camphorated tincture of opium
3. Synthetic narcotics are those man-made analgesics with properties and actions similar to the natural opioids.

4. a) methadone b) levorphanol c) remifentanil
   d) meperidine
5. a) drug b) dose c) route of administration d) type of
   pain e) patient f) length of time the drug has been
   administered
6. Narcotic analgesics may be used preoperatively to
   lessen anxiety and sedate the patient.
7. a) levomethadyl b) methadone
8. A major hazard of narcotic administration is
   respiratory depression with a decrease in the
   respiratory rate and depth.
9. a) blood pressure b) pulse c) respiratory rate
10. a) A significant decrease in the respiratory rate or a
    respiratory rate of 10 per minute or less.
    b) A significant increase or decrease in the pulse rate
    or change in pulse quality.
    c) A significant decrease in blood pressure (systolic or
    diastolic) or a systolic pressure below 100 mm Hg.

MULTIPLE CHOICE
1. b   2. a   3. d   4. a   5. d   6. b   7. a   8. c
9. a   10. c

DOSAGE PROBLEMS
1. 0. 8 milliliters
2. 0. 67 milliliters (round-up)
3. 0. 75 milliliters
4. 1. 33 milliliters

CROSSWORD SOLUTION
Across
1. Levo-Dromoran
5. Ultiva
10. Pain
11. PCA
13. Antitussive
14. Demerol
15. Enkephalins

Down
2. Epidural
3. Opioid
4. Methadone
6. Dolophine
7. Morphine
8. Fentanyl
9. Narcotic
12. Codeine

20 Narcotic Antagonists

MATCHING
1. C   2. E   3. A   4. D   5. B

FILL IN THE BLANKS
1. A drug that is an antagonist has an affinity for a cell
   receptor, and by binding to it, prevents the cell from
   responding.

2. The two narcotic antagonists in use today are
   naloxone (Narcan) and naltrexone (ReVia).
3. Naltrexone is used primarily to block the euphoric
   effects experienced in opiate dependence.
4. Administration of naloxone prevents or reverses the
   effects of the opiates.
5. Naloxone is used for complete or partial reversal of
   narcotic depression, including respiratory depression.
6. Abrupt reversal of narcotic depression may result in
   nausea, vomiting, sweating, tachycardia, increased
   blood pressure, and tremors.
7. Patients taking naltrexone on a scheduled basis will
   not experience any narcotic effects if they use an
   opioid.
8. The expected outcome for the patient with respiratory
   depression is a return to normal respiratory rate,
   rhythm, and depth.

MULTIPLE CHOICE
1. b   2. a   3. c   4. b   5. a   6. c   7. a   8. d

DOSAGE PROBLEMS
1. 680 micrograms or 0.68 milligrams
2. a) ½ tablet   b) 3 tablets
3. 2.5 milliliters

CROSSWORD SOLUTION
Across
1. Narcotic antagonist
3. Respirator
5. Methadone
6. Depression

Down
1. Naloxone
2. Naltrexone
4. Narcan

21 Drugs That Affect the Musculoskeletal System

MATCHING
1. E   2. I   3. B   4. D   5. L   6. K
7. O   8. C   9. G   10. N   11. A   12. H
13. M   14. J   15. F

FILL IN THE BLANKS
1. a) gold compounds b) antigout drugs c) skeletal
   muscle relaxants d) bisphosphonates e) corticosteroids
   f) miscellaneous drugs (1) penicillamine,
   (2) methotrexate, (3) hydroxychloroquine
2. a) gold sodium thiomalate (Aurolate) b)
   aurothioglucose (Solganal) c) auranofin (Ridaura)
3. a) dermatitis b) stomatitis
4. Colchicine reduces inflammation associated with the
   deposit of urate crystals in the joints.
5. a) allopurinol (Zyloprim) b) sulfinpyrazone
   (Anturane) c) probenecid (Benemid) d) colchicine
6. a) exfoliative dermatitis b) Stevens-Johnson syndrome

7. a) carisoprodol (Soma) b) baclofen (Lioresal)
c) chlorzoxazone (Paraflex) d) cyclobenzaprine
(Flexeril) e) diazepam (Valium)

8. Adverse reactions seen with the administration of
diazepam would include <u>drowsiness</u>, <u>sedation</u>,
<u>sleepiness</u>, <u>lethargy</u>, <u>constipation</u> or <u>diarrhea</u>,
<u>bradycardia</u> or <u>tachycardia</u>, and <u>rash</u>.

9. Cyclobenzaprine is contraindicated in patients with
recent <u>myocardial</u> <u>infarction</u>, <u>cardiac</u> <u>conduction</u>
disorders, and <u>hyperthyroidism.</u>

10. a) alendronate (Fosamax) b) etidronate (Didronel)
c) risedronate (Actonel)

11. Adverse reactions with the bisphosphonates include
<u>nausea</u>, <u>diarrhea</u>, <u>increased</u> or <u>recurrent</u> <u>bone</u> <u>pain</u>,
<u>headache</u>, <u>dyspepsia</u>, <u>acid</u> <u>regurgitation</u>, <u>dysphagia</u>,
and <u>abdominal</u> pain.

12. Corticosteroids may be used to treat rheumatic
disorders such as <u>ankylosing spondylitis</u>, <u>rheumatoid</u>
<u>arthritis</u>, <u>gout</u>, <u>bursitis</u>, and <u>osteoarthritis.</u>

13. Hydroxychloroquine is contraindicated in patients
with <u>porphyria</u>, <u>psoriasis</u>, and <u>retinal</u> disease.

14. a) appearance of the skin over the joints
b) evidence of joint deformity
c) mobility of the affected joint

MULTIPLE CHOICE

1. a 2. d 3. b 4. c 5. b 6. d 7. b 8. c
9. b 10. b 11. a 12. d 13. a 14. b

CROSSWORD SOLUTION

Across

2. Analgesic
7. Zyloprim
8. Benemid
12. Anti-inflammatory
13. Rheumatoid
14. Tinnitus
15. Methotrexate
16. Musculoskeletal

Down

1. Osteoarthritis
3. Alendronate
4. Chrysiasis
5. Soma
6. Gold
9. Synovitis
10. Antipyretic
11. Gout

DOSAGE PROBLEMS

1. 3 tablets
2. a) 1 tablet b) 3 tablets c) increase to 2.5 to 3 liters a
day
3. 2 tablets
4. a) 1½ milliliters b) before 9 A.M.

22 Adrenergic Drugs

MATCHING

1. H 2. A 3. N 4. O 5. B 6. M 7. J 8. D
9. K 10. F 11. P 12. I 13. G 14. L 15. E 16. C

LABELING

1. Brain
2. Spinal cord
3. Somatic nervous system
4. Peripheral nervous system
5. Autonomic nervous system
6. Sympathetic nervous system
7. Parasympathetic nervous system

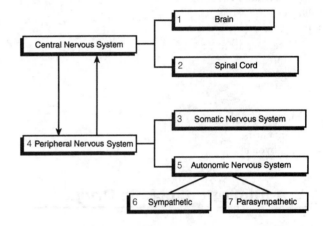

FILL IN THE BLANKS

1. The primary effects of the adrenergic drugs occur on
the <u>heart</u>, the <u>blood</u> <u>vessels</u>, and the <u>smooth</u> <u>muscles</u>,
such as the <u>bronchi</u>.

2. Adrenergic drugs mimic the activity of the <u>sympathetic</u>
<u>nervous</u> <u>system</u>.

3. a) metaraminol (Aramine) b) isoproterenol (Isuprel) c)
ephedrine

4. The adrenergic drugs are important in <u>treatment</u> and
<u>management</u> of patients in <u>shock</u>.

5. a) relaxation of the smooth muscles of the bronchi
b) constriction of blood vessels and sphincters of the
stomach
c) dilation of coronary blood vessels
d) decrease in gastric motility

6. Adrenergic drugs are used to improve <u>hemodynamic</u>
status during shock, by improving <u>myocardial</u>
contractility and <u>increasing</u> heart <u>rate</u>, which results in
<u>increased</u> cardiac <u>output.</u>

7. Some of the more common adverse reactions seen
with the adrenergic drugs would include <u>cardiac</u>
<u>arrhythmias</u> such as <u>bradycardia</u> and <u>tachycardia</u>,
<u>headache</u>, <u>insomnia</u>, <u>nervousness</u>, <u>anorexia</u>, and
<u>increased</u> blood pressure.

8. Although adrenergic drugs are potentially dangerous,
proper <u>supervision</u> and <u>management</u> before, during,
and after <u>administration</u> will <u>minimize</u> the occurrence
of any serious problems.

9. Initial <u>pharmacological</u> intervention for shock is aimed at supporting the <u>circulation</u> with <u>vasopressors.</u>
10. a) dobutamine (Dobutrex) b) dopamine (Intropin) c) norepinephrine (Levophed)

MULTIPLE CHOICE
1. b   2. a   3. d   4. c   5. a   6. c   7. c   8. a
9. d   10. a   11. b   12. c

DOSAGE PROBLEMS
1. 0.3 milliliters
2. 0.25 milliliters
3. 4 milliliters
4. a) ½ tablet b) 1 tablet c) 1½ tablet

CROSSWORD SOLUTION
Across
2. Shock
4. Norepinephrine
6. Hypoxia
7. Neurotransmitters
8. Septic

Down
1. Epinephrine
3. Hypovolemic
5. Neurogenic

23 Adrenergic Blocking Drugs

MATCHING
1. E   2. D   3. G   4. J   5. B   6. K   7. I   8. L
9. H   10. F   11. C   12. A

LABELING
A. Nerve ending
B. Receptor site on cell surface
C. Epinephrine and norepinephrine
D. Beta-adrenergic blocking drug

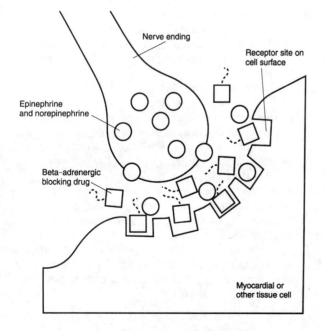

FILL IN THE BLANKS
1. a) alpha-adrenergic blocking drugs
   b) beta-adrenergic blocking drugs
   c) alpha/beta-adrenergic blocking drugs
   d) antiadrenergic drugs
2. Alpha-adrenergic blocking drugs produce their greatest effect on the <u>alpha-receptors</u> of the adrenergic nerves that control the <u>vascular</u> <u>system.</u>
3. Beta-adrenergic blocking drugs produce their greatest effect on the <u>beta-receptors</u> of the <u>heart</u>.
4. Administration of an alpha-adrenergic blocking drug may result in the adverse reactions of <u>weakness</u>, <u>orthostatic</u> <u>hypotension</u>, <u>cardiac</u> <u>arrhythmias</u>, <u>hypotension</u>, and <u>tachycardia.</u>
5. Stimulation of <u>beta-receptors</u> of the <u>heart</u> results in an <u>increase</u> in the heart rate. Blocking the stimulation causes the heart rate to <u>decrease</u> and the vessels to <u>dilate</u>.
6. Beta-adrenergic blocking ophthalmic drugs <u>reduce</u> the production of <u>aqueous</u> <u>humor</u> in the <u>anterior</u> <u>chamber</u> of the eye, to relieve the <u>intraocular</u> <u>pressure</u> of <u>glaucoma.</u>
7. Beta-adrenergic blocking drugs are used mainly in the treatment of <u>hypertension</u> and certain <u>cardiac</u> <u>arrhythmias</u>.
8. More serious adverse reactions that may be seen with the beta-adrenergic blocking drugs can include symptoms of <u>congestive</u> <u>heart</u> <u>failure</u>, which are <u>dyspnea</u>, <u>weight</u> <u>gain</u>, and <u>peripheral</u> <u>edema</u>.
9. Some of the adverse reactions observed with the administration of beta-adrenergic blocking drugs include <u>orthostatic</u> <u>hypotension</u>, <u>bradycardia</u>, <u>dizziness</u>, <u>vertigo</u>, <u>bronchospasm</u>, <u>hyperglycemia</u>, <u>nausea</u>, <u>vomiting</u>, and <u>diarrhea</u>.
10. The nurse should withhold the <u>beta-adrenergic</u> <u>blocking</u> drug propranolol (Inderal) if the patient has a heart rate of less than <u>60</u> beats/minute and notify the <u>physician</u>.

CROSSWORD SOLUTION
Across
1. Propranolol
3. First-dose effect
4. Bronchospasm
6. Postural
7. Phentolamine
8. Pheochromocytoma

Down
1. Orthostatic
5. Dyspnea

MULTIPLE CHOICE
1. d   2. b   3. a   4. a   5. c   6. b   7. d   8. c
9. d   10. b

DOSAGE PROBLEMS
1. a) 1½ tablets b) 0.6 milligrams daily
2. a) 2 tablets b) One time
3. 2 capsules
4. a) 2 tablets b) 12.5 milligrams c) 25 milligrams
   d) 50 milligrams

24 Cholinergic Drugs

MATCHING
1. C   2. G   3. E   4. I   5. A   6. H
7. J   8. B   9. F   10. D

FILL IN THE BLANKS
1. a) severe abdominal cramping
   b) diarrhea
   c) excessive salivation
   d) muscle weakness
   e) rigidity and spasm
   f) clenching of the jaw
2. a) rapid fatigability of the muscles
   b) drooping of the eyelids
   c) difficulty breathing
3. a) slowing the heart rate
   b) digesting food
   c) eliminating body waste
4. a) glaucoma b) myasthenia gravis c) urinary retention
5. a) carbachol b) pilocarpine (Isopto Carpine) c)
   temporary reduction in visual acuity d) headache
6. a) ambenonium (Mytelase) b) pyridostigmine
   (Mestinon)
7. a) bethanechol (Urecholine) b) ambenonium
   (Mytelase) c) pyridostigmine (Mestinon)

MULTIPLE CHOICE
1. a   2. c   3. b   4. d   5. b   6. c   7. d   8. a
9. a   10. b   11. c

DOSAGE PROBLEMS
1. a) 1½ tablet b) 60 milligrams
2. a) 0.5 milliliters b) 2 vials
3. ½ milliliter

CROSSWORD SOLUTION
Across
2. Myasthenia gravis
6. Cholinergic crisis
10. Micturation
11. Acetylcholinesterase

Down
1. Glaucoma
3. Ambenonium
4. Acetylcholine
5. Drooling
7. Seven
8. Miosis
9. Palpates

25 Cholinergic Blocking Drugs

MATCHING
1. E   2. D   3. A   4. C   5. B

MULTIPLE CHOICE
1. b   2. a   3. b   4. d   5. c   6. b   7. a   8. d
9. c   10. a

FILL IN THE BLANKS
1. a) perform frequent mouth care
   b) keep drinking fluid handy
   c) sip fluids throughout the day and with meals
   d) take sips of water before taking oral drugs
   e) suck on ice chips or frozen ices
   f) chew gum
   g) suck on sugar-free hard candy
   h) avoid alcohol-based mouthwash
2. The nurse should contact the primary health care
   provider if the elderly patient taking a cholinergic
   blocking drug experiences excitement, agitation,
   mental confusion, drowsiness, or urinary retention.
3. The anesthesiologist must be notified if the
   preoperative medications are given late.
4. a) eyes b) respiratory tract c) gastrointestinal tract
   d) heart e) bladder
5. The cholinergic blocking drug clidinium bromide is
   used only to treat peptic ulcer.
6. a) fever b) tachycardia c) flushing d) warm, dry skin
   e) mental confusion
7. a) meperidine (Demerol) b) flurazepam (Dalmane)
   c) diphenhydramine (Benadryl) d) phenothiazines
   e) tricyclic antidepressants

CROSSWORD SOLUTION
Across
3. Cycloplegia
10. Idiosyncratic

Down
1. Anticholinergic
2. Dry
4. Photophobia
5. Scopolamine
6. Glaucoma
7. Mydriasis
8. Atropine
9. Inhibit

DOSAGE PROBLEMS
1. 0. 6 milliliter
2. a) 2 tablets b) 800 milligrams
3. ½ tablet

26 Sedatives and Hypnotics

MATCHING
1. G   2. B   3. H   4. D   5. A   6. J
7. E   8. I   9. F   10. C

FILL IN THE BLANKS

1. Sedatives make the patient <u>drowsy,</u> but usually do not produce <u>sleep</u>.
2. Hypnotics allow the patient to <u>fall</u> <u>asleep</u> and <u>stay</u> <u>asleep</u>.
3. Sedatives are given during <u>daytime</u> hours and hypnotics are given at <u>night</u>.
4. a) ultra short-acting, 20 minutes or less
   b) short-acting, 3 to 4 hours
   c) intermediate-acting, 6 to 8 hours
   d) long-acting, 10 to 16 hours
5. Sedatives and hypnotics have an <u>additive</u> effect when administered with <u>alcohol, antidepressants, narcotic analgesics, antihistamines,</u> or <u>phenothiazines.</u>
6. Assessment of the patient receiving a <u>sedative</u> or <u>hypnotic</u> drug depends on the <u>reason</u> for administration and whether the drug is given <u>routinely</u> or as <u>needed</u>.
7. Barbiturates, when given in the presence of pain, may cause <u>restlessness, excitement</u> and <u>delirium</u>.
8. Patients who have been taking a <u>sedative</u> or <u>hypnotic</u> for several weeks should be gradually <u>withdrawn</u> from the drug to prevent <u>withdrawal</u> symptoms.

MULTIPLE CHOICE

1. b   2. a   3. b   4. d   5. c   6. a   7. c   8. b·
9. a   10. d   11. c   12. b

CROSSWORD SOLUTION
Across

4. Dalmane
6. Hypnotic
9. Sedative
10. Ataxia
12. Caffeine

Down

1. Soporific
2. Detoxify
3. Secobarbital
5. Additive
7. Melatonin
8. Valerian
11. REM

DOSAGE PROBLEMS

1. 1 tablet
2. 2 capsules
3. 0.75 milliliter
4. 1.8 milliliters

27 Central Nervous System Stimulants

MATCHING

1. B   2. D   3. G   4. I   5. A   6. E   7. H   8. C
9. F

FILL IN THE BLANKS

1. a) analeptics b) anorexiants c) amphetamines
2. a) doxapram (Dopram) b) caffeine c) modafinil
3. Caffeine has mild <u>analeptic</u> activity and also results in <u>cardiac</u> stimulation, dilation of <u>coronary</u> and <u>peripheral</u> blood vessels, constriction of <u>cerebral</u> blood vessels, and <u>skeletal</u> muscle stimulation.
4. Amphetamines and anorexiants should not be given <u>during</u> or <u>within</u> 14 days after administration of <u>monoamine oxidase inhibitors</u>, because the patient may develop <u>hypertensive crisis</u> and <u>intracranial hemorrhage</u>.
5. When CNS stimulants are prescribed for respiratory depression, nursing assessment should include the <u>depth</u> of <u>respirations</u> and any pattern to the <u>respiratory rate</u>, such as <u>shallow</u> respirations or alternating <u>deep</u> and <u>shallow</u> respirations.
6. When amphetamines are prescribed for any reason, the nurse <u>weighs</u> the patient and takes the <u>blood pressure, pulse,</u> and <u>respiratory rate</u> before starting <u>drug therapy.</u>
7. After administration of an analeptic, the nurse carefully monitors <u>respiratory rate</u> and <u>pattern</u> until <u>respirations</u> return to normal.

CROSSWORD SOLUTION
Across

1. ADD
6. Narcolepsy
7. Exogenous

Down

1. Amphetamines
2. Anorexiants
3. Phentermine
4. Analeptics
5. Doxapram
6. NoDoz

MULTIPLE CHOICE

1. b   2. d   3. b   4. c   5. a   6. d   7. c   8. b

DOSAGE PROBLEMS

1. 25 milligrams
2. 3 capsules
3. Three 10-milligram tablets or one 10-milligram and one 20-milligram tablet

28 Anticonvulsants

MATCHING

1. G   2. I   3. M   4. A   5. H   6. L
7. C   8. F   9. K   10. N   11. D   12. B
13. J   14. E

FILL IN THE BLANKS

1. An anticonvulsant drug possesses the ability to <u>depress</u> abnormal <u>neural discharges</u> in the central nervous system, resulting in an <u>inhibition</u> of <u>seizure</u> activity.

2. Patients being treated with anticonvulsants may find their <u>dosage</u> of medication may have to be <u>increased</u> or <u>decreased</u> during the <u>initial</u> period of <u>treatment</u>.
3. a) barbiturates b) benzodiazepines c) hydantoins d) oxazolidinediones e) succinimides
4. With phenobarbital, <u>agitation</u> rather than <u>sedation</u> may occur in some patients.
5. The adverse reactions seen with the benzodiazepines include <u>sedation</u>, <u>anorexia</u>, <u>constipation</u>, or <u>diarrhea</u>.
6. <u>Phenytoin</u> is the most commonly prescribed anticonvulsant.
7. a) pancytopenia b) leukopenia c) aplastic anemia d) thrombocytopenia
8. When the hydantoins are administered with the <u>succinimides</u> there may be an <u>increase</u> in the <u>hydantoin</u> blood level.
9. a) electroencephalogram b) computed tomographic scan c) complete blood count d) hepatic function test e) renal function test
10. An anticonvulsant drug must never be <u>abruptly</u> <u>discontinued</u> or have its <u>doses</u> <u>omitted.</u>

MULTIPLE CHOICE
1. c   2. d   3. a   4. d   5. c   6. a   7. d   8. a
9. a   10. b   11. c   12. b

CROSSWORD SOLUTION
Across
1. Diazepam
6. Ethosuximide
8. Gingival
10. Nystagmus
11. Clonic
12. Pancytopenia

Down
2. Ataxia
3. Anticonvulsants
4. Absence
5. Convulsion
7. Tonic
9. Epilepsy

DOSAGE PROBLEMS
1. 4 milliliters
2. 1 tablet
3. 11.25 milliliters
4. ½ tablet

29 Antiparkinsonism Drugs

MATCHING
1. C   2. G   3. D   4. F   5. A   6. B
7. E   8. H

FILL IN THE BLANKS
1. <u>Parkinson's</u> disease is characterized by fine <u>tremors</u> and <u>rigidity</u> of some muscle groups and <u>weakness</u> of others.
2. The symptoms of <u>parkinsonism</u> are caused by a <u>depletion</u> of dopamine in the <u>CNS</u>.

3. a) choreiform movements b) dystonic movements
4. Foods high in <u>pyridoxine</u> or <u>vitamin B₆</u> preparations <u>reverse</u> the effect of levodopa.
5. <u>Tolcapone</u>, a COMT inhibitor, is associated with <u>liver</u> damage and <u>liver</u> failure.
6. a) Information regarding symptoms of the disorder.
   b) Length of time symptoms have been present.
   c) The ability of patient to complete activities of daily living.
   d) Patient's present mental condition.

MULTIPLE CHOICE
1. d   2. b   3. a   4. a   5. d   6. c   7. b   8. d
9. a   10. c

DOSAGE PROBLEMS
1. a) 2 tablets b) 50 milligrams carbidopa and 200 milligrams levodopa c) 150 milligrams carbidopa and 600 milligrams levodopa
2. 10 milliliters
3. 10 milliliters
4. ½ tablet

CROSSWORD SOLUTION
Across
2. Pyridoxine
4. Choreiform
6. Chicken
7. Achalasia
8. Benztropine
9. Ataxia

Down
1. Levodopa
2. Parkinson's
3. Amantadine
5. Dystonia

30 Antianxiety Drugs

MATCHING
1. B   2. D   3. E   4. H   5. C   6. A
7. F   8. G

FILL IN THE BLANKS
1. a) increased anxiety
   b) concentration difficulties
   c) tremor
   d) sensory disturbances
      1) paresthesias
      2) photophobia
      3) hypersomnia
      4) metallic taste
2. a) antianxiety drugs (tranquilizers) b) antidepressant drugs c) antipsychotic drugs
3. a) benzodiazepines b) nonbenzodiazepines
4. Long-term treatment with the <u>antianxiety</u> drugs may result in <u>drug</u> <u>dependence</u> and <u>serious</u> <u>withdrawal</u> <u>symptoms.</u>

5. Ingestion of <u>alcohol</u> with the antianxiety drugs can cause <u>convulsions</u> and <u>coma</u>.
6. Preadministration assessment <u>before</u> starting therapy with the <u>antianxiety</u> drugs would include complete <u>medical history</u> with <u>mental</u> status and <u>anxiety</u> level.
7. a) increased blood pressure
   b) increased pulse rate
   c) increased rate and depth of respirations
   d) increased muscle tension
   e) cool, pale skin
8. Benzodiazepine toxicity causes <u>sedation</u>, <u>respiratory depression</u>, and <u>coma</u>.
9. Flumazenil (Romazicon) is an <u>antidote</u> for benzodiazepine <u>toxicity</u> and acts within <u>6</u> to <u>10</u> minutes after <u>intravenous</u> administration.
10. When <u>discontinuing</u> an antianxiety drug in patients who have used these drugs for <u>prolonged</u> periods, the <u>physician</u> will prescribe a <u>decrease</u> of <u>dosage</u> gradually over <u>4</u> to <u>8</u> weeks to <u>avoid</u> the possibility of <u>withdrawal</u> symptoms.

MULTIPLE CHOICE
1. d   2. b   3. c   4. d   5. a   6. b   7. d   8. a

DRUG MATCHING
1. F   2. A   3. E   4. D   5. C   6. H
7. G   8. B

CROSSWORD SOLUTION
Across

3. Buspirone
5. Anxiolytics
6. Hypothalamus
7. Psychotropic

Down

1. Tolerance
2. Depressant
4. Anxiety

DOSAGE PROBLEMS
1. 1/2 tablet
2. 0.5 milliliter
3. 1.5 milliliters
4. 3 milliliters

31 Antidepressant Drugs

MATCHING
1. B   2. D   3. A   4. H   5. C   6. G
7. E   8. F

FILL IN THE BLANKS
1. a) depressed mood
   b) diminished interest in activities of life
   c) significant weight loss or gain (without dieting)
   d) insomnia or hypersomnia
   e) psychomotor agitation or retardation
   f) fatigue or loss of energy
   g) feelings of worthlessness
   h) excessive or inappropriate guilt
   i) diminished ability to think or concentrate, or indecisiveness
   j) recurrent thoughts of death or suicide
2. a) ricyclic antidepressants
   b) monoamine oxidase inhibitors
   c) selective serotonin reuptake inhibitors
   d) miscellaneous, unrelated drugs
3. a) fluoxetine (Prozac) b) fluvoxamine (Luvox)
   c) paroxetine (Paxil) d) sertraline (Zoloft)
4. The most common adverse reactions seen with the TCAs are <u>sedation</u> and <u>dry</u> <u>mouth</u>.
5. <u>Orthostatic</u> hypotension is seen with both the <u>TCAs</u> and the <u>MAOIs</u>.
6. A serious <u>adverse</u> <u>reaction</u> associated with the use of MAOIs is <u>hypertensive</u> <u>crisis</u>, which may occur when <u>foods</u> containing <u>tyramine</u> are eaten.
7. a) occipital headache b) stiff or sore neck c) nausea
   d) vomiting e) sweating f) fever g) chest pain h) dilated pupils i) bradycardia or tachycardia
8. There is a <u>decreased</u> <u>effectiveness</u> of fluoxetine in patients who <u>smoke</u> <u>cigarettes</u> during administration of the drug.

MULTIPLE CHOICE
1. b   2. c   3. a   4. d   5. b   6. c   7. a   8. c
9. c   10. c   11. a   12. d

CROSSWORD SOLUTION
Across

7. Amitriptyline
9. Maprotiline
14. Sertraline
15. Tricyclic
16. Monoamine oxidase
17. Trazodone

Down

1. SSRI
2. Bupropion
3. Priapism
4. Surmontil
5. Dysphoric
6. Hypertensive crisis
8. Fluoxetine
10. Venlafaxine
11. Paroxetine
12. Depression
13. Imipramine

DOSAGE PROBLEMS
1. 2 capsules
2. 10 milliliters
3. 2 tablets
4. 4 tablets

32 Antipsychotic Drugs

MATCHING
1. J 2. D 3. F 4. B 5. K 6. I
7. C 8. E 9. O 10. H 11. M 12. A
13. N 14. G 15. L

FILL IN THE BLANKS
1. The most common adverse reactions that may occur with lithium carbonate include <u>tremors</u>, <u>nausea</u>, <u>vomiting</u>, <u>thirst</u>, and <u>polyuria.</u>
2. The <u>dosage</u> of lithium is <u>individualized</u> according to <u>serum</u> levels and <u>clinical</u> response to the drug.
3. Adverse reactions that indicate bone marrow suppression would include <u>lethargy</u>, <u>weakness</u>, <u>fever</u>, <u>sore</u> <u>throat</u>, <u>malaise</u>, <u>mucous</u> <u>membrane</u> <u>ulcerations</u>, and <u>flulike</u> <u>complaints</u>.
4. Signs of lithium toxicity would include <u>diarrhea</u>, <u>vomiting</u>, <u>nausea</u>, <u>drowsiness</u>, <u>muscular</u> <u>weakness</u>, and lack of <u>coordination</u>.

MULTIPLE CHOICE
1. c 2. a 3. b 4. c 5. d 6. b 7. a 8. b
9. d 10. d

CROSSWORD SOLUTION
Across
1. Alzheimer's
5. Delusions
6. Neuroleptic
7. Flattened affect
8. Extrapyramidal
10. Akathisia
11. Photophobia
12. Tardive dyskinesia

Down
2. Hallucinations
3. Anhedonia
4. Bipolar
9. Dystonia

DOSAGE PROBLEMS
1. 3 tablets
2. a) 10 milliliters
   b) 2 containers
3. 5 milliliters
4. 7.5 milliliters
5. 1.5 milliliters

33 Cholinesterase Inhibitors

MATCHING
1. D 2. F 3. B 4. E 5. A 6. C

FILL IN THE BLANKS
1. Drugs used to treat Alzheimer's disease do not <u>cure</u> the disease, but are aimed at <u>slowing</u> the <u>progression.</u>
2. a) donepezil (Aricept)
   b) galantamine hydrobromide (Reminyl)
   c) rivastigmine tartrate (Exelon)
   d) tacrine hydrochloride (Cognex)
3. The cholinesterase inhibitors act to <u>increase</u> the level of <u>acetylcholine</u> in the <u>CNS</u> by inhibiting its <u>breakdown</u>.
4. In the patient with Alzheimer's disease, <u>cognitive</u> ability and <u>functional</u> ability are assessed <u>before</u> and <u>during</u> therapy.
5. a) confusion b) agitation c) impulsive behavior d) speech e) ability to perform activities of daily living f) self-care ability

MULTIPLE CHOICE
1. b 2. a 3. b 4. c 5. b 6. d 7. c 8. d

CROSSWORD SOLUTION
Across
2. Cognex
4. Dementia
8. Alanine aminotransferase
9. Ginseng

Down
1. Acetylcholine
3. Ginkgo biloba
5. Exelon
6. Aricept
7. Reminyl

DOSAGE PROBLEMS
1. 2 tablets
2. a) 1.5 milliliters b) 4.5 milliliters
3. a) 16 milligrams b) 4 tablets

34 Antiemetic and Antivertigo Drugs

MATCHING
1. B 2. C 3. E 4. I 5. G 6. A
7. J 8. F 9. H 10. D

FILL IN THE BLANKS
1. Vertigo is usually accompanied by <u>light-headedness</u>, <u>dizziness</u>, and <u>weakness</u>.
2. Dronabinol is a derivative of the active substance found in <u>marijuana</u> and is a second-line <u>antiemetic</u> used after <u>treatment</u> with other <u>antiemetics</u> has failed.
3. Antivertigo drugs are essentially <u>antiemetics</u> because they have <u>direct</u> or <u>indirect</u> <u>antiemetic</u> properties.
4. Thiethylperazine is classified as a Pregnancy Category <u>X</u> drug and is <u>contraindicated</u> during pregnancy.
5. <u>Antacids</u> decrease absorption of the <u>antiemetics</u>.

6. Preadministration <u>assessment</u> for the patient with nausea and vomiting should include the <u>number</u> of times the patient has <u>vomited</u> and approximate amount of <u>fluid</u> lost.
7. The nurse notifies the <u>physician</u> if the drug <u>fails</u> to <u>relieve</u> or <u>diminish</u> symptoms.
8. The nurse instructs the patient to take buclizine by placing the <u>tablet</u> in the <u>mouth</u> and allowing it to <u>dissolve</u> or to <u>chew</u> or <u>swallow</u> the <u>tablet</u> whole.
9. a) dolasetron mesylate (Anzemet)
   b) dronabinol (Marinol)
   c) granisetron hydrochloride (Kytril)
   d) metoclopramide (Reglan)
   e) ondansetron hydrochloride (Zofran)
10. a) dry mucous membranes
    b) decreased urinary output
    c) concentrated urine
    d) restlessness
    e) confusion (especially in older patients)

MULTIPLE CHOICE
1. c   2. a   3. b   4. d   5. b   6. c   7. b   8. a
9. b   10. c

CROSSWORD SOLUTION
Across
2. Ondansetron
6. Thiethylperazine
8. Anzemet
11. Inhibit
12. Zofran
13. Promethazine
16. Marinol
17. Dronabinol

Down
1. Vestibular neuritis
3. Thorazine
5. Antivertigo
7. Antiemetic
9. CTZ
10. Ménière's
14. Nausea
15. Kytril

DOSAGE PROBLEMS
1. 0. 75 milliliter
2. 2 tablets
3. 0. 25 milliliter
4. 0. 5 or ½ milliliter
5. 3 milliliters

35 Anesthetic Drugs

MATCHING
1. H   2. I   3. B   4. J   5. E   6. C
7. A   8. D   9. G   10. F

FILL IN THE BLANKS
1. There are two types of anesthesia: <u>local</u> anesthesia and <u>general</u> anesthesia.
2. In some instances, a <u>topical</u> anesthetic may be applied by a nurse
3. The nurse usually gives a <u>preanesthesia</u> drug before the administration of <u>general</u> <u>anesthesia.</u>
4. The narcotic or antianxiety drugs are given before surgery to decrease <u>anxiety</u> and <u>apprehension</u> immediately <u>before</u> surgery.
5. Antiemetics are administered before surgery to <u>lessen</u> the <u>incidence</u> of <u>nausea</u> and <u>vomiting</u> during the immediate <u>postoperative</u> <u>recovery</u> period.
6. Preanesthesia drugs are usually selected by the <u>anesthesiologist</u> and may consist of a <u>narcotic</u> drug, an <u>antianxiety</u> drug, and/or a <u>barbiturate</u>.
7. Antianxiety drugs have the ability to <u>potentiate</u> the <u>sedative</u> action of the <u>narcotic</u> drugs.
8. a) general physical condition of the patient
   b) area, organ, or system being operated on
   c) anticipated length of the surgical procedure
9. When a nurse first sees the postoperative patient, a priority nursing task will be checking the <u>airway</u> for patency, assessing the <u>respiratory</u> status, and giving <u>oxygen</u> as needed.
10. After surgery, the nurse will monitor the patient's <u>blood</u> <u>pressure</u>, <u>pulse</u>, and <u>respiratory</u> <u>rate</u> every <u>5</u> to <u>15</u> minutes until the patient is <u>discharged</u> from the area.

MULTIPLE CHOICE
1. c   2. d   3. a   4. a   5. c   6. a   7. b   8. c
9. a   10. d

CROSSWORD SOLUTION
Across
5. General
8. Robinul
9. Anesthesia
10. Induction
11. Glycopyrrolate
12. Midazolam
14. Topical
15. Regional
16. Spinal

Down
1. Hydroxyzine
2. Preanesthesia
3. Meperidine
4. Thiopental
6. Anesthesiologist
7. Antiemetic
13. Local

DOSAGE PROBLEMS
1. 1 milliliter
2. 0. 5 milliliter
3. a) 68. 1 kilograms b) 3. 4 to 5. 4 milligrams c) yes
   d) 2. 5 milliliters

36 Antihistamines and Decongestants

MATCHING
1. B   2. E   3. G   4. A   5. C   6. I
7. H   8. J   9. D   10. F

FILL IN THE BLANKS
1. a) loratadine (Claritin)
   b) fexofenadine (Allegra)
   c) desloratadine (Clarinex)
   d) diphenhydramine (Benadryl)
   e) cetirizine (Zyrtec)
   f) chlorpheniramine maleate (Chlor-Trimeton)
2. The respiratory system consists of the upper and lower airways, the lungs, and the thoracic cavity.
3. Histamine acts on the vascular system and the smooth muscle, producing dilatation of the arterioles and an increased permeability of capillaries and venules.
4. The body produces histamine and releases it in response to injury, allergic reactions, and hypersensitivity reactions.
5. Antihistamines are drugs used to counteract the effects of histamine on body organs and structures.
6. Drowsiness and sedation are adverse reactions seen with the use of many of the antihistamines.
7. Decongestants are used for the temporary relief of nasal congestion due to the common cold, hay fever, sinusitis, and other respiratory allergies.
8. Decongestants are used as adjunctive therapy of middle ear infections to decrease congestion around the eustachian tube.
9. Hypertensive crisis can result from the use of decongestants with the MAOIs.
10. Overuse of the topical form of decongestants can cause rebound nasal congestion.

MULTIPLE CHOICE
1. b   2. c   3. a   4. b   5. d   6. b   7. a   8. c
9. b   10. a

CROSSWORD SOLUTION
Across
1. Basophil
4. Fexofenadine
6. Histamine
7. Respiratory
8. Loratadine
11. Desloratadine
12. Drowsiness

Down
2. Antihistamine
3. Phenylephrine
5. Decongestant
9. Benadryl
10. Zyrtec

DOSAGE PROBLEMS
1. a) 5 milliliters b) 100 milligrams
2. a) 10 milliliters b) 2. 68 milligrams
3. a) 2. 5 or 2½ milliliters

37 Bronchodilators and Antiasthma Drugs

MATCHING
1. B   2. K   3. L   4. E   5. I   6. O
7. N   8. C   9. G   10. J   11. A   12. D
13. H   14. F   15. M

FILL IN THE BLANKS
1. a) sympathomimetics b) xanthine derivatives
2. Use of a bronchodilating drug opens the bronchi and allows more air to enter the lungs, which in turn completely or partially relieves respiratory distress.
3. a) restlessness b) anxiety c) increased blood pressure d) palpitations e) cardiac arrhythmias f) insomnia
4. a) aminophylline b) dyphylline c) oxtriphylline d) theophylline
5. a) budesonide (Pulmicort) b) beclomethasone (Beclovent) c) flunisolide (AeroBid) d) fluticasone (Flonase) e) triamcinolone (Azmacort)
6. Leukotriene receptor antagonists include zafirlukast (Accolate) and montelukast sodium (Singulair). Zileuton (Zyflo) is classified as a leukotriene formation inhibitor.
7. The leukotriene receptor antagonists inhibit leukotriene receptor sites in the respiratory tract, preventing airway edema and facilitating bronchodilation.
8. a) cromolyn sodium (Intal) b) nedocromil sodium (Tilade)
9. The patient taking theophylline may complain of heartburn because the drug relaxes the lower esophageal sphincter, allowing gastroesophageal reflux.
10. a) hyperglycemia b) hypotension c) cardiac arrhythmias d) tachycardia e) seizures f) brain damage

MULTIPLE CHOICE
1. c   2. a   3. c   4. a   5. b   6. d   7. c   8. b
9. c   10. b   11. d   12. a   13. c   14. a   15. b

CROSSWORD SOLUTION
Across
1. Leukotrienes
3. Asthma
5. Pulmicort
6. Mixed
7. Beclomethasone
8. Azmacort
10. Salmeterol
11. Prophylaxis
13. Intrinsic
15. Zileuton
16. Emphysema
17. Bronchodilator

Down

2. Terbutaline
4. Aminophylline
9. Fluticasone
12. Singulair
14. COPD

DOSAGE PROBLEMS

1. a) 400 milligrams b) 2 tablets
2. a) 10 milliliters b) 8 milligrams
3. a) 20 milligrams b) 1 tablet
4. 12.5 milliliters

38 Antitussives, Mucolytics, and Expectorants

MATCHING

1. C   2. G   3. E   4. I   5. B   6. F
7. D   8. H   9. J   10. A

FILL IN THE BLANKS

1. a) centrally acting antitussive b) peripherally acting antitussive
2. Terpin hydrate is classified as both an <u>antitussive</u> and an <u>expectorant</u>.
3. The centrally acting antitussives <u>depress</u> the <u>cough center</u> located in the <u>medulla</u>.
4. Depression of the cough <u>reflex</u> can cause a <u>pooling</u> of <u>secretions</u> in the lungs.
5. Acetylcysteine is an example of a <u>mucolytic</u> drug.
6. Expectorants <u>increase</u> the production of <u>respiratory</u> secretions, which in turn appears to <u>decrease</u> the <u>viscosity</u> of the mucus.

MULTIPLE CHOICE

1. b   2. c   3. a   4. d   5. b   6. c   7. b   8. d
9. b   10. a

CROSSWORD SOLUTION

Across

1. Benzonatate
4. Nonproductive
6. Antitussive
9. Productive
10. Nebulization
11. Cough
12. Viscosity
13. Robitussin

Down

2. Expectorant
3. Depress
5. Guaifenesin
7. Mucolytic
8. Mucomyst

DOSAGE PROBLEMS

1. 7.5 milliliters
2. 10 milliliters
3. 2 capsules

39 Cardiotonics and Miscellaneous Inotropic Drugs

MATCHING

1. I   2. D   3. G   4. B   5. C   6. K
7. E   8. L   9. F   10. O   11. H   12. J
13. A   14. M   15. N

FILL IN THE BLANKS

1. a) shortness of breath with exercise
   b) dry, hacking cough or wheezing
   c) orthopnea (difficulty breathing when lying flat)
   d) restlessness and anxiety
2. a) swollen ankles, legs, or abdomen, leading to pitting edema
   b) anorexia
   c) nausea
   d) nocturia (the need to urinate frequently at night)
   e) weakness
   f) weight gain as the result of fluid retention
3. <u>Left</u> <u>ventricular</u> <u>dysfunction</u> is the most common form of <u>heart</u> <u>failure</u> and results in <u>decreased</u> cardiac output and <u>decreased</u> ejection fraction.
4. Diastolic heart failure occurs as the <u>ventricles</u> do not <u>fill</u> adequately, becoming <u>dilated</u> and unable to <u>relax</u> during diastole.
5. a) angiotensin-converting enzyme (ACE) inhibitors
   b) beta blockers
6. <u>Digoxin</u> <u>(Lanoxin)</u> is the most commonly used cardiotonic drug.
7. Miscellaneous drugs with <u>positive</u> inotropic action, such as <u>amrinone</u> and <u>milrinone</u>, are nonglycosides used in the <u>short-term</u> management of heart failure.
8. a) Increase cardiac output through positive inotropic activity
   b) Decrease the conduction velocity through the SA and AV nodes of the heart
9. a) heart failure
   b) atrial fibrillation
10. a) hypersensitivity to the drug
    b) ventricular failure
    c) ventricular tachycardia
    d) AV block
    e) presence of digitalis toxicity

MULTIPLE CHOICE

1. d   2. c   3. b   4. a   5. c   6. b   7. d   8. a
9. c   10. d   11. b   12. c

CROSSWORD SOLUTION
Across

3. Digitalization
4. Hypokalemia
7. Lanoxin
8. IV
12. Digibind
13. Cardiotonics

Down

1. Bigeminy
2. Antacid
5. Anorexia
6. Milrinone
9. Diuretics
10. Trigeminy
11. Digoxin

DOSAGE PROBLEMS

1. 2.5 milliliters
2. 0.5 or ½ milliliter
3. 0.4 milliliter

40 Antiarrhythmic Drugs

MATCHING
1. C   2. F   3. B   4. H   5. A   6. J
7. E   8. I   9. G   10. D

FILL IN THE BLANKS

1. a) atrial flutter
   b) atrial fibrillation
   c) premature ventricular contraction
   d) ventricular tachycardia
   e) ventricular fibrillation
   f) premature atrial contraction
   g) paroxysmal atrial tachycardia
2. An arrhythmia that results from heartbeats originating in the ventricles instead of the SA node and causes the ventricles to contract before the atria is identified as a premature ventricular contraction.
3. Atrial flutter is the rapid contraction of the atria at a rate too rapid for the ventricles to pump efficiently.
4. Ventricular tachycardia is a rapid heartbeat with a rate of more than 100 beats per minute, usually originating in the ventricles.
5. An ECG provides a graphical record of the electrical activity of the heart.
6. The goal of antiarrhythmic drug therapy is to restore normal cardiac function and to prevent life-threatening arrhythmias.
7. a) light-headedness b)weakness c) hypotension d) bradycardia e) drowsiness
8. a) quinidine b) procainamide
9. a) signs of respiratory depression
   b) bradycardia
   c) changes in mental status
   d) respiratory arrest
   e) convulsions
   f) hypotension

10. a) quinidine b) procainamide c) mexiletine d) tocainide e) verapamil

MULTIPLE CHOICE
1. a   2. b   3. d   4. a   5. c   6. a   7. b   8. c
9. d   10. c   11. a   12. b

CROSSWORD SOLUTION
Across

3. Lidocaine
5. Half-life
7. Bretylium
10. Diastole
11. Depolarization
12. Arrhythmia
13. Cinchonism

Down

1. Polarization
2. Threshold
4. ECG
6. Proarrhythmic
8. Refractory
9. Myocardium

DOSAGE PROBLEMS

1. a) 40 milligrams/hour b) 0.66 milligram or 0.6 milligram/minute
2. a) 176 milligrams/hour b) 2.93 milligrams or 2.9 milligrams/minute
3. a) 120 milligrams/hour b) 2 milligrams/minute
4. a) 180 milligrams/hour b) 3 milligrams/minute
5. 150 milligrams per dose
6. 1 tablet

41 Antianginal and Peripheral Vasodilating Drugs

MATCHING
1. C   2. G   3. B   4. I   5. E   6. H
7. J   8. A   9. F   10. D

FILL IN THE BLANKS

1. The antianginal and peripheral vasodilating drugs' primary purpose is to increase blood supply to an area by dilating blood vessels.
2. Antianginal drugs relieve chest pain or pressure by dilating coronary arteries, increasing the blood supply to the myocardium.
3. a) nitrates b) calcium channel blockers
4. The nitrates have a direct relaxing effect on the smooth muscle layer of blood vessels.
5. The calcium channel blockers dilate coronary arteries and arterioles, which, in turn, deliver more oxygen to cardiac muscle.
6. The nitrates are used to treat angina pectoris.
7. Calcium channel blockers are primarily used to prevent anginal pain associated with certain forms of angina.

8. a) sublingual b) transmucosal c) translingual spray d) transdermal pad e) topical ointment f) oral sustained-release g) IV
9. Cilostazol (Pletal) inhibits <u>platelet</u> <u>aggregation</u> and <u>dilates</u> vascular beds, particularly in the <u>femoral</u> area.
10. Peripheral vasodilating drugs are chiefly used in the treatment of <u>peripheral</u> <u>vascular</u> <u>diseases</u>, such as <u>atherosclerosis</u> <u>obliterans</u>, <u>Raynaud's</u> <u>phenomenon</u>, and <u>spastic</u> <u>peripheral</u> <u>vascular</u> <u>disorders</u>.

MULTIPLE CHOICE

1. c   2. b   3. c   4. b   5. a   6. d   7. a   8. c
9. d   10. b   11. c

CROSSWORD SOLUTION

Across

3. Angina
4. Verapamil
5. Vasodilation
9. Sublingual
10. Atherosclerosis
12. Buccal
13. Topical
14. Lumen

Down

1. Calan
2. Cilostazol
6. Isosorbide
7. Isoxsuprine
8. Diltiazem
11. Calcium

DOSAGE PROBLEMS

1. a) 90 milligrams b) 1 tablet
2. a) 120 milligrams/day b) yes, within safe range
3. a) 1 tablet b) 120 milligrams

42 Antihypertensive Drugs

MATCHING

1. E   2. I   3. O   4. C   5. F   6. N
7. K   8. A   9. J   10. G   11. D   12. L
13. B   14. H   15. M

FILL IN THE BLANKS

1. a) vasodilating drugs
   b) beta-adrenergic blocking drugs
   c) antiadrenergic drugs (centrally acting)
   d) antiadrenergic drugs (peripherally acting)
   e) alpha-adrenergic blocking drugs
   f) calcium channel blocking drugs
   g) angiotensin-converting enzyme (ACE) inhibitors
   h) angiotensin II receptor antagonists
   i) diuretics
2. a) adrenergic blocking drugs
   b) antiadrenergic blocking drugs

   c) calcium channel blocking drugs
   d) vasodilating drugs
3. Antihypertensive drugs are used cautiously in patients with <u>renal</u> or <u>hepatic</u> impairment, or <u>electrolyte</u> imbalances, during <u>lactation</u> and <u>pregnancy</u>, and in <u>older</u> patients.
4. The hypotensive effects of most antihypertensive drugs are <u>increased</u> when administered with <u>diuretics</u> and other <u>antihypertensives</u>.
5. Administration of <u>potassium-sparing</u> diuretics or <u>potassium</u> supplements concurrently with the ACE inhibitors may cause <u>hyperkalemia</u>.
6. Before therapy with an antihypertensive drug is started, the nurse obtains the <u>blood pressure</u> and <u>pulse rate</u> on both arms with the patient in <u>standing</u>, <u>sitting</u>, and <u>lying</u> positions.
7. The nurse also obtains the patient's <u>weight</u>, especially if a <u>diuretic</u> is part of therapy or if the physician prescribes a <u>weight loss</u> regimen.
8. Each time the <u>blood pressure</u> is obtained, the nurse uses the <u>same</u> arm and the patient is placed in the <u>same</u> position.
9. Sublingual nifedipine may be administered by <u>puncturing</u> the capsule with a <u>sterile</u> <u>needle</u> and then squeezing the <u>contents</u> into the <u>buccal</u> <u>pouch.</u>
10. The ACE inhibitors may cause a significant <u>drop</u> in blood pressure after the <u>first</u> dose.

MULTIPLE CHOICE

1. b   2. c   3. c   4. d   5. c   6. a   7. b   8. c
9. a   10. d   11. b   12. c

CROSSWORD SOLUTION

Across

4. Postural
5. Minoxidil
8. Hyponatremia
9. Aldoril
10. Furosemide
11. Hypokalemia
12. Endogenous

Down

1. Vasodilation
2. Orthostatic
3. Aldosterone
6. Hypertension
7. Enalapril

DOSAGE PROBLEMS

1. 10 milliliters
2. 2 tablets
3. a) 15 milligrams b) (one 10-mg and one 5-mg tablet) or (1½ 10-mg tablet) or (three 5-mg tablets)

43 Antihyperlipidemic Drugs

MATCHING
1. E   2. I   3. L   4. B   5. O   6. G
7. J   8. N   9. C   10. H   11. A   12. M
13. D   14. K   15. F

FILL IN THE BLANKS
1. a) cholesterol b) triglycerides
2. a) bile acid sequestrants
   b) HMG-CoA reductase inhibitors
   c) fibric acid derivatives
   d) niacin
3. Serum cholesterol levels above <u>240</u> mg/dL and triglycerides above <u>150</u> mg/dL are associated with <u>atherosclerosis.</u>
4. Elevation of the <u>low</u>-density lipoproteins <u>increases</u> the risk of heart disease.
5. HDL is known as the <u>good</u> lipoprotein.

MULTIPLE CHOICE
1. a   2. c   3. b   4. c   5. a   6. b   7. d   8. c

CROSSWORD SOLUTION
Across
1. Catalyst
7. Lopid
10. Cholestyramine
11. Lipids

Down
1. Cholesterol
2. Hyperlipidemia
3. VLDL
4. Chylomicron
5. Triglycerides
6. Fluvastatin
8. Lipoprotein
9. Colestid

DOSAGE PROBLEMS
1. a) 40 milligrams b) 1 capsule
2. 1 tablet

44 Anticoagulant and Thrombolytic Drugs

MATCHING
1. B   2. E   3. I   4. J   5. H   6. D
7. G   8. A   9. C   10. F

FILL IN THE BLANKS
1. a) prevention and treatment of deep vein thrombosis
   b) prevention and treatment of atrial fibrillation with embolism
   c) prevention and treatment of pulmonary embolus
   d) as part of the treatment of myocardial infarction
   e) prevention of thrombus formation after valve replacement
2. A positive Homans' sign is suggestive of <u>deep vein thrombosis.</u>
3. a) blood in the stool
   b) petechiae
   c) oozing blood from superficial injuries
   d) bleeding from the gums after oral care
   e) excessive menstrual bleeding
4. Heparin cannot be taken <u>orally</u> because it is <u>inactivated</u> by <u>gastric acid</u> in the <u>stomach.</u>
5. <u>Hemorrhage</u> is the chief complication of heparin administration.
6. The most commonly used test to monitor heparin therapy is <u>activated partial thromboplastin time.</u>
7. A patient receiving a thrombolytic will be monitored by the nurse for bleeding every <u>15</u> minutes during the first <u>60</u> minutes of therapy, every <u>15</u> to <u>30</u> minutes for the next <u>8</u> hours, and at least every <u>4</u> hours until therapy is completed.

MULTIPLE CHOICE
1. a   2. b   3. c   4. b   5. c   6. a   7. d   8. b
9. c   10. a   11. b   12. a   13. b   14. a   15. d

CROSSWORD SOLUTION
Across
2. Anticoagulant
5. Oral
7. Thrombolytic
8. PTT
9. Prophylaxis
12. Thrombus
14. Jaundice
15. Fibrin

Down
1. Dalteparin
3. APTT
4. Thrombosis
6. Prothrombin
8. PT
10. Hemostasis
11. Warfarin
13. Bleeding

DOSAGE PROBLEMS
1. 0.75 milliliter
2. 0.4 milliliter
3. 0.25 milliliter

45 Agents Used in the Treatment of Anemia

MATCHING
1. H   2. A   3. E   4. G   5. I   6. F
7. B   8. D   9. J   10. C

FILL IN THE BLANKS

1. a) antacids b) tetracyclines c) penicillamine
   d) fluoroquinolones
2. a) leafy green vegetables b) fish c) meat d) poultry
   e) whole grains (or liver, yeast)
3. a) growth
   b) cell reproduction
   c) manufacture of myelin
   d) manufacture of blood cells
4. a) fatigue b) shortness of breath c) sore tongue d)
   headache e) pallor
5. a) dyspnea b) urticaria c) rashes d) itching e) fever
6. Iron compounds are <u>contraindicated</u> in patients with
   any anemia except <u>iron</u> <u>deficiency</u> anemia.
7. a) epoetin alfa (Epogen; EPO)
   b) darbepoetin alfa (Aranesp)
8. Patients with pernicious anemia are treated with
   <u>vitamin B$_{12}$</u> by the <u>parenteral</u> route <u>weekly</u> until
   stabilized, and then are maintained with <u>monthly</u>
   injections for the rest of their life.

MULTIPLE CHOICE

1. b   2. d   3. c   4. a   5. c   6. b   7. d   8. c
9. a   10. b

CROSSWORD SOLUTION

Across

1. Pernicious
4. Epogen
5. Aranesp
7. Glossitis
9. Intrinsic factor
10. Folic acid

Down

2. Erythropoietin
3. Megaloblastic
6. Anemia
8. Iron

DOSAGE PROBLEMS

1. 1. 5 milliliters or 1½ milliliters
2. 2 milliliters

46 Diuretics

MATCHING

1. I   2. M   3. E   4. B   5. A   6. H
7. K   8. F   9. L   10. N   11. D   12. C
13. G   14. O   15. J

FILL IN THE BLANKS

1. a) carbonic anhydrase inhibitors
   b) loop diuretics
   c) osmotic diuretics
   d) potassium-sparing diuretics
   e) thiazides and related diuretics
2. a) acetazolamide (Diamox)
   b) methazolamide (Neptazane)

3. a) bumetanide (Bumex)
   b) ethacrynic acid (Edecrin, Edecrin Sodium)
   c) furosemide (Lasix)
   d) torsemide (Demadex)
4. a) amiloride hydrochloride (Midamor)
   b) spironolactone (Aldactone)
   c) triamterene (Dyrenium)
5. Before administering a diuretic, the nurse assesses the
   <u>vital</u> <u>signs</u> and <u>weighs</u> the patient.
6. If a patient has peripheral edema, the nurse inspects
   the involved <u>areas</u> and records the <u>degree</u> and <u>extent</u>
   of edema in the patient's <u>chart</u>.
7. a) reason for administration of the diuretic
   b) type of diuretic being administered
   c) route of administration
   d) condition of patient
8. a) the purpose of the drug
   b) when diuresis may be expected to occur
   c) how long diuresis will last

MULTIPLE CHOICE

1. b   2. c   3. d   4. a   5. a   6. b   7. a   8. d
9. c   10. d   11. b   12. d   13. c   14. a

CROSSWORD SOLUTION

Across

1. Demadex
2. Furosemide
5. Thiazide
8. Diuretic
10. Mannitol
14. Osmotic
15. Amiloride
16. Loop
17. Simple
18. Filtrate

Down

1. Dehydration
3. Spironolactone
4. Tubules
6. Triamterene
7. Acetazolamide
9. Glycosuria
11. Bumetanide
12. Edema
13. Glaucoma

DOSAGE PROBLEMS

1. 10 milliliters
2. 1½ tablets
3. 2 tablets

47 Urinary Anti-infectives and Miscellaneous Urinary Drugs

MATCHING
1. C   2. F   3. I   4. A   5. D   6. J   7. G
8. E   9. H   10. B

FILL IN THE BLANKS
1. a) cystitis—inflammation of the bladder
   b) urethritis—inflammation of the urethra
   c) prostatitis—inflammation of the prostate gland
   d) pyelonephritis—inflammation of the kidney and renal pelvis
2. Anti-infectives used in the treatment of urinary tract infections are drugs that have an effect on <u>bacteria</u> in the <u>urinary</u> tract.
3. a) cinoxacin (Cinobac)
   b) fosfomycin tromethamine (Monurol)
   c) methenamine mandelate (Mandelamine)
   d) nalidixic acid (NegGram)
   e) nitrofurantoin (Furadantin)
   f) trimethoprim (TMP) (Trimpex)
4. Nitrofurantoin may be <u>bacteriostatic</u> or <u>bactericidal</u>, depending on the <u>concentration</u> of the drug in the urine.
5. When trimethoprim is combined with <u>sulfamethoxazole (Septra)</u>, the <u>adverse</u> effects associated with a <u>sulfonamide</u> may also occur.
6. Oxybutynin (Ditropan) acts by <u>relaxing</u> the <u>bladder</u> muscle and reducing <u>spasm</u>.
7. When nitrofurantoin is administered with <u>anticholinergics,</u> there is a delay in gastric emptying, <u>increasing</u> the <u>absorption</u> of nitrofurantoin.
8. Phenazopyridine treats the <u>symptoms</u> of <u>pain</u> but does not treat the <u>cause</u> of the <u>disorder</u>.
9. When a patient is diagnosed with a UTI, the nurse assesses for and documents <u>pain</u>, urinary <u>frequency</u>, bladder <u>distention</u>, or other symptoms associated with the <u>urinary</u> system.
10. a) dyspnea b) chest pain c) cough d) fever e) chills

MULTIPLE CHOICE
1. b   2. c   3. a   4. b   5. d   6. b   7. b   8. c
9. d   10. d   11. a   12. c

CROSSWORD SOLUTION
Across

4. Mandelamine
7. Bacteriostatic
9. Phenazopyridine
11. Urethritis
12. Urge
14. Cystitis
15. Pyelonephritis

Down

1. Prostatitis
2. UTI
3. Sulfamethizole
5. Anti-infectives
6. Oxybutynin

8. Furadantin
10. Pyridium
13. Dysuria

DOSAGE PROBLEMS
1. 2 tablets
2. a) 5 milliliters b) 3 doses
3. a) 15 milliliters b) 300 milligrams

48 Drugs That Affect the Gastrointestinal System

MATCHING
1. L   2. B   3. C   4. D   5. M   6. N
7. O   8. F   9. E   10. K   11. H   12. A
13. J   14. I   15. G

FILL IN THE BLANKS
1. The antacids containing <u>magnesium</u> and <u>sodium</u> have a <u>laxative</u> effect and produce diarrhea.
2. a) aluminum b) magnesium c) calcium d) sodium bicarbonate
3. Antacids containing <u>aluminum</u> and <u>calcium</u> tend to produce constipation.
4. a) increase gastric pH
   b) absorb or bind drugs to their surface
   c) increase urinary pH, affecting the rate of drug elimination
5. <u>Magnesium</u> and <u>sodium</u> increase the motility of the upper gastrointestinal tract.
6. a) itching b) difficulty breathing c) urticaria
7. a) cimetidine (Tagamet)
   b) ranitidine (Zantac)
   c) famotidine (Pepcid)
   d) nizatidine (Acid Pulvules)
8. Charcoal is an <u>absorbent</u> that reduces the amount of <u>intestinal</u> gas.
9. The emetic, ipecac, causes <u>vomiting</u> because of its local <u>irritating</u> effect on the <u>stomach</u> and by stimulation of the <u>vomiting</u> center in the <u>medulla</u>.
10. a) esomeprazole (Nexium)
    b) omeprazole (Prilosec)

MULTIPLE CHOICE
1. c   2. a   3. d   4. b   5. a   6. a   7. d   8. c
9. d   10. a   11. a   12. c   13. b   14. a   15. d

CROSSWORD SOLUTION
Across

4. Maalox
6. Zantac
9. Esomeprazole
11. Emetic
12. Cimetidine

Down

1. Diphenoxylate
2. Pancreatin
3. Hydrochloric
4. Magaldrate
5. Antacid
7. Omeprazole
8. Pepcid
10. GERD

DOSAGE PROBLEMS

1. 5 milliliters
2. 2 milliliters
3. 3 capsules

49 Antidiabetic Drugs

MATCHING

1. L	2. J	3. E	4. H	5. B	6. G
7. K	8. A	9. F	10. I	11. D	12. C

FILL IN THE BLANKS

1. a) unexplained hyperventilation
   b) myalgia
   c) malaise
   d) gastrointestinal symptoms
   e) unusual somnolence
2. a) onset b) peak c) duration
3. a) rapid-acting b) intermediate-acting c) long-acting
4. a) when the patient eats too little food
   b) when insulin dose is greater than prescribed because of incorrect measuring
   c) when patient drastically increases physical activity
5. a) when patient eats too much food
   b) when too little or no insulin is given
   c) when patient experiences emotional stress or physical stress (illness, infection, surgery, pregnancy)
6. a) name of insulin
   b) source of insulin
   c) number of units per milliliter
   d) the expiration date
7. a) orange juice or fruit juice
   b) hard candy, honey
   c) commercial glucose products
   d) glucagon by the SC, IM, or IV route
   e) glucose 10% or 50 % IV
8. a) blood glucose levels >200 mg/mL
   b) headache
   c) increased thirst
   d) epigastric pain
   e) nausea
   f) hot, dry, flushed skin
   g) restlessness
   h) diaphoresis
   i) vomiting

MULTIPLE CHOICE

1. a	2. b	3. d	4. b	5. c	6. a	7. c	8. d
9. b	10. d	11. b	12. a	13. c	14. a	15. b	

CROSSWORD SOLUTION
Across

1. Hyperglycemia
2. Secondary
3. Metformin
4. Glucagon
7. Lipodystrophy
8. Glucometer
9. Diabetes mellitus
10. Sulfonylurea

Down

1. Hypoglycemia
5. Glyburide
6. Insulin

DOSAGE PROBLEMS

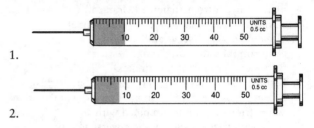

1.

2.

3. 2 tablets

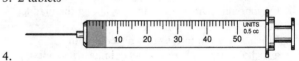

4.

50 Pituitary and Adrenocortical Hormones

MATCHING

1. L	2. N	3. C	4. I	5. F	6. K
7. H	8. A	9. M	10. O	11. J	12. G
13. E	14. B	15. D			

FILL IN THE BLANKS

1. a) abdominal pain b) sudden ovarian enlargement c) ascites
2. a) increased hunger b) increased thirst c) frequent urination
3. Excessive <u>urination</u> and excessive <u>thirst</u> characterize diabetes insipidus.
4. a) blood pressure b) pulse c) respiratory rate d) weight
5. a) blood pressure b) pulse c) respiratory rate d) abdominal sounds e) abdominal girth
6. Patients taking lypressin for treatment of diabetes insipidus learn to adjust their medication dosage based on the <u>frequency</u> of urination and <u>increase</u> of thirst.
7. a) dry mucous membranes b) concentrated urine c) poor skin turgor d) flushed, dry skin e) confusion
8. a) cortisone b) hydrocortisone c) prednisone d) prednisolone e) triamcinolone

9. a) buffalo hump b) moon face c) oily skin d) acne
   e) osteoporosis f) purple striae on abdomen and hips
   g) skin pigmentation h) weight gain i) hirsutism
10. a) chorionic gonadotropin b) clomiphene c)
    menotropins d) urofollitropin

MULTIPLE CHOICE

1. a 2. c 3. b 4. a 5. a 6. c 7. d 8. b
9. d 10. b 11. c 12. b 13. d 14. c 15. d

CROSSWORD SOLUTION

Across

1. Fludrocortisone
8. Mineralocorticoids
9. ACTH
10. Gonads
11. Cushing's

Down

2. Somatropin
3. Neurohypophysis
4. Rhynile
5. Anovulatory
6. Vasopressin
7. Cryptorchism

DOSAGE PROBLEMS

1. a) 30 kilograms b) 3 milligrams c) 0. 6 milliliter
2. 0.25 milliliters
3. 6 milliliters

51 Thyroid and Antithyroid Drugs

MATCHING

1. K 2. M 3. J 4. G 5. H 6. B
7. L 8. E 9. N 10. F 11. C 12. A
13. D 14. I 15. O

FILL IN THE BLANKS

1. Thyroid hormones are used as <u>replacement</u> therapy
   when the patient is <u>hypothyroid</u>.
2. The <u>full</u> effects of <u>thyroid</u> <u>hormone</u> <u>replacement</u> therapy
   may not be apparent for <u>several</u> weeks or <u>more</u>, but
   <u>early</u> effects may be apparent in as little as <u>48</u> hours.
3. Thyroid hormones are administered <u>once</u> a day, <u>early</u> in
   the <u>morning</u> and preferably before <u>breakfast</u>.
4. a) metallic taste in the mouth
   b) swelling and soreness of the parotid glands
   c) burning of the mouth and throat
   d) sore teeth and gums
   e) symptoms of a head cold
   f) gastrointestinal upset (occasional)
5. Iodine solutions should be <u>drunk</u> through a <u>straw</u>
   because they may cause <u>tooth</u> discoloration.

MULTIPLE CHOICE

1. d 2. d 3. a 4. a 5. c 6. a 7. b 8. c
9. a 10. b

CROSSWORD SOLUTION

Across

1. Levothyroxine
4. Iodism
6. Goiter
9. Euthyroid
10. Triiodothyronine
11. Iodine
12. Agranulocytosis

Down

2. Hypothyroidism
3. Thyrotoxicosis
5. Thyroid storm
7. Thyroid
8. Myxedema

DOSAGE PROBLEMS

1. 1 tablet
2. ½ tablet
3. a) 100 mg TID b) 2 tablets

52 Male and Female Hormones

MATCHING

1. C 2. D 3. E 4. H 5. I 6. N
7. K 8. O 9. M 10. L 11. J 12. B
13. F 14. A 15. G

FILL IN THE BLANKS

1. a) estrogen b) progesterone
2. a) estradiol b) estrone c) estriol
3. The synthetic <u>progestins</u> are usually preferred for
   medical use because of the <u>decreased</u> effectiveness of
   <u>progesterone</u> when administered <u>orally</u>.
4. a) regulating the menstrual cycle
   b) decreased blood loss during menstruation
   c) decreased incidence of iron deficiency anemia
   d) decreased dysmenorrhea
5. a) orally b) IM c) IV d) intravaginally e) transdermally
6. The anabolic steroids are <u>synthetic</u> drugs chemically
   related to the <u>androgens</u>.
7. The transdermal <u>testosterone</u> system is used as
   <u>replacement</u> therapy when endogenous <u>testosterone</u> is
   <u>deficient</u> or <u>absent</u>.

MULTIPLE CHOICE

1. b 2. a 3. d 4. c 5. a 6. d 7. c 8. a
9. c 10. d 11. b 12. b 13. d 14. a 15. d

CROSSWORD SOLUTION

Across

3. Cholasma
6. Menarche
7. Gynecomastia
12. Saw palmetto
13. Estradiol
14. Testosterone

Down

1. Catabolism
2. Progestin
4. Testoderm
5. Finasteride
9. Virilization
10. Endogenous
11. Anabolism

DOSAGE PROBLEMS

1. 1.5 mL
2. ½ tablet

53 Drugs Acting on the Uterus

MATCHING

1. D   2. F   3. A   4. H   5. G   6. B
7. E   8. C

FILL IN THE BLANKS

1. Oxytocic drugs are given after the delivery of the placenta and are used to prevent postpartum and postabortal hemorrhage due to uterine atony.
2. Immediately before starting an infusion of oxytocin, the nurse assesses the fetal heart rate and the mother's blood pressure, pulse, and respiratory rate.
3. The nurse assesses and records the activity of the uterus, which includes the strength, duration, and frequency of any contractions.
4. a) drowsiness b) confusion c) headache d) listlessness e) wheezing f) coughing g) rapid breathing
5. a) ritodrine (Yutopar)
   b)   terbutaline (Brethine)
6. Yutopar and Brethine are used a uterine relaxants in the management of preterm labor.
7. a) obtains vital signs
   b) monitors fetal heart rate
   c) checks IV infusion rate
   d) examines IV insertion site
   e) monitors uterine contractions (frequency, intensity, duration)
8. a) ergonovine (Ergotrate)
   b) methylergonovine (Methergine)
   c) oxytocin (Pitocin)

MULTIPLE CHOICE

1. c   2. a   3. a   4. c   5. a   6. c   7. d   8. b
9. c   10. a

CROSSWORD SOLUTION

Across

2. Oxytocic
4. Terbutaline
8. Uterine atony
9. Methergine
10. Preeclampsia

Down

1. Eclampsia
3. Antepartum
5. Ergotism
6. Ritodrine
7. Oxytocin

DOSAGE PROBLEMS

1. ¼ mL or 0. 25 mL

54 Immunologic Agents

MATCHING

1. P   2. O   3. A   4. L   5. F   6. N
7. B   8. G   9. J   10. Q   11. M   12. C
13. D   14. H   15. R   16. I   17. E   18. K

FILL IN THE BLANKS

1. a) Helper T4—Identify and destroy antigens
   b) Helper T1—Increase B-lymphocyte antibody production
   c) Helper T2—Increases the activity of cytotoxic (killer) T cells
   d) Suppressor T cells —Suppresses the immune response
2. Immunity refers to the ability of the body to identify and resist microorganisms that are potentially harmful.
3. a) Naturally acquired b) Artificially acquired
4. Before administration of any vaccine, the nurse obtains an allergy history.
6. a. Date of vaccination
   b. Route and site, vaccine type, manufacturer
   c. Lot number and expiration date
   d. Name, address, title of individual administering the vaccine
7. VAERS collects and analyzes information from reports of adverse reactions following immunizations.

MULTIPLE CHOICE

1. c   2. b   3. b   4. c   5. c   6. c   7. b   8. b
9. a   10. b

CROSSWORD SOLUTION

Across

2. Antigen
3. Toxin
5. Booster
9. Attenuated
11. Globulins

Down

1. Immunity
2. Antibody
4. Active
6. Toxoid
7. Passive
8. Humoral
10. Vaccine

55 Antineoplastic Drugs

MATCHING

1. E   2. H   3. J   4. A   5. F   6. M
7. K   8. N   9. G   10. B   11. C   12. I
13. L   14. D   15. O

FILL IN THE BLANKS

1. a) alkylating drugs
   b) antibiotics
   c) antimetabolites
   d) hormones
   e) mitotic inhibitors
   f) miscellaneous drugs
2. Cancer cells have no biological <u>feedback</u> controls that <u>stop</u> their aberrant <u>growth</u> or <u>proliferation.</u>
3. Chemotherapy is administered at the time the cell is <u>dividing</u> as part of a <u>strategy</u> to optimize <u>cell</u> <u>death.</u>
4. a) cells lining the oral cavity
   b) cells lining the gastrointestinal tract
   c) cells of the gonads
   d) bone marrow cells
   e) hair follicle cells
   f) lymph tissue cells
5. a) busulfan (Myleran, Busulfex)
   b) chlorambucil (Leukeran)
6. a) bleomycin (Blenoxane)
   b) doxorubicin (Adriamycin)
   c) plicamycin (Mithracin)
7. a) methotrexate (Folex)
   b) 5-fluorouracil (Adrucil)
8. a) testolactone (Teslac)
   b) megestrol (Megace)
   c) conjugated estrogens
9. a) paclitaxel (Taxol)
   b) vincristine (Oncovin)
10. a) cisplatin (Platinol)
    b) hydroxyurea (Hydrea)
11. a) swelling
    b) stinging, burning, pain at injection site
    c) redness
    d) lack of blood return

MULTIPLE CHOICE

1. b   2. b   3. d   4. c   5. a   6. b   7. d   8. c
9. b   10. d

MATCHING: ANTINEOPLASTIC DRUG

1. B   2. D   3. A   4. B   5. C   6. F
7. G   8. A   9. E   10. C

CROSSWORD SOLUTION

Across

4. Stomatitis
7. Aberrant
8. Mucositis
9. Anemia
11. Leukopenia
13. Palliative
14. Thrombocytopenia

15. Vincristine
16. Alopecia

Down

1. Vesicant
2. Metastasis
3. Chemotherapy
5. Antineoplastics
6. Antimetabolite
10. Alkylating
12. Anorexia

56 Topical Drugs Used in the Treatment of Skin Disorders

MATCHING

1. H   2. F   3. C   4. A   5. E   6. B
7. M   8. G   9. K   10. L   11. J   12. D
13. I

FILL IN THE BLANKS

1. a) antibiotic
   b) antifungal
   c) antiviral
2. a) bacitracin (Baciguent)
   b) gentamicin (G-mycin)
   c) erythromycin (Emgel)
   d) neomycin (Myciguent)
3. a) acyclovir (Zovirax)
   b) penciclovir (Denavir)
4. Benzalkonium solutions are <u>bacteriostatic</u> or <u>bactericidal</u> depending on their <u>concentrations.</u>
5. Topical <u>antiseptics</u> and <u>germicides</u> are primarily used to <u>reduce</u> the number of <u>bacteria</u> on skin <u>surfaces.</u>
6. a) amcinonide (Cyclocort)
   b) betamethasone dipropionate (Diprosone)
   c) fluocinolone acetonide (Flurosyn)
   d) hydrocortisone (Cort-Dome)
   e) triamcinolone acetate (Aristocort)
7. An example of a topical enzyme is <u>collagenase (Santyl).</u>
8. a) second- and third-degree burns
   b) pressure ulcers
   c) ulcers caused by peripheral vascular disease
9. a) masoprocol (Actinex)
   b) diclofenac (Solarase)
10. Topical anesthetics temporarily <u>inhibit</u> the conduction of <u>impulses</u> from <u>sensory</u> nerve fibers.

MULTIPLE CHOICE

1. c   2. a   3. c   4. d   5. a   6. c

CROSSWORD SOLUTION

Across

3. Purulent
4. Antiseptic
7. Dermis
8. Acyclovir
9. Immunocompromised

10. Allergic
11. Keratolytic
12. Epidermis
13. Necrotic

Down

1. Superinfection
2. Germicide
5. Proteolysis
6. Psoriasis

57 Otic and Ophthalmic Preparations

MATCHING

1. E   2. B   3. J   4. C   5. H   6. I
7. D   8. A   9. F   10. G

FILL IN THE BLANKS

1. a) antibiotics b) antibiotic and steroid combinations c) miscellaneous preparations
2. Otic preparations are instilled in the external auditory canal and may be used to relieve pain, treat infection and inflammation, and aid in the removal of earwax.
3. The nurse documents a description of any drainage or the presence of impacted cerumen.
4. a) angle-closure glaucoma b) open-angle, or chronic, glaucoma
5. Alpha$_2$-adrenergic drugs act to reduce aqueous humor production and increase the outflow of aqueous humor.
6. Sympathomimetic drugs lower the intraocular pressure by increasing the outflow of aqueous humor in the eye and are used to treat glaucoma.

MULTIPLE CHOICE

1. a   2. b   3. d   4. c   5. b   6. a   7. c   8. a
9. c   10. b   11. d   12. a   13. b

CROSSWORD SOLUTION

Across

1. Mydriasis
4. Myopia
10. Miosis
11. Cycloplegia

Down

2. IOP
3. Mydriatic
5. Antibiotic
6. Ophthalmic
7. Uveitis
8. Otic
9. Ptosis

58 Fluids and Electrolytes

MATCHING

1. E   2. C   3. B   4. G   5. F   6. I
7. H   8. D   9. J   10. L   11. A   12. K

FILL IN THE BLANKS

1. IV solutions are used to replace fluid and electrolytes that have been lost and provide calories by their carbohydrate content.
2. Normal saline contains 0.9 % NaCl; half-normal saline contains 0.45 % NaCl
3. a) Pedialyte b) Rehydralyte
4. TPN may be administered through a peripheral vein or through a central venous catheter.
5. At no time should any IV solution be infused at a rapid rate, unless there is a specific written order to do so.
6. During the first 30 minutes of infusion of a fat solution, the nurse carefully observes the patient for difficulty breathing, headache, flushing, vomiting, or signs of a hypersensitivity reaction.
7. Systemic overloading of calcium in the systemic circulation results in acute hypercalcemic syndrome. Symptoms of this syndrome include elevated plasma calcium, weakness, lethargy, severe nausea and vomiting, coma, and, if left untreated, death.
8. The knee jerk reflex is tested before each dose of magnesium sulfate.
9. The maximum recommended concentration of potassium is 80 mEq/1000 mL of IV solution.
10. A too rapid infusion of an amino acids—-carbohydrate mixture may result in hyperglycemia, glycosuria, mental confusion, and loss of consciousness.

MULTIPLE CHOICE

1. c   2. d   3. b   4. a   5. d   6. c   7. a   8. c
9. a   10. d   11. b   12. c   13. b   14. a   15. d   16. c

CROSSWORD SOLUTION

Across

2. Extravasation
8. Plasma
9. Electrolyte
10. Expanders
11. Hyponatremia

Down

1. Dextrose
3. Substrates
4. Bicarbonate
5. Infiltration
6. Hypokalemia
7. Calcium

DOSAGE PROBLEMS

1. 5 mL/bag
2. a) 100 mL b) 33 gtt/minute